Behavior and Mood Disorders

Behavior and Mood Disorders

Edited by Peter Garner

hayle medical

New York

Hayle Medical,
750 Third Avenue, 9th Floor,
New York, NY 10017, USA

Visit us on the World Wide Web at:
www.haylemedical.com

ISBN: 978-1-63241-459-5

The publisher's policy is to use permanent paper from mills that operate a sustainable forestry policy. Furthermore, the publisher ensures that the text paper and cover boards used have met acceptable environmental accreditation standards.

Printed in China.

Cataloging-in-Publication Data

Behavior and mood disorders / edited by Peter Garner.
p. cm.
Includes bibliographical references and index.
ISBN 978-1-63241-459-5
1. Affective disorders. 2. Behavior evolution. 3. Psychology, Pathological.
4. Evolutionary psychology. I. Garner, Peter.
RC537 .B44 2017
616.852 7--dc23

Table of Contents

Preface ... IX

Chapter 1 **Meta-analysis of diffusion tensor imaging studies shows altered fractional anisotropy occurring in distinct brain areas in association with depression** ... 1
Melissa L Murphy and Thomas Frodl

Chapter 2 **Mapping anhedonia onto reinforcement learning: a behavioural meta-analysis** ... 13
Quentin JM Huys, Diego A Pizzagalli, Ryan Bogdan and Peter Dayan

Chapter 3 **Neural temporal dynamics of stress in comorbid major depressive disorder and social anxiety disorder** ... 29
Christian E Waugh, J Paul Hamilton, Michael C Chen, Jutta Joormann and Ian H Gotlib

Chapter 4 **Sleep quality and neural circuit function supporting emotion regulation** ... 44
Jared D Minkel, Kristin McNealy, Peter J Gianaros, Emily M Drabant, James J Gross, Stephen B Manuck and Ahmad R Hariri

Chapter 5 **Anterior cingulate cortex and insula response during indirect and direct processing of emotional faces in generalized social anxiety disorder** ... 53
Heide Klumpp, David Post, Mike Angstadt, Daniel A Fitzgerald and K Luan Phan

Chapter 6 **An fMRI study of unconditioned responses in post-traumatic stress disorder** ... 62
Clas Linnman, Thomas A Zeffiro, Roger K Pitman and Mohammed R Milad

Chapter 7 **Emotion regulation in social anxiety disorder: behavioral and neural responses to three socio-emotional tasks** ... 74
Michal Ziv, Philippe R Goldin, Hooria Jazaieri, Kevin S Hahn and James J Gross

Chapter 8 **Genetic moderation of the association between regulatory focus and reward responsiveness: a proof-of-concept study** ... 91
Elena L Goetz, Ahmad R Hariri, Diego A Pizzagalli and Timothy J Strauman

Chapter 9 **Imaging the pathophysiology of major depressive disorder - from localist models to circuit-based analysis** ... 101
Michael T Treadway and Diego A Pizzagalli

Chapter 10 **Increased ratio of anti-apoptotic to pro-apoptotic Bcl2 gene-family members in lithium-responders one month after treatment initiation.................... 114**
Lori Lowthert, Janine Leffert, Aiping Lin, Sheila Umlauf, Kathleen Maloney, Anjana Muralidharan, Boris Lorberg, Shrikant Mane, Hongyu Zhao, Rajita Sinha, Zubin Bhagwagar and Robert Beech

Chapter 11 **Habenula volume in post-traumatic stress disorder measured with high-resolution MRI.. 125**
Jonathan B Savitz, Omer Bonne, Allison C Nugent, Meena Vythilingam, Wendy Bogers, Dennis S Charney and Wayne C Drevets

Chapter 12 **Increased default mode network activity in socially anxious individuals during reward processing.. 130**
Erin L Maresh, Joseph P Allen and James A Coan

Chapter 13 **Correlations between psychological tests and physiological responses during fear conditioning and renewal.. 142**
Karen G Martínez, Melissa Castro-Couch, José A Franco-Chaves, Brenda Ojeda-Arce, Gustavo Segura, Mohammed R Milad and Gregory J Quirk

Chapter 14 **Sex differences, gonadal hormones and the fear extinction network: implications for anxiety disorders..150**
Kelimer Lebron-Milad and Mohammed R Milad

Chapter 15 **Diminished rostral anterior cingulate cortex activation during trauma-unrelated emotional interference in PTSD... 162**
Reid Offringa, Kathryn Handwerger Brohawn, Lindsay K Staples, Stacey J Dubois, Katherine C Hughes, Danielle L Pfaff, Michael B VanElzakker, F Caroline Davis and Lisa M Shin

Chapter 16 **Effects of genetic deletion of the Kv4.2 voltagegated potassium channel on murine anxiety-, fear- and stress-related behaviors................................168**
Carly Kiselycznyk, Dax A Hoffman and Andrew Holmes

Chapter 17 **Reconceptualizing major depressive disorder as an infectious disease.....................178**
Turhan Canli

Chapter 18 **Neurocognitive therapeutics: from concept to application in the treatment of negative attention bias...183**
David M Schnyer, Christopher G Beevers, Megan T deBettencourt, Stephanie M Sherman, Jonathan D Cohen, Kenneth A Norman and Nicholas B Turk-Browne

Chapter 19 **Brain white matter integrity and association with age at onset in pediatric obsessive-compulsive disorder...187**
Isabelle M Rosso, Elizabeth A Olson, Jennifer C Britton, S Evelyn Stewart, George Papadimitriou, William DS Killgore, Nikos Makris, Sabine Wilhelm, Michael A Jenike and Scott L Rauch

Chapter 20 **Aberrant amygdala functional connectivity at rest in pediatric anxiety disorders.................197**
Lisa L Hamm, Rachel H Jacobs, Meghan W Johnson, Daniel A Fitzgerald, Kate D Fitzgerald, Scott A Langenecker, Christopher S Monk and K Luan Phan

Permissions

List of Contributors

Index

Preface

Mood disorders are characterized by disturbances in the person's mood. The objective of this book is to give a general view of the different areas of mood disorders, its relation to individual and social behaviour and its varied aspects. Most of the topics introduced in this book cover new techniques of treating the patients with mood disorders. It aims to provide a plethora of topics ranging from the causes of mood disorders and asocial behaviors to its different strategies of treatment. This book is a vital tool for all researching and studying this field. It includes contributions of experts and scientists which will provide innovative insights into this area of study.

The researches compiled throughout the book are authentic and of high quality, combining several disciplines and from very diverse regions from around the world. Drawing on the contributions of many researchers from diverse countries, the book's objective is to provide the readers with the latest achievements in the area of research. This book will surely be a source of knowledge to all interested and researching the field.

In the end, I would like to express my deep sense of gratitude to all the authors for meeting the set deadlines in completing and submitting their research chapters. I would also like to thank the publisher for the support offered to us throughout the course of the book. Finally, I extend my sincere thanks to my family for being a constant source of inspiration and encouragement.

Editor

Meta-analysis of diffusion tensor imaging studies shows altered fractional anisotropy occurring in distinct brain areas in association with depression

Melissa L Murphy and Thomas Frodl*

Abstract

Fractional anisotropy anomalies occurring in the white matter tracts in the brains of depressed patients may reflect microstructural changes underlying the pathophysiology of this disorder. We conducted a meta-analysis of fractional anisotropy abnormalities occurring in major depressive disorder using voxel-based diffusion tensor imaging studies. Using the Embase, PubMed and Google Scholar databases, 89 relevant data sets were identified, of which 7 (including 188 patients with major depressive disorder and 221 healthy controls) met our inclusion criteria. Authors were contacted to retrieve any additional data required. Coordinates were extracted from clusters of significant white matter fractional anisotropy differences between patients and controls. Relevant demographic, clinical and methodological variables were extracted from each study or obtained directly from authors. The meta-analysis was carried out using Signed Differential Mapping. Patients with depression showed decreased white matter fractional anisotropy values in the superior longitudinal fasciculus and increased fractional anisotropy values in the fronto-occipital fasciculus compared to controls. Using quartile and jackknife sensitivity analysis, we found that reduced fractional anisotropy in the left superior longitudinal fasciculus was very stable, with increases in the right fronto-occipital fasciculus driven by just one study. In conclusion, our meta-analysis revealed a significant reduction in fractional anisotropy values in the left superior longitudinal fasciculus, which may ultimately play an important role in the pathology of depression.

Introduction

Major depressive disorder (MDD) is one of the most common human diseases, with a lifetime prevalence of 16% and an annual incidence of 6.6% [1]. It is a major cause of long-term disability, with approximately 800,000 individuals worldwide dying each year as a result of suicide, a high proportion of whom have or had MDD [2]. The World Health Organization (WHO) estimates that more people die each year as a result of suicide than in all the armed conflicts worldwide [2]. Even with treatment, approximately 40% of patients do not respond to the first antidepressant prescribed, and 20% experience chronic depression [3]. Many theories exist regarding the pathophysiological basis of MDD, though it remains unresolved. However, recent studies have highlighted many interesting neuronal processes occurring concurrently in the brains of patients with MDD, and these processes may interact with one another to increase or decrease an individual's susceptibility to depression. MDD is believed to originate from a combination of a susceptible genotype, chronic stress and an adverse developmental environment, leading to alterations in the biochemistry, neuroplasticity and structure in the brain [3-7]. Recent advances in neuroimaging techniques have allowed us to study the microstructural changes occurring both prior to and as a result of this disorder.

Magnetic resonance diffusion tensor imaging (DTI) is a novel neuroimaging technique that can evaluate both the orientation and the diffusion characteristics of white matter (WM) tracts *in vivo* [8]. DTI is sensitive to the diffusion patterns of water molecules and produces a three-dimensional image of the brain as a function of this water diffusion [9]. By measuring the direction and magnitude of restricted tissue water motility (diffusion anisotropy), the orientation of WM tracts in the brain

* Correspondence: thomas.frodl@tcd.ie
Department of Psychiatry and Institute of Neuroscience, School of Medicine, Trinity College Dublin, University of Dublin, College Green, Dublin 2, Ireland

can be determined [10], allowing the investigator to assess microstructural changes occurring in response to individual genotypes and environmental factors. This water diffusion occurs in three dimensions and is represented by the three eigenvectors (λ1, λ2 and λ3), with the major eigenvector reflecting the direction of maximum diffusivity, thus revealing the orientation of that fibre tract [8]. Factors that cause reduced water motility include the parallel arrangement of adjacent WM fibres within bundles, myelination, axonal filaments and neurofibrils [8]. Fractional anisotropy (FA) is a scalar value between 0 and 1 that measures the directionality of this water diffusion and serves as an important index of structural connectivity [9,10]. Finally, using tractography or region of interest (ROI) analysis, the structural characteristics of WM bundles in an area of interest can be determined [8]. Reduced FA in the absence of gross pathological findings may represent microstructural abnormalities diminishing the integrity of the WM tracts [11].

Numerous studies conducted using DTI in psychiatric patients have found FA abnormalities in certain brain regions, suggesting that WM structural anomalies exist in diseases such as bipolar disorder [12,13], schizophrenia [14,15] and depression [16,17]. Recent DTI studies have suggested that there is a strong correlation between depression and reduced FA, with the nature of this relationship being a topic of great interest. A study comparing 13 patients with late-life depression to age-matched healthy controls found a reduction in FA in both the frontal and temporal lobes of depressed patients [10]. In addition, an inverse relationship was established between FA values and symptom severity [10]. Another recent study conducted in MDD patients using whole-brain DTI analysis found reduced FA in the left sagittal stratum, the right cingulate cortex and the posterior body of the corpus callosum, areas of the brain believed to play an important role in emotional regulation [18]. Importantly, reductions in FA have also been associated with early-life stress (ELS) in the form of disrupted mother-infant attachment and correlate with an increased risk of both anxiety and depression [11]. A study comparing 12 maternally deprived adult male macaques to 9 normally reared controls found significant reductions in FA in the anterior limb of the internal capsule in the maternally deprived macaques [11]. This is another brain region important in emotional regulation and is involved in the medial and basolateral limbic circuits [11]. Thus, disruption of this region may alter functional connectivity between the frontal and temporal lobes, conferring an increased risk of MDD [11]. Another study demonstrating the microstructural implications of ELS found significantly reduced FA within the genu of the corpus callosum among those exposed to high levels of ELS [19]. DTI represents the forefront of neuroimaging techniques in the characterisation of microstructural alterations occurring in the brain, both as an antecedent to and as a consequence of depression [9].

The aims of this meta-analysis were to identify whether and where FA is altered in patients with MDD compared to healthy controls and to examine the impact that disease variables such as severity, treatment and duration have on these parameters.

Methods

Inclusion studies

An extensive search of databases, including Google Scholar, Embase and PubMed was carried out using keywords including 'DTI + depression' and 'Diffusion tensor imaging + major depressive disorder/MDD'. Inclusion criteria were studies that (1) conducted voxel-based analysis of magnetic resonance imaging scans, (2) compared FA value differences between depressed patients and healthy controls, (3) reported whole-brain analysis in stereotactic coordinates and (4) produced results corrected for multiple comparisons. Exclusion criteria for the final meta-analysis were (1) studies of depression in the context of other diseases, such as Huntington's disease, Parkinson's disease, mania, bipolar disorder, HIV and traumatic brain injury (TBI); (2) studies that measured antidepressant efficacy in depression; (3) studies that used ROI or tractography analysis; (4) studies that used uncorrected methods of analysis; and (5) literature reviews. We also contacted authors for additional information on their studies. This resulted in seven studies' being included in the meta-analysis, and these are summarised in Table 1. However, 21 studies using DTI that investigated patients with MDD or ELS compared to controls were taken into account in our discussion. With respect to depression severity, different studies used different psychopathological measurements. These were translated into a standardised depression severity score whereby 0 indicates healthy, 1 indicates mild depression, 2 indicates medium depression, 3 indicates severe depression and 4 indicates very severe depression http://www.ids-qids.org/index2.html#table2. None of the studies of late-life depression met our inclusion criteria, and these studies are discussed separately.

Meta-analysis of studies

Meta-analytical regional differences in FA values of WM tracts were calculated using mean and threshold probability procedures with Signed Differential Mapping (SDM) software http://www.sdmproject.com/. This software uses restricted maximum likelihood estimation of the variance with the reported peak coordinates to

Table 1 Demographic and clinical characteristics of the seven voxel-based diffusion tensor imaging studies included in our meta-analysis[a]

Characteristics	Kieseppä *et al.* [18]	Blood *et al.* [24]	Zhu *et al.* [58]	Wu *et al.* [25]	Korgaonkar *et al.* [60]	Jia *et al.* [26]	Abe *et al.* [59]
Number of patients	16	22	25	23	29	52	21
Number of controls	20	22	25	21	39	52	42
Mean age of patients, years	48.4	36.3	20.6	31.4	40.5	34.5	48.1
Mean age of controls, years	42	35.3	20.3	30.4	29.6	37.1	48
Patient sex, % female	87.5	54.5	60	65.5	58.7	51.9	47.6
Control sex, % female	50	54.5	60	56.5	53.8	54	47.6
Late-life depression	0	0	0	0	0	0	0
Major depressive disorder	1	1	1	1	1	1	1
Anxiety in patients (0 = no, 1 = yes)	NA	0	0	0	NA	0	0
Treatment, % patients receiving medication at time of study	81	31.8	0	0	0	0	90.5
Mean illness duration, years	14.1	NA	13.6	2.2	NA	3.3	6
Mean BDI score	26.3	NA	NA	NA	NA	NA	NA
Hamilton score	NA	NA	NA	21.8	19.1	23	9.2
IDS-SR score	NA	36	NA	NA	NA	NA	NA
Mean CES-D score	NA	NA	35.48	NA	NA	NA	NA
Illness severity	2	2	3	3	3	3	1

[a]BDI, Beck Depression Inventory; IDS-SR, Inventory of Depressive Symptoms-Self-Rated; CES-D, Center for Epidemiologic Studies Depression Scale. NA, not applicable.

recreate maps of the positive and negative FA differences between patients and controls rather than just assessing the probability or likelihood of a peak [20]. This allowed us to accurately compare patients and controls without biasing the results towards brain regions that showed high variability between studies [21].

SDM converts DTI coordinates to Talairach space with cluster peaks from DTI studies represented on an SDM or MRIcron brain map http://www.cabiatl.com/mricro/mricron/main.html, highlighting areas of the brain where FA alterations reach significant values. Peak coordinates of FA differences between patients and controls are extracted from each data set. Peaks that are not statistically significant at the whole-brain level are excluded from these maps. This is done to ensure that the same statistical threshold throughout the brain is used within each study. Therefore, bias towards liberally thresholded brain regions is avoided, as it is not uncommon in neuroimaging studies for the statistical threshold of some ROIs to be more liberal than those in the rest of the brain. Next, a standard Talairach map of the differences in WM is recreated separately for each study by means of a Gaussian kernel that assigns higher values to the voxels closer to peaks. This includes (1) limiting voxel values to a maximum to avoid bias towards studies reporting various coordinates in close proximity and (2) reconstructing both increases and decreases in WM volume in the same map. Mean analysis, which calculates the mean value of each voxel, was carried out in our meta-analysis, with studies containing a larger sample size having more weight. Jackknife analysis was also carried out on the included studies to ensure that one study did not significantly affect our results and that the FA values obtained were highly replicable throughout all of the studies. Moreover, descriptive analyses of quartiles were used to find the actual proportion of studies reporting results in a particular brain region. Statistical significance was determined by using standard randomization tests, thus creating null distributions from which P values could be obtained directly [22]. We focus on results with $P < 0.001$ for significance in the group differences and $P < 0.0002$ for the meta-regression analysis. For meta-regression analysis of illness severity, we could not use all seven studies, as two studies did not report illness duration and these variables were not available from the authors. Instead, we used five studies for meta-regression analysis of illness duration.

Results

Included studies and sample characteristics

As shown in Figure 1, an exhaustive database search conducted using the key words 'diffusion tensor imaging + depression' resulted in 89 relevant publications. Of these, 82 studies had to be excluded on the basis of being literature reviews ($n = 8$), using tractography ($n = 7$) or ROI analysis ($n = 6$), studying depression in relation to TBI ($n = 5$), ELS ($n = 3$) or in association with other diseases ($n = 25$), assessing functional or structural response to treatment ($n = 7$), using uncorrected results

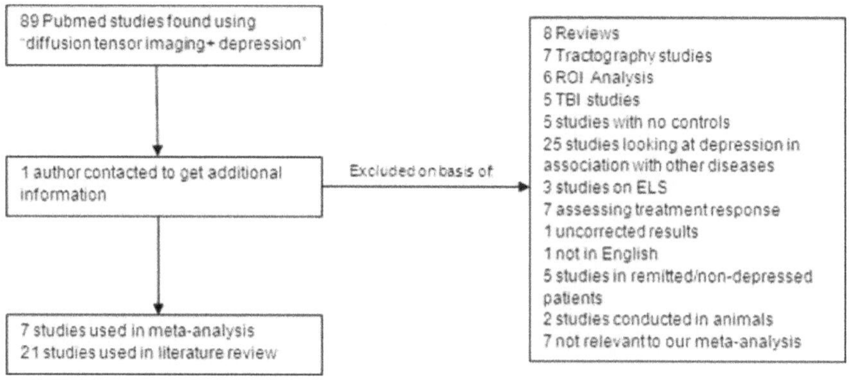

Figure 1 Summary of exclusion criteria used in finding suitable studies to be included in our meta-analysis. Seven studies were selected to be included in the meta-analysis based on extensive exclusion criteria as outlined in Methods.

(n = 1) or no controls (n = 5), not being available in English (n = 1), being conducted in remitted or nondepressed patients (n = 5), being conducted in animals (n = 2) or not being relevant for other reasons (n = 7). Contact with three researchers was made to receive additional required information, but one of the studies was later excluded from our meta-analysis as it used ROI analytical techniques [23].

This resulted in seven high-quality data sets' being selected for inclusion in the meta-analysis, all seven of which were conducted in patients with MDD and none of which were conducted in late-life individuals with MDD, as these latter studies were deemed to be unsuitable for other reasons. Combined the studies included 188 patients with MDD and 221 healthy controls. The original studies were already well matched in terms of age and sex, and no relevant differences were found between patients and controls. Illness severity was calculated by using different scoring systems in the various studies, so an electronic inventory comparing these different scoring systems was used to allow for comparisons between studies (Inventory of Depressive Symptomatology (IDS) and Quick Inventory of Depressive Symptomatology (QIDS); http://www.ids-qids.org/index2.html#table2). Using this inventory, we found that four of the studies were conducted in patients with severe depression, two in patients with moderate depression and one in patients with mild depression. Further details of each of the included studies, such as the presence of anxiety, medication status and duration of illness, are included in Table 1.

Regional differences in WM FA values

The results from the SDM analysis were converted into brain maps and visualised using MRIcron software which were then cross-compared to a Talairach map to optimally localise the brain regions most likely involved (White Matter Atlas; http://www.dtiatlas.org/). Coordinates for the SDM meta-analysis were obtained from all of the seven studies as shown in Table 2 and Figure 2.

Table 2 Significant regional differences in fractional anisotropy values of the left superior longitudinal fasciculus and right inferior fronto-occipital fasciculus were found in patients with major depressive disorder compared to controls[a]

Region	Talairach coordinates	SDM value	Uncorrected *P* value	Voxel number	Breakdown (number of voxels)
Left SLF, inferior parietal lobe	-38, -38, 26	-0.271	0.00023	179	Inferior parietal lobe (63) Subgyral parietal lobe (70) Insula (25) Supramarginal gyrus (12) Extranuclear (6) Subgyral frontal lobe (1) Superior temporal gyrus (2)
Right inferior fronto-occipital fasciculus	30, -56, 2	0.125	0.000097	33	Subgyral occipital lobe (8) Subgyral temporal lobe (11) Lingual gyrus occipital lobe (4) Middle occipital gyrus (4) Extranuclear (5) Middle occipital gyrus (1)

[a]SDM, Signed Differential Mapping; SLF, superior longitudinal fasciculus.

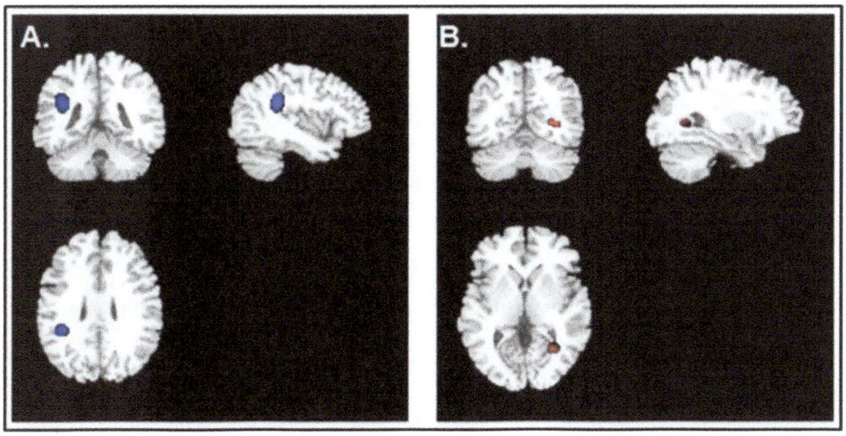

Figure 2 Signed Differential Mapping-generated MRIcron map of the areas of the brain showing fractional anisotropy alterations in association with depression. **(A)** Fractional anisotropy (FA) regional differences in patients compared to controls in right fronto-occipital fasciculus. **(B)** FA regional differences in patients compared to controls in left superior longitudinal fasciculus.

Patients with depression had significantly smaller FA values in the left superior longitudinal fasciculus (SLF) of the inferior parietal lobe as well as larger FA values in the right inferior fronto-occipital fasciculus (FOF) of the temporo-occipital region.

Descriptive analysis of quartiles

Large decreases in FA were detected in the SLF in the first quartile analysis (maximum at Talairach -38, -38 and 30; SDM = -0.746, including several nearby clusters). In the median analysis, these decreases were also detected (maximum at Talairach -30, -44 and 22; SDM = -0.159), indicating that in most of the studies we had found some decrease in FA values in this region. Increases in FA were not detected in the quartile analysis, which was related to the fact that only one study showed an increase in FA [24].

Sensitivity analysis

Whole-brain jackknife sensitivity analysis detected that decreased FA values in the left SLF inferoparietal lobe were present in six of the seven possible combinations and that five jackknife tests showed the posterior part of the SLF, whereas when the study from Wu *et al.* [25] was excluded, the left SLF (temporal) was found. When the study of Jia *et al.* [26] was excluded, the left posterior limb of the internal capsule was detected. Increased FA in the right FOF was reserved throughout six of the seven studies; however, when the study of Blood *et al.* [24] was excluded, this effect disappeared, which we anticipated as it was the only study that reported an increase in FA values. Overall, the results showed a reduced FA in the left SLF to be very stable, with increases in the right FOF being driven by just one study.

Linear regression analysis models

Regression analysis showed that depression severity was associated with decreased FA values in the left SLF: Talairach (-38, -38 and 26; five voxels), SDM = -0.396 per one point increase in severity scale (scale of 1 to 3), $P = 0.000168$ (Figures 3A and Figure 4). It also showed an increase of FA in the right FOF: Talairach (26, -54 and 0; 34 voxels), SDM = -0.344 per one point increase in severity scale (scale of 1 to 3), $P = 0.000017$. Moreover, decreased FA values were associated with longer duration of illness in the SLF (-40, -36 and 34; 33 voxels), SDM = 0.087, $P = 0.0001$ (Figure 3B). An interaction analysis showed that researchers in studies including just untreated patients reported significant FA decreases compared to studies with treated patients in the left SLF: Talairach (-38, -38 and 28; 9 voxels), SDM = 0.416, $P = 0.00077$. Moreover, studies with treated subjects had significantly larger FA in the right FOF compared to studies without treated subjects: Talairach (22, -56 and -6; 84 voxels), SDM = 0.478, $P = 0.00018$.

Discussion

The *Diagnostic and Statistical Manual of Mental Disorders, Fourth Edition* (DSM-IV) [27] defines MDD as the persistence of a depressed mood or loss of interest and pleasure (anhedonia) in association with at least four of the following symptoms: inattention, fatigue, self-depreciation or suicidal thoughts, and disturbances in sleep, appetite, psychomotor activity and weight. The annual incidence of MDD ranges from 12% in women to 7% in men [28], with the WHO ranking MDD as the second

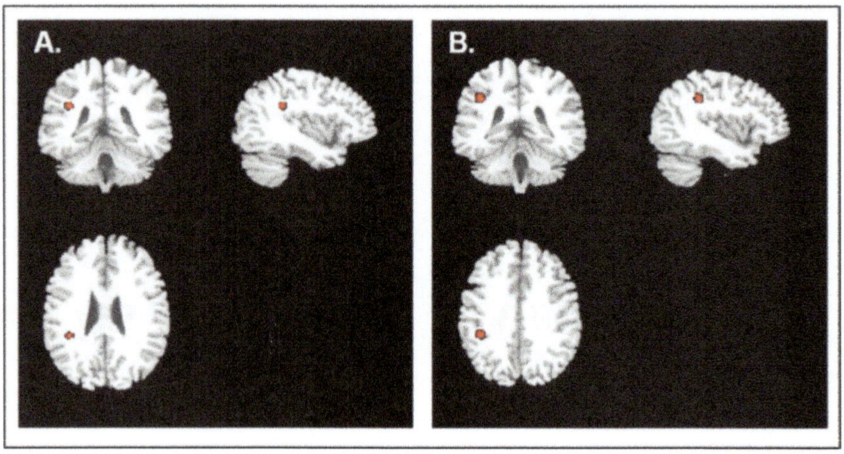

Figure 3 Reduced FA correlates with increased severity and duration of illness. **(A)** Reduced FA values were seen in the areas highlighted in red in association with increased severity of depression. **(B)** Reduced FA values were seen in the areas highlighted in red in association with increased duration of illness.

leading cause of disability-adjusted life-years in the age category 15 to 44 years for both sexes combined [29]. There is great interest in finding associations between the risk, severity and prognosis of this disease in response to specific changes in certain regions of the brain.

The relationship between FA alterations and depression varies according to different studies

Seven studies were included in the meta-analysis, resulting in a reasonable sample size (Table 3). Our meta-analysis showed significantly decreased FA values in the SLF in patients with MDD compared to healthy subjects. This effect was significantly more pronounced in studies that included only untreated patients compared to those that included treated patients. FA values in the SLF were also smaller in studies that included patients with a longer illness duration and more severe depression. Studies that consisted solely of untreated patients were also the studies that reported the most severe depressive symptoms. Therefore, it is difficult to distinguish whether this effect is due to treatment or to a more severe depressive illness. With respect to the illness duration, however, there was no difference between treated and untreated patients. Longer, more severe, untreated depressive episodes seemed to be associated with larger FA decreases in the SLF. In the studies that were included in the meta-analysis using DTI brain atlases, the coordinates of significant FA changes were within the SLF region in four of the seven studies, which is in line with our findings [18,24-26]. Interestingly, a recent study identified a reduction of the SLF in healthy adolescents at familial risk for unipolar depression compared to healthy subjects, which provides further support for the previously underestimated importance of SLF in depression [30].

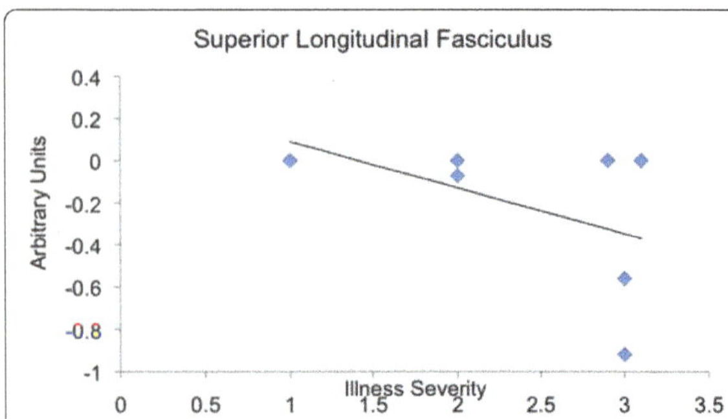

Figure 4 Correlation between superior longitudinal fasciculus FA values as determined by Signed Differential Mapping (SDM) and illness severity (SDM = -0.396, *P* = 0.000168).

The association between smaller FA values and illness duration is consistent with findings that show that brain structures decline in volume during ongoing depression [31] and with studies showing a negative correlation between cumulative illness duration and hippocampal volume [32,33]. Aside from the studies included in our meta-analysis, nine additional DTI studies were carried out: seven in late-life depression, six using ROIs and two using tractography analysis (Table 4). Prefrontal regions, the cingulate cortex and the temporal lobe areas were the most commonly used ROIs in these studies. The studies in late-life depression consistently reported reduced FA values in prefrontal brain regions

Table 3 Summary of diffusion tensor imaging studies included in our meta-analysis conducted in patients with major depressive disorder using corrected whole-brain voxel-based analysis[a]

Study	Method	Participants	Results	Comments
Kieseppä *et al.* [18]	Voxel-based analysis 1.5 Tesla 12 non-colinear directions	16 middle-aged MDD patients and 20 controls	Reduced FA in the left sagittal stratum, cingulate cortex and posterior corpus callosum	Reduced FA in left SLF (temporoparietal) and in the right cingulum in patients with MDD
Zhu *et al.* [58]	TBSS 1.5 Tesla 13 non-colinear directions	25 young first-episode MDD patients and 25 matched controls	Reduced FA in the left anterior limb of the internal capsule, right parahippocampal gyrus and left posterior cingulate cortex	FA values in the left anterior limb of the internal capsule and right cingulum (hippocampus) and left cingulum (dorsal part) were negatively correlated with symptom severity
Abe *et al.* [59]	Voxel-based analysis 1.5 Tesla 6 non-colinear directions	21 young MDD patients and 42 controls	No significant difference between groups for FA and WM volume	Negative correlation between FA and total days depressed in both the right anterior cingulate and the left frontal WM
Blood *et al.* [24]	Voxel-based analysis 3.0 Tesla 6 non-colinear directions	22 MDD patients and 22 controls	Increased FA in the right ventral tegmental area and reduced FA in DLPFC WM in MDD subjects	Increased FA in right corticospinal tract, decreased FA in left corticospinal tract, right inferior FOF (frontal lobe), bilateral DLPFC, left SLF (temporal)
Wu *et al.* [25]	Voxel-based analysis 3.0 Tesla 13 non-colinear directions	23 single-episode, medication-naive MDD subjects and 21 controls	FA reduction in right SLF, right middle frontal and left parietal WM with MDD	Reduced FA in left SLF (parietal lobe) and right frontal WM with MDD
Jia *et al.* [26]	Voxel-based analysis 3.0 Tesla 15 non-colinear directions	52 MDD patients, 16 with and 36 without a history of suicide attempts, and 52 matched controls	Reduced FA in the left anterior limb of the internal capsule in suicide attempters relative to both nonattempters and controls	Reduced FA in bilateral SLF (parietal lobe) and cerebellum
Korgaonkar *et al.* [60]	Voxel-based analysis 3.0 Tesla 42 different diffusion orientations	29 MDD subjects and 39 controls	7.8% reduction in FA in the limbic system, DLPFC, thalamic projection fibres, and corpus callosum	Limbic-DLPFC-thalamic axis Dysfunction may be involved in MDD

[a]MDD, major depressive disorder; FA, fractional anisotropy; SLF, superior longitudinal fasciculus; TBSS, tract-based spatial statistics; FOF, fronto-occipital fasciculus; DLPFC, dorsolateral prefrontal cortex; WM, white matter.

[10,17,34-37]. Reduced FA in the cingulate cortex was also detected [23,36,38]. In addition, Yang *et al.* [17] and Murphy *et al.* [36] reported a reduction in FA values in the parahippocampal gyrus. Aside from the study by Nobuhara *et al.* [10], posterior brain regions were not analysed in these studies. Interestingly, in a combined tractography and voxel-based morphometry study, Cullen *et al.* [38] found reduced FA in connections between the subgenual anterior cingulate cortex to amygdala in the right hemisphere and between the right and left uncinate to supragenual cingulum. However, the sample size was small, with 14 patients and 14 controls. On the other hand, using tractography analysis, Lu *et al.* [39] detected an increase in FA values in patients with MDD in areas of the brain associated with mood regulation, such as the right superior frontal gyrus to right pallidum and the left superior parietal gyrus to right superior occipital gyrus.

FA changes occurring in individuals exposed to ELS may underlie subsequent psychiatric sequelae

DTI studies conducted in individuals exposed to high levels of ELS commonly show reduced FA values compared to controls matched for age and gender (Table 5). Paul *et al.* [19] showed a significant reduction in the genu of the corpus callosum in women subjected to high levels of ELS compared to controls matched for age, gender and education and these changes were also seen in the absence of psychiatric symptoms. A study by Choi *et al.* [40] reported a significant decrease in FA in

Table 4 Diffusion tensor imaging studies excluded from meta-analysis conducted in patients with both major depressive disorder and late-life depression (age >65 years) using other forms of analysis such as regions of interest or tractography[a]

Study	Method	Participants	Results	Comments
Lu *et al.* [39]	Tractography 1.5 Tesla 13 non-colinear directions	23 MDD patients, 24 controls	Increased neural connections between areas involved in mood regulation in MDD subjects, such as right superior frontal gyrus to right pallidum and left superior parietal gyrus to right superior occipital gyrus	Increased neural connections in MDD patients in brain areas associated with mood regulation
Cullen *et al.* [38]	Tractography and voxel-based analysis 3.0 Tesla 30 non-colinear directions	14 healthy MDD adolescents, 14 controls	Reduced FA in WM tracts connecting subgenual ACC to amygdala in right hemisphere and right and left uncinate to supragenual cingulum	Altered frontolimbic neural pathways in adolescent depression
Shimony *et al.* [37]	ROI analysis superficial: superior, middle and inferior frontal gyri, medial and lateral orbital frontal, dorsal, ventral and ACC, mesial frontopolar cortex, motor cortex, medial temporal gyrus, fusiform gyrus, auditory cortex, somatosensory cortex and posterolateral intraparietal sulcus, occipital pole and visual cortex Deep: ventral, dorsal, and posterior frontal lobes, temporal and parietal lobes 1.5 Tesla 6 directions	73 LLD subjects, 23 controls	Reduced FA in prefrontal regions compared to controls	DTI abnormalities may be correlated with reduced cognitive processing speed
Yang *et al.* [17]	ROI analysis: DLPFC, parahippocampal gyrus and genu and body of corpus callosum 1.5 Tesla 25 diffusion-weighted directions	31 LLD subjects, 15 controls	Significantly reduced FA values in superior and middle frontal gyrus and right parahippocampal gyrus	Microstructural abnormalities in temporal and frontal areas of brain are associated with LLD
Nobuhara *et al.* [10]	ROI analysis: frontal WM 8 mm above AC-PC, on AC-PC, 8 mm below AC, genu and splenium Bilaterally: temporal WM, parietal WM and occipital WM 1.5 Tesla 6 non-colinear directions	13 LDD patients, matched controls	Significantly reduced FA in the WM of frontal, temporal and occipital brain regions and corpus callosum of LLD individuals	Frontal, temporal and orbitofrontal WM deficits may play a role in symptom severity in LLD
Li *et al.* [35]	ROI analysis: prefrontal WM at 4 mm inferior to and at 0, 4, 8, 12, 16 and 20 mm superior to AC-PC plane 1.5 Tesla 13 non-colinear directions	51 LDD individuals	Significantly reduced FA values in prefrontal WM at bilateral 20 mm, right 16 mm and right 12 mm above AC-PC. No significant correlation between FA and illness course or severity	Prefrontal WM abnormalities may occur early in the course of MDD and may play a role in the pathophysiology
Murphy *et al.* [36]	Voxel-based analysis 1.5 Tesla 8 diffusion sensitization directions	51 LDD individuals, no controls	Reduced FA in WM lateral to ACC and posterior cingulate cortex and in prefrontal, insular and parahippocampal regions	Alterations in the frontostriatal-limbic networks may be associated with executive dysfunction of LLD as measured on the Stroop task
Bae *et al.* [34]	ROI analysis: WM of superior and middle frontal gyri of DLPFC, anterior corpus callosum and anterior limb of internal capsule 1.5 Tesla 6 diffusion-weighted directions	106 LLD subjects, 84 elderly euthymic controls	Significantly reduced FA in WM of the right ACC, bilateral superior frontal gyri, and left middle frontal gyrus	Reduced FA in dorsolateral prefrontal cortex and ACC suggests altered brain connections are associated with LLD
Taylor *et al.* [16]	ROI analysis bilaterally: periventricular WM, frontal WM, anterior parietal WM, posterior parietal WM and caudate thalamus 1.5 Tesla 6 non-colinear directions	29 LLD patients and 20 controls	Depressed nonremitting subjects showed fewer changes in ACC	Nonremitting subjects showed fewer FA changes, which may reflect antidepressant failure

[a]MDD, major depressive disorder; FA, fractional anisotropy; WM, white matter; ROI, region of interest; LLD, late-life depression; DTI, diffusion tensor imaging; DLPFC, dorsolateral prefrontal cortex; ACC, anterior cingulate cortex; AC, anterior commissure; PC, posterior commissure.

Table 5 Diffusion tensor imaging studies conducted in individuals exposed to high levels of early-life stress reporting fractional anisotropy alterations[a]

Study	Method	Participants	Results	Comments
Paul *et al.* [19]	ROI analysis 1.5 Tesla 12 non-colinear directions	116 healthy subjects older than 18 years of age	Reduced FA within genu of corpus callosum in female subjects only who were exposed to significant ELS	ELS causes microstructural changes in brain that also occur in absence of clinically significant psychiatric symptoms
Eluvathingal *et al.* [42]	ROI and tractography 1.5 Tesla 6 non-colinear directions	Seven right-handed children with history of early, severe socioemotional deprivation, seven matched controls	Significantly reduced FA values in left uncinate fasciculus in individuals exposed to ELS compared to controls	Structural changes in left uncinate fasciculus may contribute to cognitive and behavioural problems seen in ELS children
Choi *et al.* [40]	TBSS 3 Tesla 12 encoding directions	16 unmedicated individuals with history of high-level exposure to PVA but no other form of maltreatment, 16 matched controls	Reduced FA in arcuate fasciculus in left superior temporal gyrus, cingulum bundle by posterior tail of left hippocampus and left body of fornix	PVA exposure may cause alterations in integrity of neural pathways with consequences for language development and psychopathology
Tomoda *et al.* [41]	Voxel-based whole-brain analysis 3 Tesla	21 unmedicated, right-handed subjects ages 18 to 25 years with histories of PVA, 19 controls	An increase in grey matter volume by 14.1% in the left superior temporal gyrus	PVA exposure may affect development of auditory association cortex involved in language processing
Jackowski *et al.* [43]	ROI analysis 1.5 Tesla 6 non-colinear directions	17 maltreated children with PTSD, 15 controls	Reduced FA in medial and posterior corpus callosum of maltreated children	Alterations in areas of brain important in processing of emotional stimuli and memory function is associated with ELS

[a]ELS, early-life stress; ROI, region of interest; FA, fractional anisotropy; TBSS, tract-based spatial statistics; PVA, parental verbal abuse; PTSD, posttraumatic stress disorder.

the left superior temporal gyrus in association with parental verbal abuse (PVA), whereas Tomoda *et al.* [41] reported a 14.1% increase in the grey matter of this area. Despite their conflicting evidence, both studies concluded that PVA causes alterations in the neural pathways responsible for language processing and development. A ROI and tractography study conducted in seven socioeconomically deprived children and controls found significant reductions in FA values of the uncinate fasciculus and suggested these changes might underlie the cognitive and behavioural changes that occur in children exposed to high levels of ELS [42]. A study of the effects of posttraumatic stress disorder (PTSD) in children reported reduced FA in the medial and posterior corpus callosum compared to controls matched for age, sex, race, IQ and handedness, areas of the brain involved in emotional processing [43].

Environmental factors experienced during the early neonatal period appear to have powerful and enduring influences on an organism's physiology and behaviour [44]. Childhood abuse has been associated with increased rates of depression, anxiety, suicide, panic disorder, PTSD, attention-deficit/hyperactivity disorder and other behavioural disorders [45,46]. A community-based study of 1,931 women found larger increases in the rates of depression, anxiety and suicide attempts in women with a history of childhood physical and sexual abuse than in women who were victims of rape and assault in adulthood [47]. The psychiatric sequelae seen in adulthood have been linked to structural changes that occur in the brain secondary to increased levels of stress hormones that result from abuse [48]. Childhood abuse and neglect lead to a decrease in cell proliferation and neurogenesis in the dentate gyrus of the hippocampus in adult brains [49]. This inhibition of neuroplasticity caused by glucocorticoid hypersensitivity leads to diminished stress coping mechanisms in adulthood, conferring a higher risk for the development of MDD [49]. Numerous preclinical studies have shown that ELS induces long-lasting hyperactivity of corticotropin-releasing hormone (CRH) with subsequent increased levels of cortisol and corticosterone as well as alterations in other neurotransmitter systems [46]. A number of studies conducted in children who experienced ELS at different developmental stages found increases in salivary cortisol levels as well as a loss in the normal circadian rhythm of cortisol secretion, suggesting a persistent sensitization of stress-responsive neural circuits [46].

Biological basis for the microstructural alterations seen in MDD

The role of the immune system

Cytokines such as IL-1, IL-6 and TNF-α play important roles in peripheral inflammation, provide neurotrophic support and enhance neurogenesis in the central nervous system and contribute to normal cognitive processes such as memory formation in laboratory animals [50]. In contrast, reduced neurogenesis, increased glutamatergic transmission, increased oxidative stress, glial apoptosis and dysregulation of neuronal and/or glial interactions have all been reported when these cytokine levels become chronically elevated [50].

The role of hypothalamic-pituitary-adrenal axis dysfunction

Hypothalamic-pituitary-adrenal (HPA) axis dysfunction is a common finding in both human and animal models of MDD [49,51,52], and restoration of normal function is a prerequisite for effective MDD treatment [5]. This dysfunction is believed to be due in part to hyperactive CRH neurons, which leads to overactivity of the HPA axis and produces symptoms of anxiety and depression [53]. The resultant increase in glucocorticoid secretion leads to an increase in excitatory amino acid neurotransmitters such as glutamate, with initial reversible remodelling and eventual cell death in the hippocampus, a highly stress-sensitive area of the brain [4]. Glucocorticoids also eliminate activity-dependent increases in brain-derived neurotrophic factor, a growth factor that is important in the formation of neural connections and inhibits dendritic branching in response to stimuli [4].

The role of epigenetics

'Epigenetics' refers to the diversity in gene regulation that occurs during development and alters an organism's behavioural and physiological responses to its environment [54]. Epigenetic regulation of the glucocorticoid receptor (GR) gene may have an important role in predisposing an individual to developing MDD and has been proposed as a mechanism involved in stress-induced neural toxicity [51]. Weaver *et al.* [55] reported that increased maternal rat pup-licking, pup-grooming and arched back pup-nursing influenced hippocampal GR expression and thus HPA axis function through epigenetic regulation of NGFI-A binding to the exon 17 promoter. Importantly, this was reversed by cross-fostering pups from low-maternal-care mothers to high-maternal-care mothers and *vice versa*, suggesting that this alteration in HPA axis regulation was not hereditary and was due purely to environmental epigenetic regulation [55]. Changes in the epigenetic status of the GR gene were also observed by MacGowan *et al.* [54] in response to alterations in parental care during the early postnatal period in rat pups. In a study of suicide victims with or without a history of child abuse as well as healthy controls, hypermethylation of the GR gene was found only in individuals with a history of child abuse [51]. Recently, we demonstrated that subjects carrying the risk short (S) allele of the polymorphism in the promoter region of the serotonin transporter 5-HTTLPR had smaller hippocampal volumes when they had a history of ELS compared to subjects who only carried the genetic risk or compared to those who had a history of ELS but did not carry the risk S allele [56]. This suggests that epigenetic mechanisms may affect brain structure.

Incredibly, new evidence exists that suggests that increased resilience to depression may be due to stronger neural connections in the prefrontal or orbitofrontal, temporal and parietal areas of the brain [9]. A study comparing 21 healthy relatives of MDD patients to 24 healthy volunteers without such a family history found higher FA values in these brain regions in individuals with a positive family history [9]. As a family history of MDD normally confers a higher risk of developing this disease [5,53], these findings suggest that individuals who manage to stay healthy have increased resilience in the form of stronger neural connections (as indicated by higher FA), which may be secondary to epigenetic regulation [9].

None of the nine excluded studies reported significant FA alterations in the SLF or FOF, and Li *et al.* [35] reported no correlation between FA values and illness course or severity. Thus these ROI and tractography studies provide some evidence that there may also be changes in diffusivity in tracts connecting prefrontal, cingulate and medial temporal lobe (amygdala and parahippocampal) regions. Also, it is difficult to distinguish the effects of illness duration from the effects of illness severity in our sample, and this is a potential area for further research. Meta-analytical methods need to include strict inclusion criteria to ensure that the studies sampled are of high quality. However, this limits the extrapolation of results, since more naturalistic studies and explorations are not taken into consideration. We tried to overcome this issue by reviewing all other DTI studies that used ROI approaches, tractography or whole-brain voxel analysis without correcting for multiple comparisons in the discussion.

Conclusion

In conclusion, MDD is a serious and occasionally life-threatening disease that is a result of many complex, interconnected processes occurring in tandem within the brain. Factors such as inherited genotype, epigenetic regulatory processes, developmental experiences and chronic stress all affect the functional and structural integrity of limbic brain regions involved in emotional processing to increase or decrease an individual's vulnerability to depression. Our meta-analysis found decreased WM FA values in the SLF and increased FA values in the FOF. The increase in the FA value of the FOF was driven by only one study, whereas the FA reduction in the SLF was consistently reported throughout all of the various analyses. The SLF is believed to be the major association fibre pathway that connects the parietotemporal association areas with the frontal lobe [57]. Although to our knowledge no previous studies have focused specifically on the relationship between the SLF pathway and depression, our meta-analysis found a significant reduction in the FA value of this tract in association with depression. Indeed, disease variables such as increased severity and duration of illness produced further reductions in FA, suggesting a direct association between disease progression and tract abnormality. Our study further strengthens the concept that microstructural abnormalities as determined by DTI analysis may underpin many of the features of psychiatric illness, in particular depression.

Acknowledgements
Financial support was provided by the Science Foundation Ireland (SFI, Stokes Professor Grant, to TF) and a Trinity College scholarship grant (to MLM).

Authors' contributions
Both authors made substantial contributions to the study's conception and design, as well as to the acquisition and analysis of data. They were involved in drafting the manuscript and gave their final approval of the version to be published.

Competing interests
The authors declare that they have no competing interests.

References
1. Kessler R, Berglund P, Demler O, Jin R, Koretz D, Merikangas K, Rush A, Walters EE, Wang PS, National Comorbidity Survey Replication: **The epidemiology of major depressive disorder: results from the National Comorbidity Survey Replication (NCS-R).** *JAMA* 2003, **289**:3095-3105.
2. McKenzie K, Serfaty M, Crawford M: **Suicide in ethnic minority groups.** *Br J Psychiatry* 2003, **183**:100-101.
3. Frodl T, Jäger M, Smajstrlova I, Born C, Bottlender R, Palladino T, Reiser M, Möller H, Meisenzahl E: **Effect of hippocampal and amygdala volumes on clinical outcomes in major depression: a 3-year prospective magnetic resonance imaging study.** *J Psychiatry Neurosci* 2008, **33**:423-430.
4. Campbell S, MacQueen G: **The role of the hippocampus in the pathophysiology of major depression.** *J Psychiatry Neurosci* 2004, **29**:417-426.
5. de Kloet E, Joëls M, Holsboer F: **Stress and the brain: from adaptation to disease.** *Nat Rev Neurosci* 2005, **6**:463-475.
6. Frodl T, Möller HJ, Meisenzahl E: **Neuroimaging genetics: new perspectives in research on major depression?** *Acta Psychiatr Scand* 2008, **118**:363-372.
7. Rao U, Chen LA, Bidesi AS, Shad MU, Thomas MA, Hammen CL: **Hippocampal changes associated with early-life adversity and vulnerability to depression.** *Biol Psychiatry* 2010, **67**:357-364.
8. Sexton CE, Mackay CE, Ebmeier KP: **A systematic review of diffusion tensor imaging studies in affective disorders.** *Biol Psychiatry* 2009, **66**:814-823.
9. Frodl T, Ferguson Y, Fagan A, Lisiecka D, Carballedo A, Daly I, Meaney J: **Microstructural correlates of resilience against major depressive disorder: epigenetic mechanisms?** *J Psychiatry Neurosci* .
10. Nobuhara K, Okugawa G, Sugimoto T, Minami T, Tamagaki C, Takase K, Saito Y, Sawada S, Kinoshita T: **Frontal white matter anisotropy and symptom severity of late-life depression: a magnetic resonance diffusion tensor imaging study.** *J Neurol Neurosurg Psychiatry* 2006, **77**:120-122.
11. Coplan JD, Abdallah CG, Tang CY, Mathew SJ, Martinez J, Hof PR, Smith EL, Dwork AJ, Perera TD, Pantol G, Carpenter D, Rosenblum LA, Shungu DC, Gelernter J, Kaffman A, Jackowski A, Kaufman J, Gorman JM: **The role of early life stress in development of the anterior limb of the internal capsule in nonhuman primates.** *Neurosci Lett* 2010, **480**:93-96.
12. Beyer J, Taylor W, MacFall J, Kuchibhatla M, Payne M, Provenzale J, Cassidy F, Krishnan K: **Cortical white matter microstructural abnormalities in bipolar disorder.** *Neuropsychopharmacology* 2005, **30**:2225-2229.
13. Yurgelun-Todd DA, Silveri MM, Gruber SA, Rohan ML, Pimentel PJ: **White matter abnormalities observed in bipolar disorder: a diffusion tensor imaging study.** *Bipolar Disord* 2007, **9**:504-512.
14. Minami T, Nobuhara K, Okugawa G, Takase K, Yoshida T, Sawada S, Ha-Kawa S, Ikeda K, Kinoshita T: **Diffusion tensor magnetic resonance imaging of disruption of regional white matter in schizophrenia.** *Neuropsychobiology* 2000, **47**:141-145.
15. Okugawa G, Nobuhara K, Minami T, Tamagaki C, Takase K, Sugimoto T, Sawada S, Kinoshita T: **Subtle disruption of the middle cerebellar peduncles in patients with schizophrenia.** *Neuropsychobiology* 2004, **50**:119-123.
16. Taylor WD, Payne ME, Krishnan KR, Wagner HR, Provenzale JM, Steffens DC, MacFall JR: **Evidence of white matter tract disruption in MRI hyperintensities.** *Biol Psychiatry* 2001, **50**:179-183.
17. Yang Q, Huang X, Hong N, Yu X: **White matter microstructural abnormalities in late-life depression.** *Int Psychogeriatr* 2007, **19**:757-766.
18. Kieseppä T, Eerola M, Mäntylä R, Neuvonen T, Poutanen VP, Luoma K, Tuulio-Henriksson A, Jylhä P, Mantere O, Melartin T, Rytsälä H, Vuorilehto M, Isometsä E: **Major depressive disorder and white matter abnormalities: a diffusion tensor imaging study with tract-based spatial statistics.** *J Affect Disord* 2010, **120**:240-244.
19. Paul R, Henry L, Grieve SM, Guilmette TJ, Niaura R, Bryant R, Bruce S, Williams LM, Richard CC, Cohen RA, Gordon E: **The relationship between early life stress and microstructural integrity of the corpus callosum in a non-clinical population.** *Neuropsychiatr Dis Treat* 2008, **4**:193-201.
20. Radua J, Via E, Catani M, Mataix-Cols D: **Voxel-based meta-analysis of regional white-matter volume differences in autism spectrum disorder *versus* healthy controls.** *Psychol Med* 2011, **41**:1539-1550.
21. Ferreira LK, Busatto GF: **Heterogeneity of coordinate-based meta-analyses of neuroimaging data: an example from studies in OCD.** *Br J Psychiatry* 2010, **197**:76-77.
22. Radua J, Mataix-Cols D: **Voxel-wise meta-analysis of grey matter changes in obsessive-compulsive disorder.** *Br J Psychiatry* 2009, **195**:393-402.
23. Taylor WD, MacFall JR, Boyd B, Payne ME, Sheline YI, Krishnan RR, Murali Doraiswamy P: **One-year change in anterior cingulate cortex white matter microstructure: relationship with late-life depression outcomes.** *Am J Geriatr Psychiatry* 2011, **19**:43-52.
24. Blood AJ, Iosifescu DV, Makris N, Perlis RH, Kennedy DN, Dougherty DD, Kim BW, Lee MJ, Wu S, Lee S, Calhoun J, Hodge SM, Fava M, Rosen BR, Smoller JW, Gasic GP, Breiter HC, Phenotype Genotype Project on Addiction and Mood Disorders: **Microstructural abnormalities in subcortical reward circuitry of subjects with major depressive disorder.** *PLoS One* 2010, **5**: e13945.
25. Wu F, Tang Y, Xu K, Kong L, Sun W, Wang F, Kong D, Li Y, Liu Y: **White matter abnormalities in medication-naive subjects with a single short-duration episode of major depressive disorder.** *Psychiatry Res* 2011, **191**:80-83.
26. Jia Z, Huang X, Wu Q, Zhang T, Lui S, Zhang J, Amatya N, Kuang W, Chan RC, Kemp GJ, Mechelli A, Gong Q: **High-field magnetic resonance imaging of suicidality in patients with major depressive disorder.** *Am J Psychiatry* 2010, **167**:1381-1390.
27. American Psychiatric Association: *Diagnostic and Statistical Manual of Mental Disorders, Fourth Edition (DSM-IV)* Washington, DC: APA Press; 1994.
28. Nolen-Hoeksema S: **Sex differences in unipolar depression: evidence and theory.** *Psychol Bull* 1987, **101**:259-282.
29. **World Health Orgnization: Mental Health: Depression.** [http://www.who.int/mental_health/management/depression/definition/en/].
30. Huang H, Fan X, Williamson DE, Rao U: **White matter changes in healthy adolescents at familial risk for unipolar depression: a diffusion tensor imaging study.** *Neuropsychopharmacology* 2011, **36**:684-691.
31. Frodl TS, Koutsouleris N, Bottlender R, Born C, Jäger M, Scupin I, Reiser M, Möller HJ, Meisenzahl EM: **Depression-related variation in brain**

morphology over 3 years: effects of stress? *Arch Gen Psychiatry* 2008, **65**:1156-1165.
32. Sheline YI: **Neuroimaging studies of mood disorder effects on the brain.** *Biol Psychiatry* 2003, **54**:338-352.
33. Sheline YI, Gado MH, Price JL: **Amygdala core nuclei volumes are decreased in recurrent major depression.** *Neuroreport* 1998, **9**:2023-2028.
34. Bae JN, MacFall JR, Krishnan KR, Payne ME, Steffens DC, Taylor WD: **Dorsolateral prefrontal cortex and anterior cingulate cortex white matter alterations in late-life depression.** *Biol Psychiatry* 2006, **60**:1356-1363.
35. Li L, Ma N, Li Z, Tan L, Liu J, Gong G, Shu N, He Z, Jiang T, Xu L: **Prefrontal white matter abnormalities in young adult with major depressive disorder: a diffusion tensor imaging study.** *Brain Res* 2007, **1168**:124-128.
36. Murphy CF, Gunning-Dixon FM, Hoptman MJ, Lim KO, Ardekani B, Shields JK, Hrabe J, Kanellopoulos D, Shanmugham BR, Alexopoulos GS: **White-matter integrity predicts stroop performance in patients with geriatric depression.** *Biol Psychiatry* 2007, **61**:1007-1010.
37. Shimony JS, Sheline YI, D'Angelo G, Epstein AA, Benzinger TL, Mintun MA, McKinstry RC, Snyder AZ: **Diffuse microstructural abnormalities of normal-appearing white matter in late life depression: a diffusion tensor imaging study.** *Biol Psychiatry* 2009, **66**:245-252.
38. Cullen K, Klimes-Dougan B, Muetzel R, Mueller BA, Camchong J, Houri A, Kurma S, Lim KO: **Altered white matter microstructure in adolescents with major depression: a preliminary study.** *J Am Acad Child Adolesc Psychiatry* 2010, **49**:173-183, e1.
39. Lu CF, Teng S, Wu YT, Wang PS, Yeh TC, Su TP, Hsieh JC: **A neuronal fiber tracking study for major depressive disorder using MR diffusion tensor imaging with fiber tractography.** *2010 International Conference on Bioinformatics and Biomedical Technology (ICBBT), 16-18 April 2010* Piscataway, NJ: IEEE; 2010, 106-110.
40. Choi J, Jeong B, Rohan ML, Polcari AM, Teicher MH: **Preliminary evidence for white matter tract abnormalities in young adults exposed to parental verbal abuse.** *Biol Psychiatry* 2009, **65**:227-234.
41. Tomoda A, Sheu YS, Rabi K, Suzuki H, Navalta CP, Polcari A, Teicher MH: **Exposure to parental verbal abuse is associated with increased gray matter volume in superior temporal gyrus.** *Neuroimage* 2011, **54(Suppl 1)**: S280-S286.
42. Eluvathingal TJ, Chugani HT, Behen ME, Juhász C, Muzik O, Maqbool M, Chugani DC, Makki M: **Abnormal brain connectivity in children after early severe socioemotional deprivation: a diffusion tensor imaging study.** *Pediatrics* 2006, **117**:2093-2100.
43. Jackowski AP, Douglas-Palumberi H, Jackowski M, Win L, Schultz RT, Staib LW, Krystal JH, Kaufman J: **Corpus callosum in maltreated children with posttraumatic stress disorder: a diffusion tensor imaging study.** *Psychiatry Res* 2008, **162**:256-261.
44. Kalinichev M, Easterling KW, Plotsky PM, Holtzman SG: **Long-lasting changes in stress-induced corticosterone response and anxiety-like behaviors as a consequence of neonatal maternal separation in Long-Evans rats.** *Pharmacol Biochem Behav* 2002, **73**:131-140.
45. Brezo J, Paris J, Barker ED, Tremblay R, Vitaro F, Zoccolillo M, Hébert M, Turecki G: **Natural history of suicidal behaviors in a population-based sample of young adults.** *Psychol Med* 2007, **37**:1563-1574.
46. Heim C, Nemeroff CB: **The role of childhood trauma in the neurobiology of mood and anxiety disorders: preclinical and clinical studies.** *Biol Psychiatry* 2001, **49**:1023-1039.
47. McCauley J, Kern DE, Kolodner K, Dill L, Schroeder AF, DeChant HK, Ryden J, Derogatis LR, Bass EB: **Clinical characteristics of women with a history of childhood abuse: unhealed wounds.** *JAMA* 1997, **277**:1362-1368.
48. Spinelli S, Chefer S, Suomi SJ, Higley JD, Barr CS, Stein E: **Early-life stress induces long-term morphologic changes in primate brain.** *Arch Gen Psychiatry* 2009, **66**:658-665.
49. Mirescu C, Peters JD, Gould E: **Early life experience alters response of adult neurogenesis to stress.** *Nat Neurosci* 2004, **7**:841-846.
50. Miller AH, Maletic V, Raison CL: **Inflammation and its discontents: the role of cytokines in the pathophysiology of major depression.** *Biol Psychiatry* 2009, **65**:732-741.
51. Law AJ, Pei Q, Walker M, Gordon-Andrews H, Weickert CS, Feldon J, Pryce CR, Harrison PJ: **Early parental deprivation in the marmoset monkey produces long-term changes in hippocampal expression of genes involved in synaptic plasticity and implicated in mood disorder.** *Neuropsychopharmacology* 2009, **34**:1381-1394.
52. Oberlander TF, Weinberg J, Papsdorf M, Grunau R, Misri S, Devlin AM: **Prenatal exposure to maternal depression, neonatal methylation of human glucocorticoid receptor gene (NR3C1) and infant cortisol stress responses.** *Epigenetics* 2008, **3**:97-106.
53. Bradley RG, Binder EB, Epstein MP, Tang Y, Nair HP, Liu W, Gillespie CF, Berg T, Evces M, Newport DJ, Stowe ZN, Heim CM, Nemeroff CB, Schwartz A, Cubells JF, Ressler KJ: **Influence of child abuse on adult depression: moderation by the corticotropin-releasing hormone receptor gene.** *Arch Gen Psychiatry* 2008, **65**:190-200.
54. McGowan PO, Szyf M: **The epigenetics of social adversity in early life: Implications for mental health outcomes.** *Neurobiol Dis* 2010, **39**:66-72.
55. Weaver IC, Cervoni N, Champagne FA, D'Alessio AC, Sharma S, Seckl JR, Dymov S, Szyf M, Meaney MJ: **Epigenetic programming by maternal behavior.** *Nat Neurosci* 2004, **7**:847-854.
56. Frodl T, Reinhold E, Koutsouleris N, Donohoe G, Bondy B, Reiser M, Möller HJ, Meisenzahl EM: **Childhood stress, serotonin transporter gene and brain structures in major depression.** *Neuropsychopharmacology* 2010, **35**:1383-1390.
57. Makris N, Kennedy DN, McInerney S, Sorensen AG, Wang R, Caviness VS Jr, Pandya DN: **Segmentation of subcomponents within the superior longitudinal fascicle in humans: a quantitative, *in vivo*, DT-MRI study.** *Cereb Cortex* 2005, **15**:854-869.
58. Zhu X, Wang X, Xiao J, Zhong M, Liao J, Yao S: **Altered white matter integrity in first-episode, treatment-naive young adults with major depressive disorder: A tract-based spatial statistics study.** *Brain Research* 2011, **1369**:223-229.
59. Abe O, Yamasue H, Kasai K, Yamada H, Aoki S, Inoue H, Takei K, Suga M, Matsuo K, Kato T, Masutani Y, Ohtomo K: **Voxel-based analyses of gray/white matter volume and diffusion tensor data in major depression.** *Psychiatry Res* 2010, **181**:64-70.
60. Korgaonkar MS, Grieve SM, Koslow SH, Gabrieli JD, Gordon E, Williams LM: **Loss of white matter integrity in major depressive disorder: evidence using tract-based spatial statistical analysis of diffusion tensor imaging.** *Hum Brain Mapp* .

2

Mapping anhedonia onto reinforcement learning: a behavioural meta-analysis

Quentin JM Huys[1,2,3,4*], Diego A Pizzagalli[5], Ryan Bogdan[6] and Peter Dayan[1]

Abstract

Background: Depression is characterised partly by blunted reactions to reward. However, tasks probing this deficiency have not distinguished insensitivity to reward from insensitivity to the prediction errors for reward that determine learning and are putatively reported by the phasic activity of dopamine neurons. We attempted to disentangle these factors with respect to anhedonia in the context of stress, Major Depressive Disorder (MDD), Bipolar Disorder (BPD) and a dopaminergic challenge.

Methods: Six behavioural datasets involving 392 experimental sessions were subjected to a model-based, Bayesian meta-analysis. Participants across all six studies performed a probabilistic reward task that used an asymmetric reinforcement schedule to assess reward learning. Healthy controls were tested under baseline conditions, stress or after receiving the dopamine D_2 agonist pramipexole. In addition, participants with current or past MDD or BPD were evaluated. Reinforcement learning models isolated the contributions of variation in reward sensitivity and learning rate.

Results: MDD and anhedonia reduced reward sensitivity more than they affected the learning rate, while a low dose of the dopamine D_2 agonist pramipexole showed the opposite pattern. Stress led to a pattern consistent with a mixed effect on reward sensitivity and learning rate.

Conclusion: Reward-related learning reflected at least two partially separable contributions. The first related to phasic prediction error signalling, and was preferentially modulated by a low dose of the dopamine agonist pramipexole. The second related directly to reward sensitivity, and was preferentially reduced in MDD and anhedonia. Stress altered both components. Collectively, these findings highlight the contribution of model-based reinforcement learning meta-analysis for dissecting anhedonic behavior.

Keywords: Anhedonia, Major depressive disorder, Depression, Reinforcement learning, Reward learning, Prediction error, Computational, Meta-analysis, Reward sensitivity, Learning rate

Background

Anhedonia is one of the cardinal symptoms for a clinical diagnosis of major depressive disorder (MDD; [1-3]) and refers to an inability to experience pleasure or a diminished reactivity to pleasurable stimuli. It is typically measured by verbal reports. In people subjectively reporting anhedonia, reward feedback objectively has less impact in a variety of behavioural tasks [4-15]. However, modern accounts of decision-making distinguish structurally different ways in which this reduction might be realized, and precisely which of these is associated with anhedonia remains unclear.

Here, we attempt to distinguish two critical factors. The first factor is a reduction in the *primary sensitivity* to rewards. This is possibly the closest behavioural equivalent to the notion of a reduction in consummatory pleasure. Instruments measuring anhedonia, such as the relevant subscores of the Beck Depression Inventory [16] or the Mood and Anxiety Symptom Questionnaire (MASQ) [17] typically focus on this factor [18]. The second factor is an alteration in participants' ability to *learn* from reward feedback. This is emphasized by preclinical animal models of depression [19-22] and, because of the

*Correspondence: qhuys@cantab.net
[1] Gatsby Computational Neuroscience Unit, UCL, London, UK
[2] Wellcome Trust Centre for Neuroimaging, UCL, London, UK
Full list of author information is available at the end of the article

close association between dopamine (DA) signalling and reward learning [23-27], by neurobiological accounts linking anhedonia to DA [11,14,28-35]. It is most important to separate these factors, since they are likely to be associated with radically different ætiologies and therapeutic routes.

The distinction between these two factors is sharp in the mathematical formulation of reward learning based on prediction errors that underpins the account of DA activity [23-27], and is itself based on principles articulated in psychological [36] and engineering [37,38] theories of learning. Consider an experiment in which a reward of a given magnitude is given stochastically on some trials: where $r_t = 1$ if the participant did receive the reward on trial t, and $r_t = 0$ if it did not. We write ρ for the value the participant assigns to this reward. The participants are assumed to build and maintain an expectation ($\mathcal{Q}_t$) of the average reward it might gain on this trial, by means of a prediction error on trial t which is the difference $\delta_t = \rho r_t - \mathcal{Q}_t$ between the obtained ρr_t and expected $\mathcal{Q}_t$ reward. This prediction error can be used to improve the expectations adaptively [39] by adding the error to the previous expectation $\mathcal{Q}_{t+1} = \mathcal{Q}_t + \epsilon\delta_t$, where $0 \leq \epsilon \leq 1$ is a learning rate. This reduces the prediction error over time, at least on average.

The critical factors that might be associated with anhedonia are the two parameters ρ and ϵ in the above expressions. First, ρ is a measure of primary reward sensitivity – the larger ρ, the more sensitive the participant is to a reward of a given magnitude, or the greater the internal worth of an external reward. We comment on the difference between liking and wanting rewards later [40]. Second, the term ϵ governs how reward prediction errors influence learning. Evidence suggests that the phasic activity of DA cells is roughly proportional to δ_t; thus, alterations in the amount of DA released per spike, or in the sensitivity of postsynaptic receptors should behave like a change in the *learning rate* ϵ and affect the speed at which reward affects behaviour [41].

These quantities are formal parameters of a reinforcement learning rule. The question thus arises whether they can actually be distinguished in experimental practice. In this paper, we focus on objective measures of learning behavior. Crudely, since ρ only affects one term in δ_t, whereas ϵ controls the effect of the whole of δ_t on $\mathcal{Q}_{t+1}$, these quantities are theoretically distinguishable. A change in reward sensitivity leads to the asymptotic average value of $\mathcal{Q}_t$ being different. However, a change in learning rate alters the speed at which this asymptote is reached. More particularly, if the behavioural impacts of anhedonia were due to a DA deficit, the extent of anhedonic symptoms might correlate preferentially with the learning rate ϵ. If instead its effects were due to a change in primary reward sensitivity, then one would expect the impact to concentrate on the reward sensitivity ρ. To examine this, we re-analyzed what is perhaps the most substantial body of data on reward learning in anhedonia, namely the probabilistic reward task of (Figure 1A-B). Behaviour in this task has previously been quantified by dividing it into three blocks and examining the evolution of a response bias across the blocks (Figure 1C). However, such measures cannot easily disentangle ρ and ϵ: Figure 1D-E shows that varying both parameters can roughly qualitatively explain the observed patterns. However, there are subtle differences to do with the asymptote of learning that provide us with a window of opportunity.

The fact that varying either parameter can lead to similar qualitative patterns shows that the two parameters play partially replaceable roles and may not be fully separable [42]. Any separation is likely to require substantial amounts of data. We therefore here fitted trial-by-trial individual reinforcement learning (RL) models in a meta-analytic manner to a series of six experiments involving 392 experimental sessions across 313 different participants. Model fitting allows for comprehensive tests of the ability of each hypothesis to account for the entire dataset. Bayesian model comparison ensures that the conclusions are based on parsimonious accounts of the data, avoiding overfitting and overly complex explanations [42-46].

To maximise the chance of identifying specific contributions of learning rate and reward sensitivity, we jointly analysed a series of datasets that are likely to differentially affect the two parameters (Table 1). Three of these probed anhedonia in the context of depression; one in bipolar disorder. A further dataset probed the effect of a dopaminergic manipulation, which we expected to primarily affect ϵ. A final dataset probed the effect of stress, which is prominently involved in the pathogenesis of depression, and which we have previously suggested may reduce phasic DA bursts via an increase of tonic DA release [47].

Our main result is that measures of anhedonia and depression preferentially affected the reward sensitivity ρ, while a dopamine manipulation by pramipexole mainly affected the learning rate ϵ. Stress, however, affected both reward sensitivity and the learning rate. There was no difference in these two parameters in euthymic bipolar individuals, or those with a past history of depression.

Methods

Task and data

In this paper, we re-analyse 392 sessions of behavioural data derived from a probabilistic reward task ([10]; adapted from [55]), which is displayed schematically in Figure 1A. Central to the task is that an asymmetrical reinforcement scheme was used to induce a response bias:

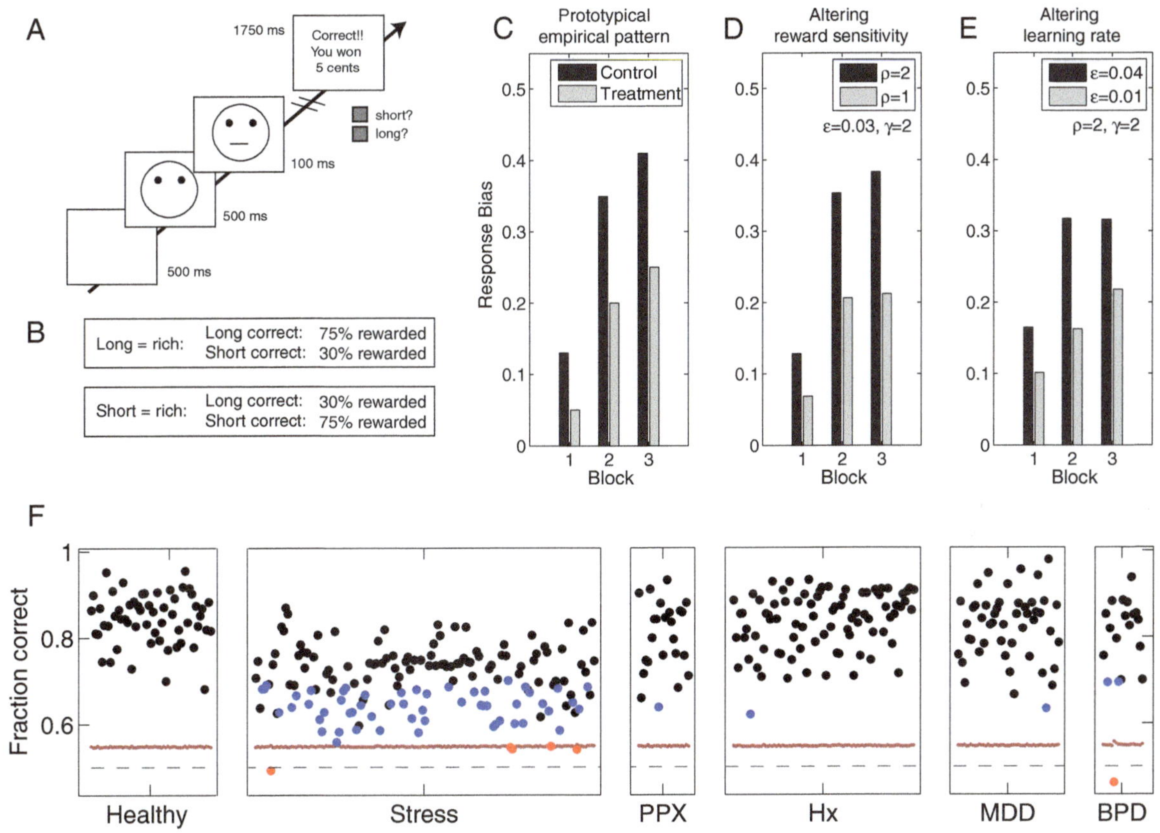

Figure 1 Task and typical behaviour. A: Task. Each trial had the following structure: 1) 500 ms presentation of a central fixation cross; 2) 500 ms presentation of face without a mouth; 3) 100 ms presentation of long (13 mm) or short (11.5 mm) mouth inside the face; 4) participants reported whether the mouth was long or short by key-press ('Z' or '/' on US keyboard, counterbalanced); 5) Face without mouth remained on screen until participant response. Short and long stimuli were each presented 50 times per block in pseudorandom sequence avoiding more than three repetitions in a row. Adapted from [10]. **B**: Reward schedule. One response (counterbalanced across participants) had a higher reward expectation. Correct identification of that "rich" stimulus was more likely to be rewarded (75% probability) than correct identification of the other, "lean", stimulus (30% probability). There was no punishment. If in doubt, choosing the more rewarded stimulus was beneficial. **C**: Surrogate simulated data showing prototypical response evolution. The dark bars show a hypothetical control group, developing a strong response bias towards the more rewarded response over the three blocks of 100 trials. The light bars show a prototypical treatment group with a reduced response bias. **D-E**: Surrogate simulated data generated from a simple reinforcement learning ('Stimulus-action') model. Both a reduction in reward sensitivity (**D**) and a reduction in learning rate (**E**) can roughly reproduce the pattern in the data (**C**). **F**: Percent correct responses for each of the 392 experimental sessions. Each black point represents one experimental session. Vertical bars demarcate datasets. Red horizontal line represents chance performance for each session. Four participants performed below chance (red). Sixty-three out of 392 experimental sessions were not fitted better than chance by model 'Belief' (binomial test; blue). Of these, 58 out of 63 were in the Stress dataset, in which performance was generally worst.

Correct responses to one stimulus, designated "rich", were more likely to be rewarded than correct responses to the other stimulus, designated "lean" (Figure 1B). No feedback was given on other trials, including incorrect trials, and no explicit information about the asymmetry was provided. Participants were explicitly encouraged to win as much money as possible, and so could benefit from reporting the rich, rather than the lean, stimulus when in doubt. One measure of the tendency to do this is the response bias [10]:

$$\frac{1}{2}\log\left(\frac{n(a_1|s_r)\,n(a_1|s_l)}{n(a_2|s_r)\,n(a_2|s_l)}\right) \qquad (1)$$

where s_r and s_l indicate presentation of the rich and lean stimulus, respectively, a_1 and a_2 are the two possible key presses, and $n(a|s)$ is the number of times a particular choice was made in response to that stimulus. Each count n was augmented by $\frac{1}{2}$ to avoid numerical instabilities. Outlier trials with very short ($<$ 150 ms) or very

Table 1 Datasets used

Name	Manipulation	Reference	Participants #
Healthy	High *vs* low BDI scores	[10]	57
	Healthy volunteers. Payment: US$5 and course credit.		
MDD	MDD *vs* controls	[48]	48
	23 participants during an episode of MDD and 25 controls matched for age, sex, education, ethnicity and marital status. MDD participants met DSM-IV criteria for MDD, had Hamilton Rating Scale for depression scores $\geq$ 17, and no other axis I comorbidities except for anxiety. Inclusion required a minimal drug-free period of 2 weeks. Payment: US$10/hour plus 5US$ average task earnings.		
Hx	History of MDD *vs* no history	[49]	85
	Currently healthy participants with and without a history of major depressive disorder (MDD). Participants received US$15/hr in compensation for their time, as well as their task "earnings" (on average, US$5).		
BPD	BPD *vs* controls	[50]	19
	Euthymic outpatients (matched to the same 25 controls as in dataset 'MDD'). The outpatients had a long-standing diagnosis of Bipolar Disorder, currently satisfying criteria on the Affective Disorder Evaluation, which contains modified SCID mood and psychosis modules. Patients were classified as euthymic if they currently Young Mania Rating Scale [51] score <12, and if their Hamilton Rating Scale for Depression [52] score was below 8. Exclusion criteria included other axis I disorders, a past history of MDD, substance abuse and ECT in the past 6 months. Participants were paid US$25 for participation and task earnings.		
PPX	Pramipexole *vs* placebo	[53]	24
	Healthy volunteers received either placebo or a single dose of the D2/D3 agonist pramipexole hydrochloride (PPX) 0.5 mg 2 hours prior to the task. At this low dose, PPX is thought to reduce phasic DA release through autoreceptor stimulation. Payment: US$ 40 for the pharmacological session and US$24.60 for the task session.		
Stress	Threat-of-shock acute *vs* no stressor	[54]	79(x2) +1
	Healthy volunteers took part in the task twice (one missing session), once in a no-stress condition and once in a stress condition. Participants were told that poor performance on the task might lead to a shock being delivered through electrodes attached to the back of their neck. In the stress condition, they were told that this was quite likely, whereas they were told that no shock would be delived in the no-stress condition. No shocks were actually delivered. Notably, the version of the task used in this study was more difficult, with the difference in size between long and short mouth being smaller. This resulted in fewer correct discriminations (see Figure 1F). Payment: either course credit or US$10/hour as well as money "won" during the task (US$10.60 on average).		

Full details of all the patient and control groups are provided in the original publications.

long (> 1500 ms) reaction times are excluded (see [10] for a full description of the 2-step procedure used to exclude trials with outlier responses). Figure 1F shows the fraction of correct responses for each of the 392 individual experimental sessions. In addition to the computer task, participants completed self-report questionnaires (see Table 2). The datasets and manipulations are shown in Table 1. Briefly, the studies examined the effect of i) depression (categorical diagnosis according to DSM-IV; continuous quantification based on self-report measures of depressive features and anhedonia; and past history of MDD); ii) bipolar disorder, currently euthymic (categorical diagnosis according to DSM-IV); iii) stress; and iv) low-dose D_2 agonist pramipexole. The low dose (0.5 mg) of pramipexole was assumed to reduce phasic DA bursts to unexpected rewards due to presynaptic (autoreceptor) activation [53,56]. We note that the dataset 'Stress' differs from the others because a more difficult version of the task was used [54].

Reinforcement learning models

Reinforcement learning models account for every choice on every trial for every participant individually. Here, we describe the model for one particular participant. 'Weights' for emitting a particular choice are updated after every trial to predict the next choice. We consider a set of factors that might affect the weights, and use complexity-sensitive model comparison methods to try to identify the importance of each. Briefly, write a_t for the participant's choice on trial t (key '/' or 'z'), and $\bar{a}_t$ for the choice not taken on that trial (key 'z' or '/'). If stimulus s_t (long or short mouth) was presented, the model assigns to a_t a probability $p(a_t|s_t)$. This probability depends on the 'weights' $\mathcal{W}_t(a_t|s_t)$ and $\mathcal{W}_t(\bar{a}_t|s_t)$ assigned to each

Table 2 Sample characteristics: psychometric measures

Measure	N	mean	median	1st quartile	3rd quartile
BDI	366	8.3	6	1	11
BDA	281	1.9	0	1	3
BDI\A	281	6.9	1	5	10
Generalized distress depression (GDD)	276	23.2	16	20	30
Generalized distress anxiety (GDA)	276	18.8	15	18	24
Anxious anxiety (AA)	276	53.7	45	53.5	65
Anhedonic Depression (AD)	276	21.1	17	20.5	25
Full (BDI + BDA + MASQ subscores)	255				

BDI is the total Beck Depression Inventory II [16]. BDA stands for the anhedonic subscore of the BDI consisting of the sum of items 4 (loss of pleasure), 12 (loss of interest), 15 (loss of energy) and 21 (interest in sex). BDI\A is the total BDI score without the anhedonic component (BDI\A = BDI - BDA). Mood and Anxiety Symptom Questionnaire (MASQ) subscores [17] were anxious arousal (AA), anhedonic depression (AD), general distress anxiety (GDA) and generalised distress depression (GDD).

choice when presented with stimulus s_t. The mapping from weight to probability is made via a 'softmax' function so that a choice a_t will be expected to be emitted more frequently the bigger the difference between its weight and the weight of the alternative choice, or more specifically:

$$p(a_t|s_t) = \frac{1}{1 + \exp\left[-(\mathcal{W}_t(a_t, s_t) - \mathcal{W}_t(\bar{a}_t, s_t))\right]} \tag{2}$$

The choice weights themselves change over time (hence the subscript on $\mathcal{W}$) and are composed of several terms, whose contributions differ for the different models. The models are variants on an underlying full model called 'Belief', for which

$$\mathcal{W}_t(a_t, s_t) = \gamma \mathcal{I}(a_t, s_t) + \zeta\, \mathcal{Q}_t(a_t, s_t) + (1-\zeta)\, \mathcal{Q}_t(a_t, \bar{s}_t) \tag{3}$$

The first of these terms, $\gamma\mathcal{I}(a_t, s_t)$, depends on instructions: $\mathcal{I}(a_t, s_t) = 1$ if a_t is the instructed choice for stimulus s_t (for instance pressing 'z' for the long mouth) and is zero otherwise. The parameter γ thus determines the participants' ability to follow the instructions. The bigger γ, the larger the contribution from $\mathcal{I}(a_t, s_t)$, and hence the instructed response contributes more to choice. Importantly, this instructed choice is symmetric between rich and lean stimulus; thus this term leaves the asymmetry to the other terms.

The second and the third term depend on the expected reward $\mathcal{Q}_t(a_t, s_t)$. This captures the effect of the experienced rewards on previous trials, just as described in the introduction (except allowing different predictions for the different actions and stimuli). $\mathcal{Q}_t(a_t, s_t)$ depends on four factors: the binary sequence r_t up to that point in time, which indicates whether a reward was delivered or not, an initial $\mathcal{Q}_0$ value, the learning rate ϵ and the subjective (i.e. internal to the participant as opposed to the external magnitude in a fixed number of cents) effect size of a reward ρ, which we identify with reward sensitivity.

After every choice, this $\mathcal{Q}$ value is updated according to the prediction error $\delta_t = \rho r_t - \mathcal{Q}_t(a_t, s_t)$ as follows:

$$\mathcal{Q}_{t+1}(a_t, s_t) = \mathcal{Q}_t(a_t, s_t) + \epsilon\delta_t \tag{4}$$

That is, after every trial, the expected reward $\mathcal{Q}(a, s)$ for choice a for stimulus s is increased towards the subjective reward size ρ if a reward is received ($r_t = 1$) but the expectation $\mathcal{Q}$ was lower than ρ, and it is decreased towards zero if no reward was received ($r_t = 0$). The larger ρ, the larger the effect of rewards on choice propensities. As the learning rate ϵ approaches 1, learning is so fast that the $\mathcal{Q}$ values are simply the last experienced outcome for each choice-action pair. For $0 < \epsilon < 1$, expectations represent exponentially weighted averages over the recent outcome history. A multiplicative change to δ is equivalent to a change in ϵ.

In the task, the mouth is only shown for a very short period of time. Thus participants cannot be sure which stimulus was actually presented, and, as experimenters, we cannot know what the participants perceived. This uncertainty has two consequences. First, it implies that the factor γ which governs the effect of the instructions, should be less than ∞. Second, the participants will not be sure which value $\mathcal{Q}_t(a_t, \text{long})$ or $\mathcal{Q}_t(a_t, \text{short})$ and instruction weight $\mathcal{I}(a_t, s_t)$ to employ in their choice, or which $\mathcal{Q}$ value to update using Equation 4. We capture this effect by assuming that they *know* which stimulus-choice pair to update in terms of learning (Equation 4), but that when choosing, they use a form of Bayesian decision theory [57] to combine estimates based on both possibilities. That is, we use a parameter $0 \leq \zeta \leq 1$ to represent participants' average uncertainty about which stimulus was actually presented. Assume participants expected .75 unit reward for pressing button 'z' given the long mouth ($\mathcal{Q}(z, \text{long}) = 0.75$), and 0 given the short stimulus ($\mathcal{Q}(z, \text{short}) = 0$). If they now believed with a probability ζ that they had seen stimulus s and with a probability $1 - \zeta$ that they had seen stimulus $\bar{s}$, then their expectation for pressing button 'z' would be $\zeta\,\mathcal{Q}(z,\text{long}) + (1-\zeta)\mathcal{Q}(z,\text{short}) = .75\zeta$. This is the contribution of $\mathcal{Q}$ in Equation 3. We write ζ as applying to the $\mathcal{Q}$ term only. We could also apply it to the instruction term $\mathcal{I}(a,s)$, but this would be equivalent to rescaling γ (see Additional file 1).

Equations 3 and 4 comprise the full model 'Belief'. We also considered two simpler variants, both of which had one fewer free parameter, and one more complicated variant, with an extra parameter. First, at $\zeta = 1$, participants are certain, and use the correct stimulus-action value to guide their choice. The model in which this value is forced is called 'Stimulus-action'. At $\zeta = 0.5$, they are indiscriminate between the two stimuli. This is model 'Action' because they learn only about the values of choices, independently of stimuli. Finally, the more complex model 'Punishment' is based on the possibility that participants might treat a non-reward as a punishment, so making $\delta_t = \rho r_t + \rho^-(1-r_t) - \mathcal{Q}_t(a_t, s_t)$, where $\rho > 0$. We mention other possible models in the discussion.

Model fitting & comparison

Bayesian model comparison at the group level and model fitting procedures are described in detail in [58]. The key equations are provided in the Additional file 1. Briefly, model fitting was performed by Expectation-Maximisation to find group priors and individual (Laplace) approximate posterior distributions for the estimates for each parameter for each participant. For models 'Action' and 'Stimulus-action', this comprised parameters $\{\mathcal{Q}_0, \rho, \epsilon, \gamma\}$; for model 'Belief' it additionally included parameter ζ, and for model 'Punishment' also ρ^-. All parameters were represented as non-linearly transformed variables with support on the real line and normally distributed group priors.

More complex models will often fit the data better because they have more freedom. However, model complexity is better assessed by methods other than counting parameters [43,59]. Bayesian model comparison is a principled way of assessing model parsimony by computing the posterior probability of each model given the entire dataset for all participants. Because exact computation of these quantities is intractable, individual parameters were integrated out by sampling from the fitted priors, and a standard Bayesian information criterion (BIC)-like approximation was employed at the group level [43]. This procedure results in a measure we term iBIC (for 'integrated BIC') which captures how well each model explains the data given how complex it is [58]. The smaller this number, the greater the model parsimony. The difference between two such values, ΔiBIC, is an approximation of the models' relative log Bayes factor.

The same principles of model comparison also apply to the categorical question whether two groups differ in terms of their parameters. That is, when asking whether group A and B differ in terms of their reward sensitivity ρ or in terms of their learning rate ϵ, the correct approach is to compute the posterior likelihood of models *incorporating* these hypotheses about group differences. That is, we computed pairs of models for each dataset: in the first model of each pair $\mathcal{M}_\rho$, which allows group differences in ρ, participants share a common prior for all parameters except for ρ, for which the two groups have separate priors. In the second model $\mathcal{M}_\epsilon$, participants similarly share a prior for all parameters except for ϵ. Computing the Bayes factors (ΔiBIC) values for these two models relative to each other indicates whether group differences in one or the other parameter provide a more parsimonious account of the *entire* dataset while taking into account the relative flexibility each parameter accords the model and interactions between parameters. The Bayes factors of these models relative to the original model with no group separation, indicate whether the groups significantly differ in either characteristic.

Regression analyses

After model validation, we first assessed inter-correlations between specific questionnaire measures (AD, BDA, GDD, BDI\A, AA, GDA) and reward sensitivity or learning rate in the entire sample using one multiple linear regression analysis for ρ and one for ϵ (`regstats.m` in Matlab V7.14). However, this analysis neglected two aspects of the data: first that the questionnaire data are likely correlated; and secondly that parameters for different participants are estimated with different degrees of confidence. We therefore ran a weighted hierarchical multivariate regression. This is equivalent to a standard hierarchical multivariate regression, except that parameters were weighted by the precisions with which they were estimated (see [60] for details). Note that parameters are represented in the transformed space throughout to avoid issues with non-Gaussianity.

Results

Model validation

We built a set of models that embody key hypotheses about the course of learning in the different groups and fitted them to the data. The models parameterize the *type* of learning performed by participants, allowing us to assess whether they attach rewards to stimulus-action pairs; or just to actions, or to a mixture of the two. We also test the status of 'no reward': do participants treat this outcome as a punishment, reducing the probability of the associated action, or do they treat it as a non-informative null outcome, as intended?

Since we are interested in understanding the characteristics of groups of individuals, we need to ascertain at the group, rather than at the individual level, which model does best [43,45,58]. We indeed found that, taking suitable account of complexity, a single model did capture all groups satisfactorily, allowing for a common and interpretable semantics for the parameters. These so-called random effects models capture inter-subject variation in a way that allows for differences in the extent to which individual participants' data constrain the parameters. When we perform correlation analyses (below), we weigh parameters according to the precision with which they were inferred.

The results are shown in Figure 2A. The most parsimonious account of the data was provided by model 'Belief'. This conclusion rests on the group-level Bayes factors iBIC (see Methods and Additional file 1 for further details). This compares the approximate posterior probability of each model given the data to that of model 'Belief'. Two key aspects of this quantity are that 1) it punishes overly complex models; 2) it assesses this at the group, rather than the individual level. The higher this number, the poorer the combination of model fit and model simplicity. Differences above 10 are typically considered to be strong evidence for one model over the other [43].

Both the standard Rescorla-Wagner model 'Stimulus-action' with separate stimulus-choice values $\mathcal{Q}(s, a)$, and model 'Punishment', which treats trials on which no reward was given as punishing, performed poorly with much worse iBIC values. This suggests that participants were not able to treat the two stimuli as entirely separate; and that they did not treat the absence of rewards as punishments with aversive properties. Model 'Action', which assumes that participants learn only action values, and thus do not separate between stimuli at all in the asymmetric component of choice ($\zeta = 0.5$) was an improvement over the basic model 'Stimulus action' ($\zeta = 1$) but came a distant second to the model 'Belief' (ζ inferred for each session). Indeed, the belief parameter ζ was broadly distributed around 0.5 (mean 0.53, standard deviation 0.13). That is, on average, participants behave as model 'Action', neglecting the stimuli when learning and forming expectations. Individually, however, there was variability in how well they were able to discriminate the stimuli.

Figure 1F shows the probability of performing a correct choice for all participants in all datasets, with those not predicted better than chance by model 'Belief' circled in blue. This model correctly predicted significantly more choices than chance (binomial test, $p < .05$) for most experimental sessions (329 out of 392; black dots). Due to a smaller difference between long and short mouth, and hence a more difficult perceptual discrimination problem (Table 1), participants in the stress dataset– whether in the stress or the no stress condition–showed on average a lower probability of correct choice. They were consequently less well predicted by all models, but model 'Belief' still gave the best account of these data too (see Additional file 1: Section S2.1). Figure 2B shows that, as intended, the overall probability correct was captured by the instruction sensitivity parameter γ (Pearson correlation 0.93, $p < 10^{-20}$), which in turn frees the other parameters to capture trial-to-trial variation in the behaviour contingent on the reward outcomes.

Finally, Additional file 1: Section S2.2 also provides the results of a resampling analysis. This shows that if the model is run on the task, it spontaneously generates data that looks similar to the experimental data.

Regression analyses

Given that model 'Belief' captured the data satisfactorily, we proceeded to analyse the relationship between model parameters and self-report questionnaire measures. Our aims were primarily to identify correlations between measures of anhedonia and learning rates or reward sensitivities. A standard, unweighted, multiple linear regression analysis revealed a significant negative correlation between ρ and anhedonic depression (AD), the most specific measure of anhedonic symptoms available to us ($p = 0.004$; uncorrected for multiple comparisons). There was no correlation between ρ and other questionnaire measures, and no correlation between the questionairre measures and the learning rate ϵ (all $p > 0.1$). Participants in the 'Stress' dataset were tested twice. Repeating this analysis using only the session without stress yielded similar results ($p = 0.007$ for the correlation ρ vs AD, all other $p > 0.09$).

As expected, questionnaire scores were substantially correlated (Figure 3A), and the parameters of different experimental sessions were inferred with varying certainty. We therefore additionally orthogonalized the three anhedonic measures (BDA, GDD, AD) with respect to all the three other measures (BDI\A, AA, GDA) and fit a weighted generalised linear model (GLM). Figure 3B shows that anhedonic depression AD remained significantly and negatively related to the reward sensitivity ρ ($p = 0.005$, Bonferroni-corrected for 8 comparisons). No other correlation survived correction for multiple comparisons (all $p > 0.1$). In particular, no measure of anhedonia was associated with the learning rate ϵ. Figure 3C shows a scatter plot of AD scores vs. reward sensitivity with dot size proportional to the weight (inverse variance) in the weighted regression analysis.

Next, there was a negative linear correlation between ρ and ϵ of -0.41 ($p < 0.0001$; Figure 3D). To further question the selectivity of the correlation between AD and ρ, we orthogonalized ρ with respect to ϵ in addition to orthogonalising as above. This again yielded an (unweighted) significant correlation of AD with ρ ($p = 0.004$, multiple weighted linear regression, uncorrected for multiple comparisons), with no other correlations significant. The

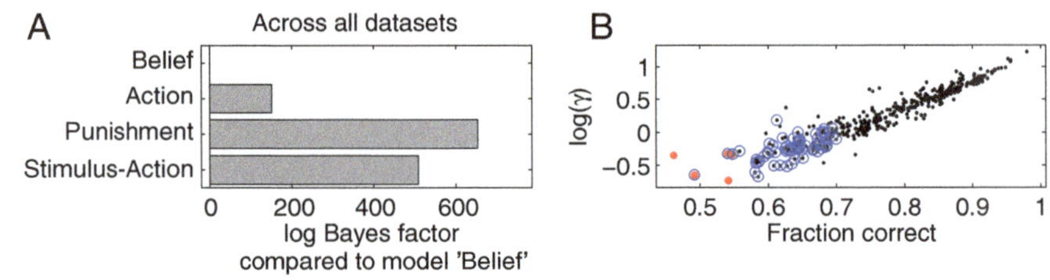

Figure 2 Model performance. A: Model comparison. Group-level log Bayes factors ΔiBIC for each model relative to model 'Belief' across all datasets. A difference $\geq$ 10 in this measure is strong evidence for the model with the lower score. **B**: The parameter γ in the model largely captures the probability with which participants made a correct choice. Note that, by design of the task, this explicitly captures the effect of symmetric instructions and perceptual difficulties, rather than the asymmetric effect of rewards.

reverse orthogonalization did not yield any significant correlations with ϵ.

At least part of the correlation between ρ and ϵ arises because the the two parameters can explain similar features of the data, i.e. alterations in one parameter can be compensated for by alterations in the other parameter (see Figure 1). To establish whether the association between AD and the reward sensitivity parameter was due to real features in the data, rather than due to inference issues, we asked whether the correlations with question-

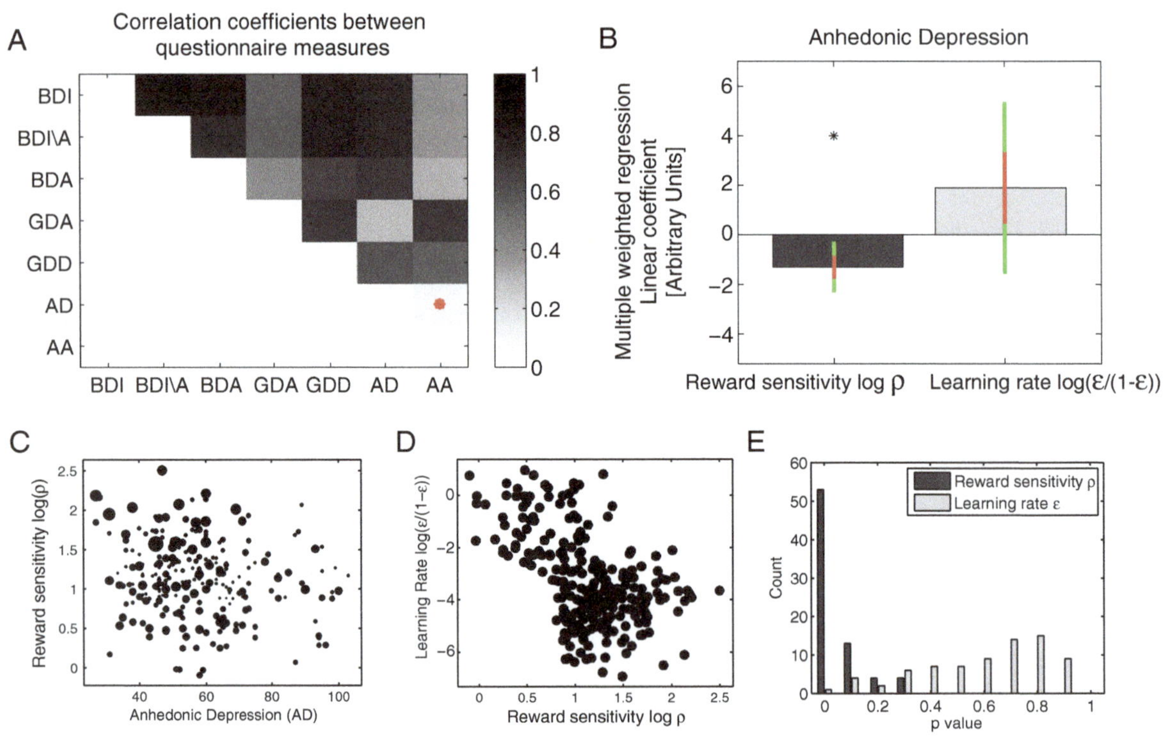

Figure 3 Correlates of anhedonia. A: Correlation coefficients for all pairwise correlations between questionnaire measures. All are highly significant ($p < .01$), except for the correlation between anhedonic depression and anxious anxiety, denoted by a red dot. **B**: Hierarchical weighted regression analysis across all datasets, involving all 255 participants with a full set of BDI, BDA and MASQ scores. The plots shows the linear coefficients between anhedonic depression (AD) score and the reward sensitivity and learning rate parameters ρ and ϵ. Each bars shows one linear coefficient; the red error bars indicate $\pm$ 1 standard error; and the green error bars indicate the 99.4% confidence interval (corresponding to a Bonferroni corrected level $p = .05/8$). AD is significantly and negatively correlated with the reward sensitivity ρ, but not significantly correlated with the learning rate ϵ. **C**: Scatter plot of anhedonic depression against reward sensitivity. Size of dots scale with weight (inference precision). **D**: Scatter plot of reward sensitivity vs. learning rate. **E**: Significance of correlations across parameter estimates from 70 surrogate datasets. There is a consistent and stably significant correlation between AD and reward sensitivity ρ, but not between AD and learning rate ϵ.

naire measures remained stable and identifiable in the surrogate data. For each of the 70 surrogate datasets of 392 experimental sessions, we repeated the standard, unweighted multiple linear regression. Figure 3E shows the distribution of p values for the correlation of AD with ρ and ϵ. While the median p value for the correlation between ρ and AD was 0.04, that for ϵ and AD was 0.71.

Finally, all correlation analyses using the reward sensitivity and learning parameters inferred from the second-best model 'Action' yielded the same results, showing that the results are not dependent on a particular model formulation.

Categorical comparisons

We next examined how learning rate and reward sensitivity were affected by the factors explored in each of the individual datasets. For each dataset, we compared two models: one which assumes that the two experimental groups differed in terms of ρ, the other in terms of ϵ.

Figure 4 shows the Bayes factors for models $\mathcal{M}_\rho$ compared with $\mathcal{M}_\epsilon$ for each of the individual datasets. Given the correlation results, we additionally performed a comparison between all participants with the 20% highest and lowest AD scores. Bayes factors above 20 (or below 1/20) are very strong evidence in favour of a hypothesis [43], while likelihood ratios of 3 to 10 (or the inverse) are weak evidence. We found strong evidence that MDD and AD were better accounted for by a change in reward sensitivity ρ, rather than learning rate ϵ. The opposite was true for pramipexole, which mainly acted by reducing the learning rate ϵ.

However, the Bayes factors comparing models $\mathcal{M}_\rho$ and $\mathcal{M}_\epsilon$ to the basic 'Belief' model without split parameters were all ≤ 3. This means that there was no strong evidence that either of these parameters categorically separates any two groups. Stress appeared most likely to have a genuinely shared effect on both parameters. Participants with a history of depression, or currently euthymic bipolar participants showed weak evidence of reductions in reward sensitivity. Note that all these ratios are by necessity numerically more modest than those in Additional file 1: Figure S1 because they are inferred from far less data.

Discussion

Our results suggest that anhedonia (as measured by AD) and MDD affect appetitive learning more by reducing the primary sensitivity to rewards ρ than by affecting the learning rates. Non-significant trends for such an effect were observed for participants with a past history of depression, and amongst euthymic bipolar disorder patients. By contrast, a dopaminergic manipulation was found to preferentially affect the speed of learning, ϵ. Acute stress had no preferential effect on reward sensitivity or learning rate. These two parameters appear to be state, rather than trait measures: Neither a past history of depression, nor one of BPD, had a significant effect on ρ or ϵ.

Anhedonia

Two self-report measures of anhedonia were used in this paper: the anhedonic depression subscore of the MASQ questionnaire, and the anhedonic subscore of the BDI. The former was clearly related to the reward sensitivity ρ. This subscore quantifies participants' verbally expressed inability to experience pleasure, and so might be expected to capture something akin to consummatory 'liking' [40].

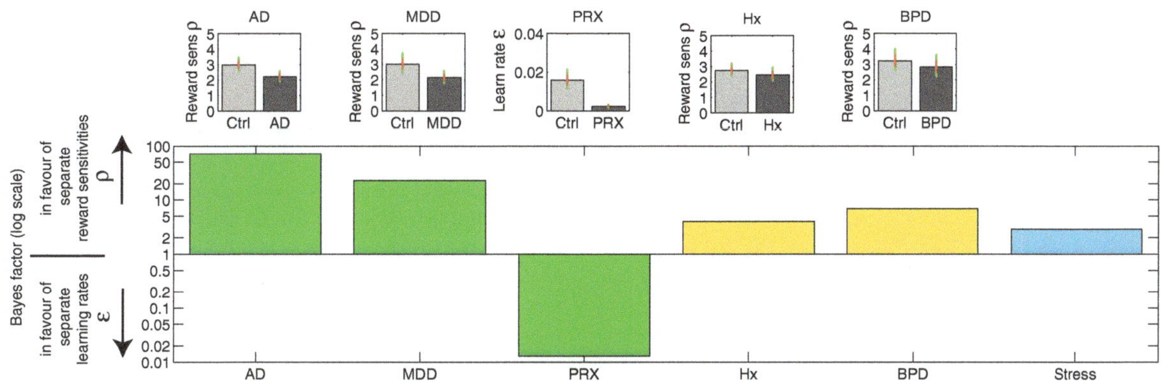

Figure 4 Comparing models incorporating hypotheses about group differences in terms of reward sensitivity ρ or learning rate ϵ. Each bar of the large panel shows the Bayes factor comparing $\mathcal{M}_\rho$ to $\mathcal{M}_\epsilon$. Green bars indicate very strong evidence for model $\mathcal{M}_\rho$ (Bayes factor $\geq$ 20), yellow bars weak evidence (Bayes factor 3 – 10) and cyan bars insufficient evidence (Bayes factor < 3). MDD and high scores of anhedonic depression (AD) result in a reduction in ρ. Pramipexole instead reduces the learning rate. Stress has no differential effect on reward sensitivity compared with learning rate. Participants with a past history of depression, or euthymic individuals with bipolar disorder, showed weak evidence for a reduction in ρ. The insets at the top show the inferred priors over the relevant parameters of the winning model for each group.

Note, however, that various studies (e.g. [18,61,62]) have failed to find a direct correlate between anhedonia measures such as those employed here and participants' ratings of how pleasant a sucrose solution is—a widely-used animal model of anhedonia [63].

By contrast, in our paradigm, ρ falls squarely within the behavioural definition of 'wanting' whereby past experiences are collated into values that influence choice. One possibility is thus that our results reflect the way that 'liking' is coupled into 'wanting', with the reward having less impact when it occurred (ρ was lower), rather than the same amount of pleasure not being translated efficiently into anticipation (which would be the consequence of lowered ϵ). Such a reduction in reward sensitivity parallels reductions in emotional reactions seen in MDD in response to appetitive, but also aversive, stimuli [64].

At a neurobiological level, 'liking', has been linked to μ-opioid signalling [40,65-67] in NAcc shell. Recent PET studies have reported prefrontal changes in μ-opioid receptors in MDD [68], and μ-opioid receptors have been found to affect the response to antidepressant medications [69]. We also note that substance abuse disorders, including of opiates, are prominently co-morbid with depressive disorders [70,71], although it is not clear whether abuse causes depression or *vice versa*. It would be interesting to examine the effect of opiates on tasks like those examined here. If the primary reward sensitivity relates to "liking" and consummatory pleasure, then one would expect a preferential impact on ρ, unlike dopamine.

Dopamine in depression

The temporal difference learning model of phasic dopamine signalling posits that DA reports the prediction error δ. As mentioned in the introduction, a multiplicative change in this signal would be equivalent to a change in the learning rate ϵ. Although an alteration in the reward sensitivity ρ necessarily also leads to an alteration in the prediction error δ, the consequences of an abnormality that arises upstream of the prediction error are subtly different from an abnormality affecting the already computed prediction error signal. It is the latter that is most closely aligned with a primary alteration in dopaminergic function.

In the current study, we report tentative findings suggesting that pramipexole reduced the learning rate rather than affecting the reward sensitivity, which might correspond to a direct reduction in the signal reported by phasic DA. Although pramipexole is a non-ergot D_2/D_3 *agonist* (and is clinically used as such in Parkinson's disease, restless leg syndrome, and occasionally in treatment-resistant MDD), it has previously been found to have behavioural effects of a DA *antagonist* at the low doses (0.5 mg) used in our dataset [72-74]. Similarly, low doses of the D_2 agonist cabergoline have been found to specifically reduce reward go learning [75]. With both drugs, it has been postulated that this may be due to activation of inhibitory [76] presynaptic D_2 receptors, which have a higher affinity for DA [77] and *reduce* phasic DA release ([78-82]; see also [56]) and DA cell firing [83]. Thus, our findings echo those of a recent study showing that dopamine agonists can reinstate prediction errors by restoring the component of the prediction error related to expected value, rather than that of reward [84]. However, we emphasize that the conclusions pertaining to dopamine rest on the contribution of only one study and that there are important technical caveats to be borne in mind (see below).

As indicated in the introduction, DA has multiple and profound involvements with depression. These range from the fact that DA manipulations affect mood [85] and that many antidepressants have pro-DA effects (including buproprion, sertraline, nomifensine, tranylcypromine amongst others; [86]), to a role in resilience [87,88], and suicidality in MDD [89,90]. Critically, depression is common in other disorders that also involve DA dysfunction, such as Parkinson's disease and schizophrenia [91,92]. However, the findings reported here speak to the specific aspects of phasic DA in learning, rather than to all the manifold ways in which DA may be involved in anhedonia and depression. Tonic DA levels, which are partially independent of phasic bursts of activity [93,94] have a profound impact on energy levels and vigour [95,96] making this feature of DA a likely candidate for the severe psychomotor retardation seen in melancholic depression [32], and to the distinction between pleasure and motivational aspects of anhedonia [18,97]. In the context of our task, this may relate to reaction times (albeit noting that these can also be affected by phasic DA signals; [98]), which were not analysed. Rather, here, we focused on the role of DA in instrumental learning of action values. Note, though, that the current design cannot completely disentangle instrumental effects from those due to Pavlovian approach [58,99]. Such Pavlovian influences involve dopamine and the nucleus accumbens (NAcc; [100-105]), and may indeed constitute one of the ways in which DA supports antidepressant function [106,107].

Overall, our findings are consistent with the fact that DA by itself is not a major target for psychopharmacological treatment of anhedonia [92], and, modulo the issues mentioned above, that DA appears to mediate 'wanting', more than 'liking' [40,108]. There has been a number of recent functional imaging investigations into reward-related decision making in MDD (e.g. [11,109-114]). Our findings have key implications for the interpretations of these studies, as it is important to separate contributions to the correlates of prediction errors that arise from changes in reward sensitivity from changes in learning rate. Because a) 'wanting' (reinforcement) and 'liking' (hedonic) aspects of tasks will often overlap; and b) both changes in ρ and ϵ would affect correlations with a regressor based on prediction errors δ, our findings do not invalidate these imaging results, but call for studies and analyses that further separate them.

Analysis methods

Our conclusions were derived from a detailed, model-based meta-analysis combining behavioural data from six datasets in 392 sessions. Several features and limitations of this analysis deserve comment.

First, the interpretability of the parameters is maximised by using rigorous model comparisons. The Bayesian approach we used prevents overfitting by *integrating out* individual subject parameters [43,45,46,58]. Rather than just comparing how careful parameter tuning can allow a model to fit the data extremely well, we extensively sampled the model's entire parameter space, and ask how well, on average, the *class* of model, independent of its particular parameters, can fit the given data (for an insightful explanation, see chapter 28 of [59]). Next, our model comparison is done at the group level, rather than at the individual level, again through sampling and Bayesian model comparison. This ensures that conclusions about the parameters do apply to the group.

Second, our approach takes individual model fits into account. The regression analyses are true random effects analyses, weighting parameters by how strongly they are constrained by each participant's own choice data, and by how well the model fits that particular participant. This, in combination with the explicit modelling of stimulus uncertainty (beliefs) and instruction weights, ensures that any non-specific performance variability does not unduly affect our parameters of interest. Furthermore, the weighted regression ensures that each participant influences the conclusions proportionally to how well they are fit by the model.

Third, it is standard practice to constrain the parameters when fitting models, for instance to avoid extreme outlier inference. We use two types of constraints. The parameter transformations generate hard constraints that force parameters to remain inside feasible regions. The empirical Bayesian inference of the group priors additionally yields the most appropriate soft constraints [59,115].

Fourth, learning rate and reward sensitivity were correlated in all models tested. To alleviate this, we enforced independence at the group level. One standard approach would have been to compare models in which one dimension is constrained by forcing the parameters for all participants along that dimension to be equal. However, this a) is an unrealistic constraint; b) fails to address the fact that parameters may not give the model equal flexibility; and c) renders parameters hard to interpret as variability from one is squeezed into all the other parameters (which further aggravates point b). To circumvent these issues, we contrasted the parsimony of models that explicitly allowed participants to fall into distinct groups. Doing this at the group level addressed the questions at the group level, which is where we sought to draw conclusions. We also performed the regression analysis in a number of ways to assess the selectivity of the relationship with ρ and its stability in the inference procedure.

Fifth, it is important to note that our failure to discover correlations between AD and learning rate, or between the effects of pramipexol and reward sensitivity might be due to limits of power. This is particularly true for the categorical comparisons on which arguments about the differential effect of dopamine and anhedonia or depression rest mainly. It will be critical to replicate these findings in larger samples, potentially requiring paradigms explicitly adapted to separating the two factors.

Sixth, we find no evidence that either learning rate of reward sensitivity clearly separates any of the groups when comparing the basic model to models $\mathcal{M}_\rho$ or $\mathcal{M}_\epsilon$ that allow for the two groups to have different means in one of the other parameter. However, our central motivation was whether anhedonia associated more with unusual ρ or unusual ϵ, because of the different psychiatric and psychological interpretations of these possibilities. The most direct test of this is to compare $\mathcal{M}_\rho$ to $\mathcal{M}_\epsilon$ rather than comparing each to a mid-point in the shape of the basic model. Furthermore, there are a number of caveats to this finding, which form the basis for reporting the more lenient comparison between models $\mathcal{M}_\rho$ and $\mathcal{M}_\epsilon$. First, the model comparison technique may be too conservative for this particular analysis. For instance, at the top level we very stringently punish according to the total number of observations. Although we have found this to overestimate the rate at which the group-level variance should drop with observations, in our hands this penalty has proven to yield the correct responses most reliably when tested on a variety of surrogate datasets (unpublished data in preparation). This is likely to be particularly important given that the power in the analyses in Figure 4 is much lower than that in the preceding analyses using the entire dataset. These considerations do not bear on comparisons between models $\mathcal{M}_\rho$ and $\mathcal{M}_\epsilon$. Furthermore, the panels showing the parameters in Figure 4 appear to show robust group differences. However, a separation in parameter space does not guarantee that the increase in fit outweighs the increase in model complexity.

Of course, even though our best fitting model did an excellent job predicting the data of a plurality of participants, there could be a model that we did not try that would do even better. This is particularly true of the participants in the Stress dataset, who were fit the worst. There is a conventional ANOVA-like procedure in these circumstances that involves assessing the extent to which responses are potentially predictable [44,116] from running the same task multiple times. Unfortunately, it is not clear how to execute this in cases involving learning which is contingent on the participants' behaviour.

Alternative models

One advantage of the simplicity of the task is that it is likely insensitive to several aspects of reinforcement learning that are under current investigation, such as goal-directed *versus* habitual decision-making [117,118]. However, one interesting direction would be to consider a more Bayesian treatment of the learning process, according to which the effective learning rate ϵ should be a function of the amount of experience that the participant has had, modulated by the participant's belief that the contingencies are constant [119-121].

This elaborate account raises an important question about the factor ϵ in the models that we did build. Here, we considered the effect on learning of manipulating the magnitude of δ_t; but noted that this is exactly confounded in the magnitude of ϵ. Neurobiologically, though, there could be an alternative realization of ϵ, notably via cholinergic influences [122-124]. It would be interesting to examine the effect of cholinergic manipulations on the basic task.

Equally, in conventional reinforcement learning models, it is common to employ a variant of Equation 2 in which the terms $\mathcal{W}$ are multiplied by another arbitrary constant which is usually written β and called an inverse temperature. The larger β, the more deterministic the choice between a_t and $\bar{a}_t$, all else being equal. Thus β is often used as a surrogate for controlling exploration, as more stochastic choices (lower β) are more exploratory. However, in our model, β can substitute *exactly* for ρ (in a very similar way that ϵ can substitute for the magnitude of δ). Thus reward insensitivity could masquerade as over-exploration or (particularly in depression) as under-exploitation. These are not differentiable in this task. Nevertheless, the neurobiological realization of the exploration constant β has been suggested as being rather different – notably involving noradrenergic neuromodulation [125] – opening up another line of experimental investigation.

Finally, two relevant findings may be important for future model development. First, positive affective responses to positive events in daily life have recently been found to be *stronger* in depressed than in non-depressed individuals [126]. Second, the impact of negative events has been found to be determined not by the strength of the immediate emotional reaction, but by the attributions made about it [127]. Thus, it may be that the effects seen here can be modified by higher-order processes in ways that are critical for the development of psychopathology, and it may be useful to extend the present methods to such interactions [60].

Conclusions

This paper presented a model-based meta-analysis of behavioural data spanning several related manipulations and adds to a growing literature of behavioural correlates of depression [64,128]. We concluded that anhedonia in depressive states was mediated by a change in reward sensitivity, which has different behavioural consequences from either stress or DA manipulations. Our analysis allowed us to draw these conclusions while taking into account as much as possible the variability between the datasets and participants; and the variability in other, unrelated aspects of task performance. We believe that similar analyses could be readily applied to other datasets. We hope that our findings will encourage the re-analysis of the dissociation between reward sensitivity and dopaminergic processes in depressive states.

Additional file

Additional file 1: Supplementary methods and results [43,63-65].

Competing interests

The authors declare that they have no competing interests.

Authors' contributions

QJMH and PD performed the computational modelling analysis. DAP and RB devised the experiment and collected the data. All authors wrote the manuscript. All authors read and approved the final manuscript.

Acknowledgements

The authors would like to thank the member of the Affective Neuroscience Laboratory for their assistance with collection of the data analysed in this manuscript.

Funding

Funding from the Gatsby Charitable Foundation (QH, PD) and Deutsche Forschungsgemeinschaft DFG GZ RA/1047/2-1 (QH). Collection of datasets presented in the current manuscript was supported by grants from the National Institute of Mental Health (R01 MH068376, R21 MH078979, R01 MH095809) and National Center for Complementary & Alternative Medicine (R21AT002974) awarded to DAP. DAP has also received consulting fees from ANT North America Inc. (Advanced Neuro Technology), AstraZeneca, Ono Pharma USA, Shire and Servier, as well as honoraria from AstraZeneca for projects unrelated to this study.

Author details

[1]Gatsby Computational Neuroscience Unit, UCL, London, UK. [2]Wellcome Trust Centre for Neuroimaging, UCL, London, UK. [3]Translational Neuromodeling Unit, University of Zurich and ETH Zurich, Switzerland. [4]Department of Psychiatry, Psychotherapy and Psychosomatics, University Hospital of Psychiatry, Zurich, Switzerland. [5]Department of Psychiatry, Harvard Medical School, MA, USA. [6]Department of Psychology and Neuroscience, Duke University, NC, USA.

References

1. American Psychiatric Association: *Diagnostic and Statistical Manual of Mental Disorders*: American Psychiatric Association Press; 1994.
2. World Health Organization: *International Classification of Diseases*: World Health Organization Press; 1990.
3. Myin-Germeys I, Peeters F, Havermans R, Nicolson NA, DeVries MW, Delespaul P, Os JV: **Emotional reactivity to daily life stress in psychosis and affective disorder: an experience sampling study.** *Acta Psychiatr Scand* 2003, **107**(2):124–131.
4. Costello CG: **Depression: Loss of reinforcers or loss of reinforcer effectiveness?.** *Behav Ther* 1972, **3:**240–247.
5. Akiskal HS, McKinney WT: **Depressive disorders: toward a unified hypothesis.** *Science* 1973, **182**(107):20–29.
6. Blaney PH: **Contemporary theories of depression: critique and comparison.** *J Abnorm Psychol* 1977, **86**(3):203–223.
7. Nelson RE, Craighead WE: **Selective recall of positive and negative feedback, self-control behaviors, and depression.** *J Abnorm Psychol* 1977, **86**(4):379–388.
8. Henriques JB, Glowacki JM, Davidson RJ: **Reward fails to alter response bias in depression.** *J Abnorm Psychol* 1994, **103**(3):460–466.
9. Henriques JB, Davidson RJ: **Decreased Responsiveness to reward in depression.** *Cogn Emotion* 2000, **14**(5):711–724.
10. Pizzagalli DA, Jahn AL, O'Shea JP: **Toward an objective characterization of an anhedonic phenotype: a signal-detection approach.** *Biol Psychiatry* 2005, **57**(4):319–327. [http://dx.doi.org/10.1016/j.biopsych.2004.11.026]
11. Steele JD, Kumar P, Ebmeier KP: **Blunted response to feedback information in depressive illness.** *Brain* 2007, **130**(Pt 9):2367–2374. [http://dx.doi.org/10.1093/brain/awm150]
12. Huys QJM: **Reinforcers and control. Towards a computational ætiology of depression.** *PhD thesis*. Gatsby Computational Neuroscience Unit, UCL, University of London 2007, [http://www.gatsby.ucl.ac.uk/ qhuys/pub.html]
13. Huys QJM, Vogelstein J, Dayan P, Bottou L: **Psychiatry: Insights into depression through normative decision-making models.** In *Advances in Neural Information Processing Systems 21*. Edited by Koller D, Schuurmans D, Bengio Y: MIT Press; 2009:729–736.
14. Chase HW, Frank MJ, Michael A, Bullmore ET, Sahakian BJ, Robbins TW: **Approach and avoidance learning in patients with major depression and healthy controls: relation to anhedonia.** *Psychol Med* 2010, **40**(3):433–440 doi:10.1017/S0033291709990468.
15. Chase HW, Michael A, Bullmore ET, Sahakian BJ, Robbins TW: **Paradoxical enhancement of choice reaction time performance in patients with major depression.** *J Psychopharmacol* 2010, **24**(4):471–479. [http://dx.doi.org/10.1177/0269881109104883]
16. Beck A, Steer R, Brown G: *Manual for the Beck Depression Inventory-II*. San Antonio: Psychological Corporation; 1996.
17. Watson D, Weber K, Assenheimer JS, Clark LA, Strauss ME, McCormick RA: **Testing a tripartite model: I. Evaluating the convergent and discriminant validity of anxiety and depression symptom scales.** *J Abnorm Psychol* 1995, **104:**3–144.
18. Treadway MT, Zald DH: **Reconsidering anhedonia in depression: lessons from translational neuroscience.** *Neurosci Biobehav Rev* 2011, **35**(3):537–555. [http://dx.doi.org/10.1016/j.neubiorev.2010.06.006]
19. Papp M, Klimek V, Willner P: **Parallel changes in dopamine D_2 receptor binding in limbic forebrain associated with chronic mild stress-induced anhedonia and its reversal by imipramine.** *Psychopharmacology* 1994, **115**(4):441–446.
20. Ichikawa J, Meltzer HY: **Effect of antidepressants on striatal and accumbens extracellular dopamine levels.** *Eur J Pharmacol* 1995, **281**(3):255–261.
21. D'Aquila PS, Collu M, Gessa GL, Serra G: **The role of dopamine in the mechanism of action of antidepressant drugs.** *Eur J Pharmacol* 2000, **405**(1-3):365–373.
22. Barr AM, Markou A, Phillips AG: **A 'crash' course on psychostimulant withdrawal as a model of depression.** *Trends Pharmacol Sci* 2002, **23**(10):475–482.
23. Montague PR, Dayan P, Sejnowski TJ: **A framework for mesencephalic dopamine systems based on predictive Hebbian learning.** *J Neurosci* 1996, **16**(5):1936–1947.
24. O'Doherty JP, Dayan P, Friston K, Critchley H, Dolan RJ: **Temporal difference models and reward-related learning in the human brain.** *Neuron* 2003, **38**(2):329–337.
25. Bayer HM, Glimcher PW: **Midbrain dopamine neurons encode a quantitative reward prediction error signal.** *Neuron* 2005, **47:**129–141. [http://dx.doi.org/10.1016/j.neuron.2005.05.020]
26. Waelti P, Dickinson A, Schultz W: **Dopamine responses comply with basic assumptions of formal learning theory.** *Nature* 2001, **412**(6842):43–48. [http://dx.doi.org/10.1038/35083500]
27. D'Ardenne K, McClure SM, Nystrom LE, Cohen JD: **BOLD responses reflecting dopaminergic signals in the human ventral tegmental area.** *Science* 2008, **319**(5867):1264–1267. [http://dx.doi.org/10.1126/science.1150605]
28. Kapur S, Mann JJ: **Role of the dopaminergic system in depression.** *Biol Psychiatry* 1992, **32:**1–17. [http://dx.doi.org/10.1016/0006-3223(92)90137-O]
29. Nutt DJ: **The role of dopamine and norepinephrine in depression and antidepressant treatment.** *J Clin Psychiatry* 2006, **67**(Suppl 6):3–8.
30. Nestler EJ, Carlezon WA: **The mesolimbic dopamine reward circuit in depression.** *Biol Psychiatry* 2006, **59**(12):1151–1159. [http://dx.doi.org/10.1016/j.biopsych.2005.09.018]
31. Dunlop BW, Nemeroff CB: **The role of dopamine in the pathophysiology of depression.** *Arch Gen Psychiatry* 2007, **64**(3):327–337. [http://dx.doi.org/10.1001/archpsyc.64.3.327]
32. Parker G: **Defining melancholia: the primacy of psychomotor disturbance.** *Acta Psychiatr Scand* 2007, **115 (Suppl 433)**(2):21–30.
33. Mathew SJ, Manji HK, Charney DS: **Novel drugs and therapeutic targets for severe mood disorders.** *Neuropsychopharmacology* 2008, **33**(9):2080–2092. [http://dx.doi.org/10.1038/sj.npp.1301652]
34. Schlaepfer TE, Cohen MX, Frick C, Kosel M, Brodesser D, Axmacher N, Joe AY, Kreft M, Lenartz D, Sturm V: **Deep brain stimulation to reward circuitry alleviates anhedonia in refractory major depression.** *Neuropsychopharmacology* 2008, **33**(2):368–377. [http://dx.doi.org/10.1038/sj.npp.1301408]
35. Bewernick BH, Hurlemann R, Matusch A, Kayser S, Grubert C, Hadrysiewicz B, Axmacher N, Lemke M, Cooper-Mahkorn D, Cohen MX, Brockmann H, Lenartz D, Sturm V, Schlaepfer TE: **Nucleus accumbens deep brain stimulation decreases ratings of depression and anxiety in treatment-resistant depression.** *Biol Psychiatry* 2010, **67**(2):110–116. [http://dx.doi.org/10.1016/j.biopsych.2009.09.013]
36. Rescorla R, Wagner A: **A theory of Pavlovian conditioning: Variations in the effectiveness of reinforcement and nonreinforcement.** In *Classical Conditioning II: Current Research and Theory*. Edited by Black AH, Prokasy WF: Appleton-Century-Crofts; 1972:64–99.
37. Widrow B, Hoff M: **Adaptive switching circuits.** In *WESCON Convention Report, Volume 4*: Institute of, Radio Engineers; 1960:96–104.
38. Sutton R, Barto A, et al: **Toward a modern theory of adaptive networks Expectation and prediction.** *Psychol Rev* 1981, **88**(2):135–170.
39. Sutton RS, Barto AG: *Reinforcement Learning: An Introduction*. Cambridge: MIT Press; 1998. [http://www.cs.ualberta.ca/~sutton/book/the-book.html]
40. Berridge KC, Robinson TE: **What is the role of dopamine in reward hedonic impact, reward learning, or incentive salience?.** *Brain Res Rev* 1998, **28**(3):209–269.
41. Smith A, Li M, Becker S, Kapur S: **A model of antipsychotic action in conditioned avoidance: a computational approach.** *Neuropsychopharm* 2004, **29**(6):1040–1049.
42. Daw N: **Decision Making, Affect, and Learning: Attention and Performance XXIII.** Edited by Delgado MR, Phelps EA, Robbins TW: OUP; 2009.
43. Kass R, Raftery A: **Bayes factors.** *J Am Stat Assoc* 1995, **90**(430):773–795.
44. Gelman A, Carlin J, Stern H, Rubin D: *Bayesian Data Analysis*: Chapman and Hall/CRC Press; 2004.
45. Stephan KE, Penny WD, Daunizeau J, Moran RJ, Friston KJ: **Bayesian model selection for group studies.** *Neuroimage* 2009, **46**(4):1004–1017. [http://dx.doi.org/10.1016/j.neuroimage.2009.03.025]
46. Huys QJM, Moutoussis M, Williams J: **Are computational models of any use to psychiatry?.** *Neural Netw* 2011, **24**(6):544–551. [http://dx.doi.org/10.1016/j.neunet.2011.03.001]

47. Bogdan R, Santesso DL, Fagerness J, Perlis RH, Pizzagalli DA: **Corticotropin-releasing hormone receptor type 1 (CRHR1) genetic variation and stress interact to influence reward learning.** *J Neurosci* 1324, **31**(37):6–13254. [http://dx.doi.org/10.1523/JNEUROSCI.2661-11.2011]
48. Pizzagalli DA, Iosifescu D, Hallett LA, Ratner KG, Fava M: **Reduced hedonic capacity in major depressive disorder: evidence from a probabilistic reward task.** *J Psychiatr Res* 2008, **43:**76–87. [http://dx.doi.org/10.1016/j.jpsychires.2008.03.001]
49. Dutra S, Brooks N, Lempert K, Guardado A, Goetz E, Pizzagalli D: **Reward responsiveness in a remitted depressed sample: Effects of gender and trait negative affect.** In *23rd Annual Meeting of the Society for Research in Psychopathology*. Minneapolis; 2009.
50. Pizzagalli DA, Goetz E, Ostacher M, Iosifescu DV, Perlis RH: **Euthymic patients with bipolar disorder show decreased reward learning in a probabilistic reward task.** *Biol Psychiatry* 2008, **64**(2):162–168. [http://dx.doi.org/10.1016/j.biopsych.2007.12.001]
51. Young RC, Biggs JT, Ziegler VE, Meyer DA: **A rating scale for mania reliability, validity and sensitivity.** *Br J Psychiatry* 1978, **133:** 429–435.
52. Hamilton M: **A rating scale for depression.** *J Neurol Neurosurg Psychiatry* 1960, **23:**56–62.
53. Pizzagalli DA, Evins AE, Schetter EC, Frank MJ, Pajtas PE, Santesso DL, Culhane M: **Single dose of a dopamine agonist impairs reinforcement learning in humans: behavioral evidence from a laboratory-based measure of reward responsiveness.** *Psychopharmacol (Berl)* 2008, **196**(2):221–232. [http://dx.doi.org/10.1007/s00213-007-0957-y]
54. Bogdan R, Pizzagalli DA: **Acute stress reduces reward responsiveness: implications for depression.** *Biol Psychiatry* 2006, **60**(10):1147–1154. [http://dx.doi.org/10.1016/j.biopsych.2006.03.037]
55. Tripp G, Alsop B: **Sensitivity to reward frequency in boys with attention deficit hyperactivity disorder.** *J Clin Child Psychol* 1999, **28**(3):366–375. [http://dx.doi.org/10.1207/S15374424jccp280309]
56. Santesso DL, Evins AE, Frank MJ, Schetter EC, Bogdan R, Pizzagalli DA: **Single dose of a dopamine agonist impairs reinforcement learning in humans: evidence from event-related potentials and computational modeling of striatal-cortical function.** *Hum Brain Mapp* 2009, **30**(7):1963–1976. [http://dx.doi.org/10.1002/hbm.20642]
57. Green DM, Swets JA, et al: *Signal Detection Theory and Psychophysics, Volume 1974*. New York: Wiley; 1966.
58. Huys QJM, Cools R, Gölzer M, Friedel E, Heinz A, Dolan RJ, Dayan P: **Disentangling the roles of approach, activation and valence in instrumental and pavlovian responding.** *PLoS Comput Biol* 2011, **7**(4):e1002028. [http://dx.doi.org/10.1371/journal.pcbi.1002028]
59. MacKay DJ: *Information Theory, Inference and Learning Algorithms*. Cambridge: CUP; 2003.
60. Huys QJM, Eshel N, O'Nions E, Sheridan L, Dayan P, Roiser JP: **Bonsai trees in your head: how the Pavlovian system sculpts goal-directed choices by pruning decision trees.** *PLoS Comput Biol* 2012, **8**(3):e1002410. [http://dx.doi.org/10.1371/journal.pcbi.1002410]
61. Berlin I, Givry-Steiner L, Lecrubier Y, Puech AJ: **Measures of anhedonia and hedonic responses to sucrose in depressive and schizophrenic patients in comparison with healthy subjects.** *Eur Psychiatry* 1998, **13**(6):303–309. [http://dx.doi.org/10.1016/S0924-9338(98)80048-5]
62. Dichter GS, Smoski MJ, Kampov-Polevoy AB, Gallop R, Garbutt JC: **Unipolar depression does not moderate responses to the Sweet Taste Test.** *Depress Anxiety* 2010, **27**(9):859–863. [http://dx.doi.org/10.1002/da.20690]
63. Willner P, Towell A, Sampson D, Sophokleous S, Muscat R: **Reduction of sucrose preference by chronic unpredictable mild stress, and its restoration by a tricyclic antidepressant.** *Psychopharmacology* 1987, **93**(3):358–364. [http://dx.doi.org/10.1007/BF00187257]
64. Bylsma LM, Morris BH, Rottenberg J: **A meta-analysis of emotional reactivity in major depressive disorder.** *Clin Psychol Rev* 2008, **28**(4):676–691. [http://dx.doi.org/10.1016/j.cpr.2007.10.001]
65. Smith KS, Berridge KC: **The ventral pallidum and hedonic reward neurochemical maps of sucrose "liking" and food intake.** *J Neurosci* 2005, **25**(38):8637–8649.
66. Pecina S, Berridge KC: **Hedonic hot spot in nucleus accumbens shell where do mu-opioids cause increased hedonic impact of sweetness?.** *J Neurosci* 1177, **25**(50):7–11786.
67. Berridge KC: **'Liking' and 'wanting' food rewards: brain substrates and roles in eating disorders.** *Physiol Behav* 2009, **97**(5):537–550. [http://dx.doi.org/10.1016/j.physbeh.2009.02.044]
68. Kennedy SE, Koeppe RA, Young EA, Zubieta JK: **Dysregulation of endogenous opioid emotion regulation circuitry in major depression in women.** *Arch Gen Psychiatry* 2006, **63**(11):1199–1208. [http://dx.doi.org/10.1001/archpsyc.63.11.1199]
69. Garriock HA, Tanowitz M, Kraft JB, Dang VC, Peters EJ, Jenkins GD, Reinalda MS, McGrath PJ, von Zastrow M, Slager SL, Hamilton SP: **Association of mu-opioid receptor variants and response to citalopram treatment in major depressive disorder.** *Am J Psychiatry* 2010, **167**(5):565–573. [http://dx.doi.org/10.1176/appi.ajp.2009.08081167]
70. Grant BF: **Comorbidity between DSM-IV drug use disorders and major depression: results of a national survey of adults.** *J Subst Abuse* 1995, **7**(4):481–497.
71. Swendsen J, Conway KP, Degenhardt L, Glantz M, Jin R, Merikangas KR, Sampson N, Kessler RC: **Mental disorders as risk factors for substance use, abuse and dependence: results from the 10-year follow-up of the National Comorbidity Survey.** *Addiction* 2010, **105**(6):1117–1128. [http://dx.doi.org/10.1111/j.1360-0443.2010.02902.x]
72. Samuels ER, Hou RH, Langley RW, Szabadi E, Bradshaw CM: **Comparison of pramipexole and amisulpride on alertness, autonomic and endocrine functions in healthy volunteers.** *Psychopharmacology (Berl)* 2006, **187**(4):498–510. [http://dx.doi.org/10.1007/s00213-006-0443-y]
73. Samuels ER, Hou RH, Langley RW, Szabadi E, Bradshaw CM: **Comparison of pramipexole and modafinil on arousal, autonomic, and endocrine functions in healthy volunteers.** *J Psychopharmacol* 2006, **20**(6):756–770. [http://dx.doi.org/10.1177/0269881106060770]
74. Samuels ER, Hou RH, Langley RW, Szabadi E, Bradshaw CM: **Comparison of pramipexole with and without domperidone co-administration on alertness, autonomic, and endocrine functions in healthy volunteers.** *Br J Clin Pharmacol* 2007, **64**(5):591–602. [http://dx.doi.org/10.1111/j.1365-2125.2007.02938.x]
75. Frank MJ, O'Reilly RC: **A mechanistic account of striatal dopamine function in human cognition: psychopharmacological studies with cabergoline and haloperidol.** *Behav Neurosci* 2006, **120**(3):497–517. [http://dx.doi.org/10.1037/0735-7044.120.3.497]
76. Grace AA: **Phasic versus tonic dopamine release and the modulation of dopamine system responsivity: a hypothesis for the etiology of schizophrenia.** *Neuroscience* 1991, **41:**1–24.
77. Cooper J, Bloom F, Roth R: *The Biochemical Basis of Neuropharmacology*. 8th edition. USA: Oxford University Press; 2003.
78. Baudry M, Martres MP, Schwartz JC: **In vivo binding of 3H-pimozide in mouse striatum: effects of dopamine agonists and antagonists.** *Life Sci* 1977, **21**(8):1163–1170.
79. Fuller RW, Clemens JA, Hynes MD: **Degree of selectivity of pergolide as an agonist at presynaptic versus postsynaptic dopamine receptors implications for prevention or treatment of tardive dyskinesia.** *J Clin Psychopharmacol* 1982, **2**(6):371–375.
80. Tissari AH, Rossetti ZL, Meloni M, Frau MI, Gessa GL: **Autoreceptors mediate the inhibition of dopamine synthesis by bromocriptine and lisuride in rats.** *Eur J Pharmacol* 1983, **91**(4):463–468.
81. Sumners C, de Vries JB, Horn AS: **Behavioural and neurochemical studies on apomorphine-induced hypomotility in mice.** *Neuropharmacology* 1981, **20**(12A):1203–1208.
82. Schmitz Y, Benoit-Marand M, Gonon F, Sulzer D: **Presynaptic regulation of dopaminergic neurotransmission.** *J Neurochem* 2003, **87**(2):273–289.
83. Piercey MF, Hoffmann WE, Smith MW, Hyslop DK: **Inhibition of dopamine neuron firing by pramipexole, a dopamine D3 receptor-preferring agonist comparison to other dopamine receptor agonists.** *Eur J Pharmacol* 1996, **312:**35–44.
84. Chowdhury R, Guitart-Masip M, Lambert, Dayan P, Huys QJM, Düzel E, Dolan RJ: **Dopamine restores reward prediction errors in older age.** *Nat Neurosci* 2013. in press.

85. Tremblay LK, Naranjo CA, Cardenas L, Herrmann N, Busto UE: **Probing brain reward system function in major depressive disorder: altered response to dextroamphetamine.** *Arch Gen Psych* 2002, **59**(5): 209–215.
86. Berton O, Nestler EJ: **New approaches to antidepressant drug discovery: beyond monoamines.** *Nat Rev Neurosci* 2006, **7**(2):137–151. [http://dx.doi.org/10.1038/nrn1846]
87. Krishnan V, Han MH, Graham DL, Berton O, Renthal W, Russo SJ, Laplant Q, Graham A, Lutter M, Lagace DC, Ghose S, Reister R, Tannous P, Green TA, Neve RL, Chakravarty S, Kumar A, Eisch AJ, Self DW, Lee FS, Tamminga CA, Cooper DC, Gershenfeld HK, Nestler EJ: **Molecular adaptations underlying susceptibility and resistance to social defeat in brain reward regions.** *Cell* 2007, **131**(2):391–404. [http://dx.doi.org/10.1016/j.cell.2007.09.018]
88. Vialou V, Robison AJ, Laplant QC, Covington HE, Dietz DM, Ohnishi YN, Mouzon E, Rush AJ, Watts EL, Wallace DL, Iñiguez SD, Ohnishi YH, Steiner MA, Warren BL, Krishnan V, BolaÃśos CA, Neve RL, Ghose S, Berton O, Tamminga CA, Nestler EJ: **DeltaFosB in brain reward circuits mediates resilience to stress and antidepressant responses.** *Nat Neurosci* 2010, **13**(6):745–752. [http://dx.doi.org/10.1038/nn.2551]
89. Pitchot W, Hansenne M, Ansseau M: **Role of dopamine in non-depressed patients with a history of suicide attempts.** *Eur Psychiatry* 2001, **16**(7):424–427.
90. Pitchot W, Reggers J, Pinto E, Hansenne M, Fuchs S, Pirard S, Ansseau M: **Reduced dopaminergic activity in depressed suicides.** *Psychoneuroendocrinology* 2001, **26**(3):331–335.
91. Tandberg E, Larsen JP, Aarsland D, Cummings JL: **The occurrence of depression in Parkinson's disease. A community-based study.** *Arch Neurol* 1996, **53**(2):175–179.
92. Gelder M, Harrison P, Cowen P: *Shorter Oxford Textbook of Psychiatry.* Oxford: Oxford University Press; 2006.
93. Floresco SB, West AR, Ash B, Moore H, Grace AA: **Afferent modulation of dopamine neuron firing differentially regulates tonic and phasic dopamine transmission.** *Nat Neurosci* 2003, **6**(9):968–973. [http://dx.doi.org/10.1038/nn1103]
94. Goto Y, Grace AA: **Dopaminergic modulation of limbic and cortical drive of nucleus accumbens in goal-directed behavior.** *Nat Neurosci* 2005, **8**(6):805–812. [http://dx.doi.org/10.1038/nn1471]
95. Salamone JD, Correa M, Farrar AM, Nunes EJ, Pardo M: **Dopamine behavioral economics, and effort.** *Front Behav Neurosci* 2009, **3**(13). [http://dx.doi.org/10.3389/neuro.08.013.2009]
96. Niv Y, Daw ND, Joel D, Dayan P: **Tonic dopamine: opportunity costs and the control of response vigor.** *Psychopharmacol(Berl)* 2007, **191**(3):507–520. [http://dx.doi.org/10.1007/s00213-006-0502-4]
97. Gard D, Gard M, Kring A, John O: **Anticipatory and consummatory components of the experience of pleasure: a scale development study.** *J Res Pers* 2006, **40**(6):1086–1102.
98. Satoh T, Nakai S, Sato T, Kimura M: **Correlated coding of motivation and outcome of decision by dopamine neurons.** *J Neurosci* 2003, **23**(30):9913–9923.
99. Guitart-Masip M, Fuentemilla L, Bach DR, Huys QJM, Dayan P, Dolan RJ, Duzel E: **Action dominates valence in anticipatory representations in the human striatum and dopaminergic midbrain.** *J Neurosci* 2011, **31**(21):7867–7875. [http://dx.doi.org/10.1523/JNEUROSCI.6376-10.2011]
100. Parkinson JA, Olmstead MC, Burns LH, Robbins TW, Everitt BJ: **Dissociation in effects of lesions of the nucleus accumbens core and shell on appetitive pavlovian approach behavior and the potentiation of conditioned reinforcement and locomotor activity by D-amphetamine.** *J Neurosci* 1999, **19**(6):2401–2411.
101. Dickinson A, Smith J, Mirenowicz J: **Dissociation of Pavlovian and instrumental incentive learning under dopamine antagonists.** *Behav Neurosci* 2000, **114**(3):468–483.
102. Parkinson JA, Dalley JW, Cardinal RN, Bamford A, Fehnert B, Lachenal G, Rudarakanchana N, Halkerston KM, Robbins TW, Everitt BJ: **Nucleus accumbens dopamine depletion impairs both acquisition and performance of appetitive Pavlovian approach behaviour: implications for mesoaccumbens dopamine function.** *Behav Brain Res* 2002, **137**(1-2):149–163.
103. Di Ciano P, Cardinal RN, Cowell RA, Little SJ, Everitt BJ: **Differential involvement of NMDA, AMPA/kainate, and dopamine receptors in the nucleus accumbens core in the acquisition and performance of pavlovian approach behavior.** *J Neurosci* 2001, **21**(23):9471–9477.
104. Murschall A, Hauber W: **Inactivation of the ventral tegmental area abolished the general excitatory influence of Pavlovian cues on instrumental performance.** *Learn Mem* 2006, **13**(2):123–126. [http://dx.doi.org/10.1101/lm.127106]
105. Lex B, Hauber W: **The role of nucleus accumbens dopamine in outcome encoding in instrumental and Pavlovian conditioning.** *Neurobiol Learn Mem* 2010, **93**(2):283–290. [http://dx.doi.org/10.1016/j.nlm.2009.11.002]
106. Sasaki-Adams DM, Kelley AE: **Serotonin-Dopamine interactions in the control of conditioned reinforcement and motor behaviour.** *Neuropsychopharm* 2001, **25**(3):440–452.
107. Iiguez SD, Warren BL, Bolaos-Guzmn CA: **Short- and long-term functional consequences of fluoxetine exposure during adolescence in male rats.** *Biol Psychiatry* 2010, **67**(11):1057–1066. [http://dx.doi.org/10.1016/j.biopsych.2009.12.033]
108. Flagel SB, Clark JJ, Robinson TE, Mayo L, Czuj A, Willuhn I, Akers CA, Clinton SM, Phillips PEM, Akil H: **A selective role for dopamine in stimulus-reward learning.** *Nature* 2011, **469**(7328):53–57. [http://dx.doi.org/10.1038/nature09588]
109. Elliott R, Sahakian BJ, Michael A, Paykel ES, Dolan RJ: **Abnormal neural response to feedback on planning and guessing tasks in patients with unipolar depression.** *Psychol Med* 1998, **28**(3):559–71.
110. Steele JD, Meyer M, Ebmeier KP: **Neural predictive error signal correlates with depressive illness severity in a game paradigm.** *Neuroimage* 2004, **23:**269–2680.
111. Knutson B, Bhanji JP, Cooney RE, Atlas LY, Gotlib IH: **Neural responses to monetary incentives in major depression.** *Biol Psychiatry* 2008, **63**(7):686–692. [http://dx.doi.org/10.1016/j.biopsych.2007.07.023]
112. Kumar P, Waiter G, Ahearn T, Milders M, Reid I, Steele JD: **Abnormal temporal difference reward-learning signals in major depression.** *Brain* 2008, **131**(Pt 8):2084–2093. [http://dx.doi.org/10.1093/brain/awn136]
113. Pizzagalli DA, Holmes AJ, Dillon DG, Goetz EL, Birk JL, Bogdan R, Dougherty DD, Iosifescu DV, Rauch SL, Fava M: **Reduced caudate and nucleus accumbens response to rewards in unmedicated individuals with major depressive disorder.** *Am J Psychiatry* 2009, **166**(6):702–710. [http://dx.doi.org/10.1176/appi.ajp.2008.08081201]
114. Smoski MJ, Felder J, Bizzell J, Green SR, Ernst M, Lynch TR, Dichter GS: **fMRI of alterations in reward selection, anticipation, and feedback in major depressive disorder.** *J Affect Disord* 2009, **118**(1-3):69–78. [http://dx.doi.org/10.1016/j.jad.2009.01.034]
115. Dempster A, Laird N, Rubin D: **Maximum likelihood from incomplete data via the EM algorithm.** *J Royal Stat Soc Series B (Methodological)* 1977, **39:**1–38.
116. Sahani M, Linden JF: **How linear are auditory cortical responses?** In *Advances in Neural Information Processing Systems, Volume 15.* Edited by Becker S, Thrun S, Obermayer K. Cambridge: MIT Press; 2003:109–116.
117. Dickinson A, Balleine B: **The role of learning in the operation of motivational systems.** In *Stevens' Handbook of Experimental Psychology, Volume 3.* Edited by Gallistel R. New York: Wiley; 2002:497–534.
118. Daw ND, Niv Y, Dayan P: **Uncertainty-based competition between prefrontal and dorsolateral striatal systems for behavioral control.** *Nat Neurosci* 2005, **8**(12):1704–1711. [http://dx.doi.org/10.1038/nn1560]
119. Sutton R: **Integrated architectures for learning, planning, and reacting based on approximating dynamic programming.** In *Proceedings of the Seventh International Conference on Machine Learning, Volume 216*; 1990:224.
120. Dayan P, Kakade S, Montague PR: **Learning and selective attention.** *Nat Neurosci* 2000, **3 Suppl:**1218–1223. [http://dx.doi.org/10.1038/81504]
121. Behrens TEJ, Woolrich MW, Walton ME, Rushworth MFS: **Learning the value of information in an uncertain world.** *Nat Neurosci* 2007, **10**(9):1214–1221. [http://dx.doi.org/10.1038/nn1954]
122. Baxter MG, Chiba AA: **Cognitive functions of the basal forebrain.** *Curr Opin Neurobiol* 1999, **9**(2):178–183.
123. Yu AJ, Dayan P: **Uncertainty, neuromodulation, and attention.** *Neuron* 2005, **46**(4):681–692. [http://dx.doi.org/10.1016/j.neuron.2005.04.026]

124. Hasselmo: **Neuromodulation: acetylcholine and memory consolidation.** *Trends Cogn Sci* 1999, **3**(9):351–359.
125. Aston-Jones G, Cohen JD: **Adaptive gain and the role of the locus coeruleus-norepinephrine system in optimal performance.** *J Comp Neurol* 2005, **493:**99–110. [http://dx.doi.org/10.1002/cne.20723]
126. Bylsma LM, Taylor-Clift A, Rottenberg J: **Emotional reactivity to daily events in major and minor depression.** *J Abnorm Psychol* 2011, **120:**155–167. [http://dx.doi.org/10.1037/a0021662]
127. Haeffel GJ, Abramson LY, Brazy PC, Shah JY, Teachman BA, Nosek BA: **Explicit and implicit cognition: a preliminary test of a dual-process theory of cognitive vulnerability to depression.** *Behav Res Ther* 2007, **45**(6):1155–1167. [http://dx.doi.org/10.1016/j.brat.2006.09.003]
128. Eshel N, Roiser JP: **Reward and punishment processing in depression.** *Biol Psychiatry* 2010, **68**(2):118–124. [http://dx.doi.org/10.1016/j.biopsych.2010.01.027]

3

Neural temporal dynamics of stress in comorbid major depressive disorder and social anxiety disorder

Christian E Waugh[1*], J Paul Hamilton[2], Michael C Chen[2], Jutta Joormann[3] and Ian H Gotlib[2]

Abstract

Background: Despite advances in neurobiological research on Major Depressive Disorder and Social Anxiety Disorder, little is known about the neural functioning of individuals with comorbid depression/social anxiety. We examined the timing of neural responses to social stress in individuals with major depression and/or social anxiety. We hypothesized that having social anxiety would be associated with earlier responses to stress, having major depression would be associated with sustained responses to stress, and that comorbid participants would exhibit both of these response patterns.

Methods: Participants were females diagnosed with pure depression (n = 12), pure social anxiety (n = 16), comorbid depression/social anxiety (n = 17), or as never having had any Axis-I disorder (control; n = 17). Blood oxygenation-level dependent activity (BOLD) was assessed with functional magnetic resonance imaging (fMRI). To induce social stress, participants prepared a speech that was ostensibly to be evaluated by a third party.

Results: Whereas being diagnosed with depression was associated with a resurgence of activation in the medial frontal cortex late in the stressor, having social anxiety was associated with a vigilance-avoidance activation pattern in the occipital cortex and insula. Comorbid participants exhibited activation patterns that generally overlapped with the non-comorbid groups, with the exception of an intermediate level of activation, between the level of activation of the pure depression and social anxiety groups, in the middle and posterior cingulate cortex.

Conclusions: These findings advance our understanding of the neural underpinnings of major depression and social anxiety, and of their comorbidity. Future research should elucidate more precisely the behavioral correlates of these patterns of brain activation.

Keywords: Depression, Anxiety, Comorbidity, FMRI, Stress, MPFC

Background

Although investigators have examined the psychological and neurobiological mechanisms that underlie Major Depressive Disorder (MDD) and Social Anxiety Disorder (SAD), most researchers have assessed these disorders separately. Over 50 percent of people diagnosed with a psychological disorder, however, have additional comorbid disorders [1]. Depression is likely to co-occur with forms of anxiety and, in particular, with social anxiety [2]. Indeed, individuals with comorbid depression/social anxiety (MDD/SAD) have poorer behavioral (e.g. strengthened negative cognitive biases) [3] and life (e.g. likelihood of suicide attempt) [4] outcomes than do people with either diagnosis alone.

These deleterious consequences of comorbid depression and social anxiety underscore the importance of elucidating the neural mechanisms that underlie this comorbidity. After decades of research, investigators now have formulated neural models of depression [5] and of social anxiety (e.g.,) [6] based on patterns of neural activation that have been found in these disorders. For example, in response to emotional stimuli, depressed participants exhibit abnormal increases in amygdala [7] and subgenual anterior cingulate cortex

* Correspondence: waughce@wfu.edu
[1]Department of Psychology, Wake Forest University, P.O. Box 7778, Winston Salem, NC 27109, USA
Full list of author information is available at the end of the article

activity, [8] and an abnormal lack of dorsolateral prefrontal cortex activity [9]. In response to emotional stimuli, participants with social anxiety exhibit hyperactivity in the amygdala (similar to depressed participants), [6] as well as hyperactivity in the rostral anterior cingulate cortex [10] and insula [11]. These neural models, however, are based on findings of studies conducted with pure, non-comorbid forms of these disorders. We know much less about the neural functioning of individuals with comorbid depression/social anxiety – whether comorbid individuals exhibit neural responses that are more similar to the responses of people with one disorder or the other, an additive combination of the disorder-specific responses, or an intermediate blend of the disorder-specific responses.

Recent studies highlight the utility of examining the neural functioning of individuals with comorbid disorders. For example, Andreescu et al. [12] found that older participants with diagnosed major depression and high scores on a self-report measure of anxiety exhibited greater activation than did depressed participants with low anxiety scores in the dorsal anterior cingulate cortex in a cognitive interference task. More recently, Etkin and Schatzberg [13] examined the neural functioning of patients diagnosed with depression and/or Generalized Anxiety Disorder while they performed an emotional conflict task and found that, whereas activation deficits in the ventral cingulate and amygdala were shared by all patient groups, activation in the lateral prefrontal cortex was unique to the non-comorbid depression group. These findings demonstrate that examining individuals with comorbid disorders can distinguish patterns of neural functioning that are common to both disorders from those that are unique to each disorder. In the present study, we both extend these findings of studies assessing other comorbid disorders to examine the neural mechanisms that underlie the comorbidity of depression and social anxiety, and advance research on neural functioning in comorbid disorders by examining the temporal dynamics of whole-brain responses to stress.

Given the importance of stress in the etiology and maintenance of both depression [14] and anxiety, [15] it is likely that examining the neural correlates of the stress response will prove critical in understanding neural aspects of comorbidity. For example, Young and colleagues found that individuals with comorbid depression and anxiety (including, but not limited to social anxiety) exhibited greater hypothalamic-pituitary-adrenal (HPA) axis responses to social stress than did individuals diagnosed with either depression or anxiety alone [16]. One potentially illustrative difference between anxious and depressed persons is the timing of their responses to stress. Anxious people are characterized by a vigilance-avoidance attentional bias in which they both engage with and disengage from threat-related stimuli relatively quickly [17-19] (although there is mixed evidence for the avoidance from threat-related stimuli in social anxiety) [20], which may be one mechanism underlying their enhanced responses during the anticipation of stressors [11]. In contrast, depressed individuals are characterized by high levels of rumination about past negative emotional stimuli, [21,22] which may underlie their more sustained responses to stress [23].

Recently, investigators have used social evaluative threat tasks to assess temporal aspects of the neural response to stress in humans. Social evaluative threat tasks induce robust changes in both hypothalamic-pituitary-adrenal axis activity [24] and peripheral nervous system activity [25]. Investigators have demonstrated that the association between social threat and these stress-induced physiological responses is mediated by the rostral medial frontal cortex [26]. This medial frontal region exhibits activation early in the stressor as well as sustained activation throughout the duration of the stressor [26,27]. Although this may represent a normal response profile to stress, the finding that the medial frontal cortex is involved in both the initial generation and subsequent maintenance of the stress response highlights this region as a possible site for activation patterns hypothesized to characterize both social anxiety and depression. Whereas the hyper-vigilance to threat in socially anxious people may affect medial frontal cortex activation early in the stressor, the sustained responses to threat in depressed people may influence medial frontal cortex activation late in the stressor.

In the current study, we examined the magnitude and timing of neural responses to social stress in participants diagnosed as having pure depression, pure social anxiety, comorbid depression/social anxiety, or as never having had any Axis-I disorder. We hypothesized that relative to participants without social anxiety, participants diagnosed with social anxiety will exhibit greater changes in medial frontal cortex activation from baseline to early in the stressor (i.e., during instructions or early speech preparation) and less activation late in the stressor (i.e., during late speech preparation or recovery). Alternatively, relative to participants without depression, participants diagnosed with depression will exhibit greater responses in the medial frontal cortex later in the stressor. Finally, it is not clear whether the effects of comorbidity are additive or interactive. We hypothesized that if comorbidity is the additive combination of depression and social anxiety, then comorbid participants should exhibit medial frontal cortex responses both early and late in the stressor.

Methods

Participants

Participants were recruited from local psychiatric outpatient clinics and through website postings. Sixty-four female individuals participated in this study: 16 participants diagnosed with social anxiety disorder; 14 participants diagnosed with major depressive disorder; 17 participants diagnosed with comorbid major depressive disorder and social anxiety disorder; and 17 never-disordered control participants. Diagnostic evaluations were based on DSM-IV-TR criteria using the Structured Clinical Interview for DSM-IV-TR Axis I (SCID-I) [28] administered by trained interviewers. Participants in the comorbid group met diagnostic criteria for both current social anxiety disorder and current major depressive disorder, but did not meet current or lifetime criteria for any other Axis-I disorder. Participants in the two non-comorbid clinical groups met diagnostic criteria for either current social anxiety disorder or major depressive disorder, but did not meet criteria for lifetime comorbidity of anxiety and depression or for any other current or lifetime Axis-I disorder. Finally, controls did not meet criteria for current or past Axis-I psychopathology. Inter-rater reliability kappas ranged from .92 to 1.0 for the above diagnoses. All participants were between 18 and 55 years of age, had no lifetime history of psychotic ideation and no reported substance abuse within the past six months. All aspects of this study complied with the ethical standards for treatment of human participants from the American Psychiatric Association and were approved by the Institutional Review Board. All participants provided informed consent. Due to equipment issues, data from two participants (both from the non-comorbid major depressive disorder group) were excluded from further analyses.

Demographic and clinical information

Participants provided demographic and clinical information, including age, education, household income, race, symptoms of social anxiety (Social Phobia Anxiety Index) [29] and depression (Beck Depression Inventory - II), [30] treatment status (Table 1), and current medications (Additional file 1: Table S1).

Social evaluative threat task

In the scanner, participants completed a social evaluative threat task (450 seconds; 7:30) [26]. All instructions were presented visually. For baseline (120 seconds), participants were instructed to relax, to clear their minds of all thoughts and feelings, and to keep their eyes on a fixation cross. In the task instructions period (80 seconds), participants were told that they would have 2 minutes to prepare a 7-minute speech on "Why you are a good friend," that they would be audiotaped, that others would evaluate their performance, and that there was a possibility that they would not have to give their speech. In the speech preparation period (120 seconds), participants were instructed to 'Prepare your speech now,' which remained on the screen for the entire period. In the recovery period (130 seconds), participants were notified that they would not have to give a speech and were instructed to wait for the next task to begin; throughout this period, participants viewed a fixation cross. This speech task has been used successfully in several studies to induce robust affective [25], cardiovascular, [25,31] and neural responses [26].

fMRI Data Acquisition

BOLD data were acquired with a 3.0 T General Electric Signa MR scanner. Following scout scanning, high order shimming was performed over the whole brain until diminishing returns on image distortion correction were met. Next, BOLD data were acquired with a single channel, whole-head imaging coil from 31 axial slices using a spiral pulse sequence [32] [repetition time = 2000 ms, echo time = 40 ms, flip angle = 70°, field of view = 220 mm, number of frames = 225]. Axial slices had 3.44 mm^2 in-plane and 4 mm through-plane resolution (with 1 mm between-slice distance). A high resolution structural scan (115 slices, 1 mm^2 in-plane and 1.5 mm through-plane resolution, echo time = min, flip angle = 15°, field of view = 22 cm) was performed following BOLD scanning runs.

fMRI Image Preprocessing

Preprocessing was performed with the AFNI imaging analysis suite [33]. BOLD images were slice-time corrected to the fifteenth axial slice and motion corrected to the middle acquisition slice using Fourier interpolation. Data were then spatially smoothed with an 8 mm Gaussian kernel and warped to Talairach template space (voxel size = 3 mm^3) [34]. Next, multiple regression was used to remove nuisance effects including six head movement parameters (estimated from motion correction procedure), whole-brain global time series, and linear drift. These images were then converted to statistical parametric mapping (SPM) analyze format and gray-matter masked with the participants' averaged structural image.

fMRI data analysis

To determine *where* and *when* the four groups differed in their brain activation during the social evaluative threat task, we conducted both standard GLM analyses and change-point analyses [27] on the preprocessed images using a combination of SPM and custom MATLAB (Mathworks, Inc.) scripts. For both analyses, each participant's data were first temporally smoothed (6 s kernel; according to published specifications) [27] with an exponentially weighted moving average.

Table 1 Demographic characteristics, clinical characteristics, and self-reported responses to the social evaluative threat task of the diagnosed groups

	Depression (n = 12)	Social Anxiety (n = 17)	Comorbid (n = 17)	Control (n = 16)	Interaction of depression and social anxiety	Main effect of having depression	Main effect of having social anxiety
			G^2				
Race (%Caucasian)	75%	71%	76%	50%	5.10	2.34	1.84
Current treatment	33%	13%	35%	0%	9.82*	7.22*	.60
			F				
Age	39.67 (11.30)	32.82 (12.34)	29.88 (10.92)	33.64 (9.36)	2.40	.28	3.36
Income[ab]	3.70 (2.11)	4.08 (1.44)	2.60 (1.55)	4.00 (1.75)	1.52	3.47	1.15
Education (years)[c]	15.80 (2.69)	16.06 (1.12)	14.92 (2.25)	17.80 (2.73)	.48	6.27*	4.32*
Depression (BDI-II)	26.58 (13.85)	11.65 (8.82)	30.35 (10.83)	2.06 (3.15)	.63	100.85*	13.88*
Social Anxiety (SPAI)	63.31 (29.67)	91.47 (26.11)	98.55 (17.81)	29.79 (28.88)	3.70	8.73*	49.71*
Anti-Depressant Load	1.75 (2.01)	.41 (1.18)	1.12 (2.12)	.00 (.00)	1.74	9.61*	.08
Anti-Anxiety Load	.33 (.65)	.12 (.33)	.18 (.39)	.00 (.00)	1.86	3.80*	.04
Perceived demands	4.78 (1.44)	5.45 (1.18)	5.45 (1.39)	3.74 (1.35)	2.31	2.29	12.09*
Perceived resources	3.94 (1.25)	3.73 (1.71)	2.96 (1.37)	5.04 (1.05)	.21	6.81*	10.39*
Positive affect during speech prep	1.98 (.94)	1.90 (.68)	1.74 (.83)	2.58 (.94)	1.03	3.05	4.40*
Negative affect during speech prep	3.02 (1.21)	3.32 (1.12)	3.45 (1.04)	2.26 (.82)	1.35	2.70	7.63*
Positive affect after speech prep	2.31 (.88)	2.30 (.82)	2.13 (.59)	2.78 (1.03)	.44	2.20	2.30
Negative affect after speech prep	1.22 (.46)	1.33 (.42)	1.53 (.64)	1.29 (.58)	.93	.20	1.60

BDI-II = Beck Depression Inventory; SPAI = Social Phobia and Anxiety Inventory; PA = positive affect; NA = negative affect. Standard deviations are in parentheses.
* $p < .05$.
[a] Income was measured on an ordinal scale (1 = less than 10 k, 2 = 10-25 k, 3 = 25-50 k, 4 = 50-75 k, 5 = 75-100 k, 6 = more than 100 k).
[b] N = 52 (Depression, n = 10; Social Anxiety, n = 13; Comorbid, n = 15; Control, n = 14).
[c] N = 50 (Depression, n = 11; Social Anxiety, n = 16; Comorbid, n = 13; Control, n = 10).

GLM analysis

We first conducted a standard GLM analysis to determine whether this simpler analysis could capture temporal differences in activation patterns as a function of diagnosis. The smoothed time-series data were regressed on activation functions that modeled each task period (i.e. 1 s during the task period of interest and 0 s everywhere else). The task periods of interest included the instructions, early speech preparation, late speech preparation, and recovery periods. The participants' beta coefficients were then submitted to a multiple regression model. Similar to factorial analyses conducted in previous fMRI studies examining the comorbidity of depression and anxiety [13], we entered into this group-level regression model mean-scaled dummy variables representing a) being diagnosed with depression or not (MDD or MDD/SAD [1] vs. CTL or SAD [−1]); b) being diagnosed with social anxiety or not (SAD or MDD/SAD [1] vs. MDD or CTL [−1]); and c) their interaction (the product of the first two predictors). We also added into our model medication covariates reflecting both antidepressant and anxiolytic/sedative loads as regressors of non-interest (See Additional file 1: Table S1) [35]. The resulting whole-brain t-maps were corrected (threshold = .0005, k = 14) to derive per-voxel corrected p-values < .05 (based on 1000 Monte Carlo simulations) [36].

Change-point analysis

The primary difference between the GLM analysis and the change-point analysis is that instead of estimating activation for an entire task period, the change-point analysis estimates activation for every time-point after baseline. To do this, we first subtracted activity during the baseline period from activity from the task periods of interest (everything after baseline). Next, we conducted weighted multiple regression (using the same group-level regression model mentioned above) on every time-point in each voxel's time-series [27]. Similar to the GLM, 'activation' still reflects changes from baseline, and 'activation differences' still reflects changes in activation between diagnostic groups. Because the change-point analysis conducted hundreds of regressions for each voxel (for each time point), we implemented family-wise error control with a Monte Carlo simulation (5000 iterations) to get corrected p-values across each voxel's time-series. A change-point in activation was defined as the longest series of consecutive time-points exhibiting suprathreshold activation levels or differences in activation as a function of our group-level regressors (minimum of 3 time-points to capture meaningful changes in activation; corrected $p < .05$). This created three separate activation maps: 1) a map of the max t within a change-point series, which corresponds roughly to standard GLM contrast maps; 2) a map of the first suprathreshold time-point of the change-point series to determine when these change-points began; and 3) a map of the duration of the change-point series. For ease of presentation, we categorized the change-point onsets as occurring during the instructions (60–100 time-points), early speech preparation (101–130 time-points), late speech preparation (131–160 time-points), or recovery period (161–225 time-points).

Next, to derive maps of the simple main effects of diagnoses that were not qualified by the interaction of the two diagnoses, we masked the main effects max-t activation maps with the interaction map. In addition, to limit diagnosis-related differences in activation to those areas that were specifically responsive to the social evaluative threat task, we masked the main effects and interaction max-t activation maps with the max-t activation map from the group intercept. These steps were not necessary for the GLM analyses because we found no main effects or interaction of diagnoses. These change-point max-t activation maps were then thresholded with the same criteria used for the GLM analyses.

For post-hoc contrasts tests, we conducted simple-slopes analyses [37] using the average of the beta-coefficients across all the suprathreshold time-points for all the voxels in each cluster. For post-hoc correlations, we averaged each participant's BOLD responses across all the suprathreshold change-point TRs for each voxel in the clusters of interest. We corrected for multiple correlations using Bonferroni correction.

Self-report responses to the social evaluative threat task

Speech appraisals

After participants exited the MRI scanner, they were asked to rate how they would feel "right now if you would have had to give the speech" on scales assessing appraisals of stress [38]. Participants provided responses from 1 (*strongly disagree*) to 7 (*strongly disagree*) on two subscales: one assessing the perceived demands of the social evaluative threat task (e.g. "The speech would have been very demanding;" "The speech would have been very stressful"), and the other assessing the participants' perceived resources available to engage in the speech (e.g. "I feel that I would have had the abilities to perform well in the speech"). The ratio of perceived demands to perceived resources has been found to underlie feelings of threat [39]. The two subscales exhibited good reliability (demands: $\alpha = .86$; resources: $\alpha = .84$).

Affect

Participants were also asked to rate how they felt "when preparing your speech" and "when you learned that you did not have to give your speech" on a shortened Positive and Negative Affect Schedule (PANAS) yielding total positive affect and negative affect scores [40]. Each of the four measures was found to be reliable (speech preparation positive affect: $\alpha = .89$; speech preparation negative affect: $\alpha = .82$; recovery positive affect: $\alpha = .88$; recovery negative affect: $\alpha = .78$).

Results

Self-report responses to the social evaluative threat task

Speech appraisals

We conducted a 2 (depression: present, absent) x 2 (social anxiety: present, absent) x 2 (appraisal type: demands, resources) mixed ANOVA with depression and social anxiety as between-subjects factors and appraisal type as the within-subject factor. This analysis yielded significant interactions of appraisal type and depression, $F(1,57) = 7.10$, $p = .01$, and appraisal type and social anxiety, $F(1,57) = 17.51$, $p < .001$. In both cases, the presence of a disorder was associated with greater perceived demands than perceived resources (Table 1), indicating that participants with depression and/or social anxiety perceived the social evaluative threat task as threatening.

Affect

We conducted separate 2 (depression: present, absent) x 2 (social anxiety: present, absent) x 2 (period: speech preparation, recovery) mixed ANOVAs on positive and negative affect, with depression and social anxiety as between-subjects factors and period as a within-subject factor. For positive affect, the ANOVA yielded significant main effects of depression, $F(1,57) = 4.14$, $p = .046$, and social anxiety, $F(1,57) = 5.12$, $p = .027$. In both cases, the presence of the disorder was associated with lower positive affect than was the absence of the disorder (Table 1). The ANOVA also yielded a significant main effect of period, $F(1, 57) = 9.87$, $p = .003$, indicating that participants reported feeling higher positive affect during recovery (Mean = 2.38, SD = .84) than during speech preparation (Mean = 2.03, SD = .85). None of the higher-order interactions was significant. The ANOVA conducted on negative affect yielded significant main effects of social anxiety and period that were qualified by a significant interaction of social anxiety and period, $F(1, 57) = 5.56$, $p = .022$. This interaction was due to participants with social anxiety reporting higher levels of negative affect (Mean = 3.40,

SD = 1.05) than did participants without social anxiety (Mean = 2.64, SD = 1.06) during speech preparation, $F(1,57) = 9.47$, $p = .003$, but not during recovery (social anxiety: Mean = 1.43, SD = .53; no social anxiety: Mean = 1.25, SD = .54; $F(1, 57) = .50$, $p = .48$).

fMRI findings – GLM analysis

Overall intercept

Medial frontal cortex. On average, participants exhibited increased medial frontal cortex activation during the early and late speech preparation periods (Table 2).

Table 2 GLM analysis of BOLD responses to the social evaluative threat task – overall intercept[1]

Region	x	y	z	voxels	vol (mm³)	Peak t
		Positive Activation				
Instructions						
Occipital cortex	4	−64	−8	3772	101844	10.78
Midbrain	8	−8	−10	153	4131	6.37
l. Amygdala	−20	−10	−10	22	594	5.10
r. Middle Temporal G.	56	−34	−2	68	1836	5.37
r. Inferior Frontal G.	44	22	22	142	3834	5.26
l. Inferior Frontal G.	−38	28	20	22	594	4.77
Early Speech Prep						
Medial Frontal G./Anterior Cingulate G.	4	22	16	1640	44280	6.61
Late Speech Prep						
l. Middle Frontal G.	−32	4	38	24	648	5.85
r. Precentral G.	32	−16	40	21	567	4.08
Medial Frontal G.	2	26	40	14	378	4.30
Recovery						
l. Middle Temporal G.	−52	−22	−8	54	1458	5.16
r. Lingual G.	26	−80	−4	15	405	4.48
Midbrain	−2	−28	4	69	1863	5.07
l. Superior Temporal G.	−50	−32	16	140	3780	4.66
l. Middle Frontal G.	−44	28	20	45	1215	4.43
Precuneus	2	−34	44	36	972	4.65
		Negative Activation				
Instructions						
l. Uncus	−32	2	−28	22	594	−5.03
Bilateral Inferior Frontal G./Middle Cingulate G.	−8	−8	28	6335	171045	−10.32
r. Middle Frontal G.	32	52	8	97	2619	−6.78
r. Middle Frontal G.	−32	52	8	102	2754	−5.53
Early Speech						
Occipital Cortex	−2	−64	2	2488	67176	−8.72
l. Middle Frontal G.	−40	22	20	132	3564	−6.18
Late Speech						
r. Parahippocampal G.	32	−26	−22	29	783	−4.39
l. Parahippocampal G.	−34	−32	−22	35	945	−4.34
Midbrain	2	−28	2	64	1728	−5.22
Recovery						
Pons	−8	−32	−28	69	1863	−4.99
Anterior Cingulate G./Caudate/Insula	8	8	14	2350	63450	−7.05

Note. [1] The GLM analysis did not yield any activation differences as a function of diagnosis. l. = left, r. = right.

Other regions. Notably, participants also exhibited decreased activation in a large region of cortex spanning bilateral inferior frontal gyrus and middle cingulate during the instructions period, as well as decreased activation in the anterior cingulate and insula during recovery.

Diagnosis differences

The GLM analysis did not yield any significant main effects of depression and social anxiety, or significant interaction of depression and social anxiety.

fMRI findings - change-point analysis

Overall intercept

Medial frontal cortex. On average, participants exhibited increased medial frontal cortex activation during the early speech preparation period (Figure 1; Table 3). **Other regions.** Notably, participants also exhibited decreased activation in the posterior cingulate during the late speech preparation period and decreased activation in the anterior cingulate during recovery.

Depression vs. No Depression

Medial frontal cortex. As hypothesized, the change-point analysis yielded a main effect of being diagnosed with depression on medial frontal cortex activation during the late speech preparation period. Whereas participants diagnosed with depression (MDD, MDD/SAD) exhibited a resurgence of medial frontal cortex activation during the late speech preparation period, participants without depression (SAD, CTL) exhibited a return to baseline during this period (Figure 2). There was also a main effect of being diagnosed with depression on medial frontal cortex activation in the instructions period; participants with diagnosed depression did not exhibit the deactivation that was evident in nondepressed participants (Figure 2; Table 4). Notably, these associations between depression and medial frontal cortex activity remained significant when controlling for depression and anxiety symptoms (both ts > 3.8, ps < .001). **Other regions.** As with the medial frontal cortex findings, participants diagnosed with depression exhibited a more extensive pattern of activation than did participants without depression during the instructions (e.g., middle cingulate, precentral gyrus) and late speech preparation (e.g., insula, caudate; Table 4) periods. In the early speech preparation period, participants with depression exhibited greater activation than did participants without depression in the inferior frontal gyrus.

Social Anxiety vs. No Social Anxiety

Medial frontal cortex. Contrary to predictions, there was no effect of social anxiety diagnosis on medial frontal cortex activation in the speech preparation period or during recovery. **Other regions.** Instead, participants diagnosed with social anxiety (SAD, MDD/SAD), relative to participants without diagnosed social anxiety (MDD, CTL), exhibited greater activation in the occipital cortex and middle temporal gyrus during instructions as well as less activation in the insula and postcentral gyrus during recovery (Table 5).

Interaction of Depression and Social Anxiety

Medial frontal cortex. There was no interaction of diagnoses of depression and social anxiety on activation in the medial frontal cortex. **Other regions.** Participants diagnosed with comorbid depression/social anxiety exhibited different patterns of activation than did participants with non-comorbid diagnoses in several regions (Figure 3; Table 6). The comorbid participants exhibited intermediate activation in the middle cingulate cortex and precentral gyrus (less than the pure depression group and more than the pure social anxiety group; Figure 3) as well as the posterior cingulate (less than the pure social anxiety group and more than the pure depression group). The comorbid participants also exhibited activation similar to that exhibited

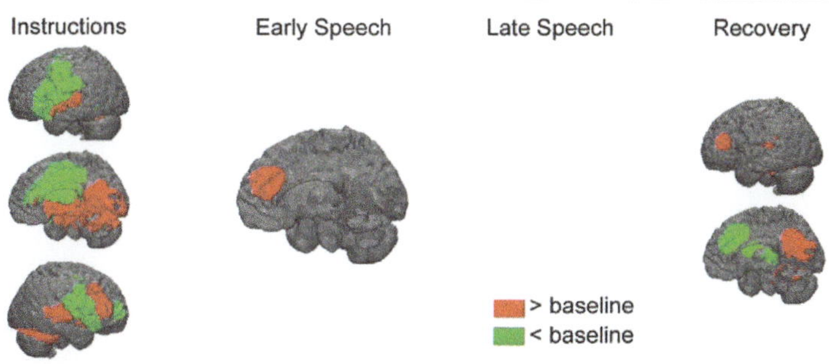

Figure 1 BOLD responses to social evaluative threat for the overall group intercept. These BOLD responses represent overall changes in activation (intercept from multiple regression equation) from baseline to the four periods of interest (instructions [60–100 time-points)], early speech preparation [101–130 time-points], late speech preparation [131–160 time-points], and recovery period [161–225 time-points]).

Table 3 Change-point analysis of the BOLD responses to the social evaluative threat – average (intercept) across all participants

Region	x	y	Z	voxels	vol (mm^3)	Peak t	Change-point onset	Change-point offset
				Activation > Baseline				
Instructions								
Occipital cortex	2	−58	−4	3811	102897	18.22	64	106
Midbrain	2	−8	−10	197	5319	7.68	63	78
l. Superior Temporal G.	−52	−4	−2	138	3726	7.89	68	82
r. Superior Temporal G. & Insula	50	−16	4	284	7668	8.44	62	80
r. Inferior Frontal G.	44	28	16	121	3267	7.16	65	82
Early Speech Prep								
Medial Frontal G.	4	38	20	73	1971	5.2	108	119
Late Speech Prep								
No suprathreshold voxels								
Recovery								
r. Fusiform G.	32	−50	−14	98	2646	6.45	164	171
l. Parahippocampal G.	−26	−40	−14	83	2241	7.32	163	171
Precuneus	8	−62	22	200	5400	8.28	163	173
Posterior Cingulate G.	−16	−52	10	28	756	7.05	163	171
l. Superior Temporal G.	−50	−32	16	40	1080	5.04	165	177
l. Middle Frontal G.	−44	34	16	15	405	5.55	164	169
				Activation < Baseline				
Instructions								
Middle Cingulate G./Bilateral Insula/Parietal Cortex	−8	−8	26	5617	151659	−11.87	63	88
r. Hippocampus	32	−22	−4	27	729	−6.09	66	71
r. Middle Temporal G.	34	52	8	24	648	−4.97	70	80
r. Caudate	22	−32	16	22	594	−5.72	65	71
r. Superior Temporal G.	40	−46	22	19	513	−5.39	63	66
Early Speech Prep								
l. Posterior Cingulate G.	−26	−44	34	33	891	−6.19	106	117
Late Speech Prep								
No suprathreshold voxels								
Recovery								
r. Thalamus	28	−26	−2	35	945	−5.82	165	169
l. Putamen	−32	−22	−2	50	1350	−5.84	165	170
r. Putamen	28	−8	8	78	2106	−6.55	164	171
l. Thalamus	−16	−22	10	25	675	−6.84	165	170
Anterior Cingulate G.	10	26	34	135	3645	−5.58	165	179

Note. vol = volume; G. = Gyrus.

by the control participants in several regions, including greater activation than participants with pure depression or pure social anxiety in the insula (instructions) and middle temporal gyrus (recovery), and less activation than the pure diagnostic groups in the cerebellum (instructions) and cuneus (instructions/recovery).

Correlations among brain activation and self-reported responses to the social evaluative threat task

Regions associated with depression

We examined whether the differential medial frontal cortex responses (MDD > No MDD) during the instructions and late speech preparation periods were related to

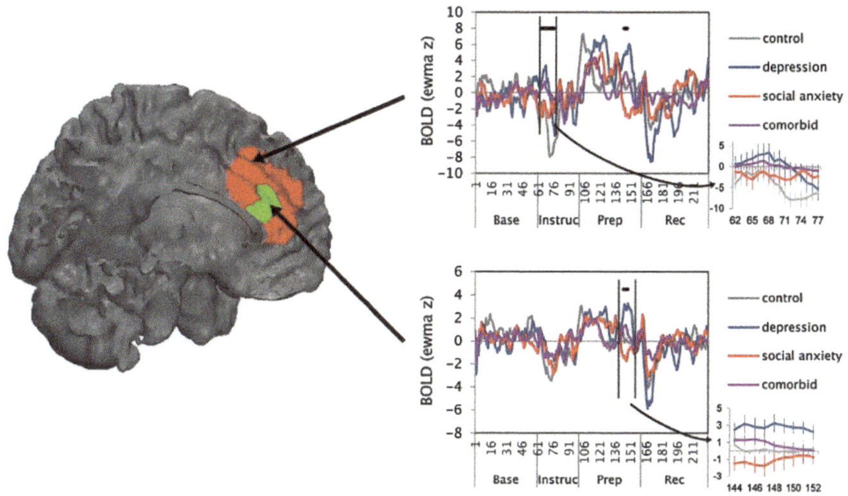

Figure 2 BOLD responses to social evaluative threat by diagnostic group in the medial frontal cortex. Each graph plots activation across time: EWMA z = exponentially weighted moving average z-statistic (temporally smoothed deviations from baseline period). Base = baseline, Instruc = instructions period, Prep = speech preparation period, and Rec = recovery period. Solid black bars designate the time-points for which there was a main effect of being diagnosed with depression vs. not having depression; insets show these data with standard error bars. BOLD = blood oxygenation level dependent.

self-reported responses to the task ($\alpha_{corr} = .05/6 = .008$). No correlations survived Bonferroni correction.

Regions associated with social anxiety

We next examined the correlations between self-reported responses to the speech task and differential responses in the lingual gyrus and superior temporal gyrus during the instructions period (SAD > No SAD) and in the insula during the recovery period (SAD < No SAD) – regions that may represent the hypothesized 'vigilance-avoidance' pattern of responding ($\alpha_{corr} = .05/6 = .008$). Across all participants, no correlations survived Bonferroni correction. Across only the participants with social anxiety, activation in the lingual gyrus during the instructions period was negatively correlated with negative affect to preparing the speech, $r(32) = -.49$, $p = .004$, and perceived demands of the speech, $r(32) = -.47$, $p = .006$. In addition, left insula activation during the recovery period was positively correlated with perceived demands of the speech, $r(32) = .48$, $p = .005$.

Discussion

The present study was designed to examine magnitude and timing of neural responses to stress in individuals diagnosed with non-comorbid depression, non-comorbid social anxiety, and comorbid depression/social anxiety. All groups exhibited increased medial frontal cortex activation during the early speech preparation, which is consistent with findings from previous studies [26], followed by decreased activation toward the middle of the speech anticipation period. As we predicted, the change-point analysis revealed that participants with depression (both pure and comorbid) exhibited greater medial frontal cortex activation than those without depression late in the stress task. Notably, whereas we had initially hypothesized that depressed participants would exhibit a sustained pattern of activation, we found instead that depressed participants exhibited a resurgence of medial frontal cortex activation late in the stress task. This late resurgence of medial frontal cortex activation suggests that participants with depression re-engaged with the stressor, although it is unclear what psychological functions subserved this re-engagement. This medial frontal cortex activation during the late speech preparation period was not significantly correlated with any self-reported responses to the speech task, suggesting that depressed participants' re-engagement with the stressor was not due to a more intense negative emotional response to the stressor. One possible explanation for this finding is that this late activation in the medial prefrontal cortex for the depressed participants was due to rumination about negative aspects of the stress task. Indeed, activation in the medial frontal cortex has been found to be associated with functions that subserve rumination about negative events: self-referential processing, [41] self-conscious emotional reactivity, [42] and extended duration of negative emotions [43]. Alternatively, this region has also been found to be associated with generating the arousal necessary for anticipated effort, [26,44] suggesting the possibility that this pattern of activation was

Table 4 Change-point analysis of the BOLD responses to the social evaluative threat task of participants with and without major depressive disorder

Region	x	y	z	voxels	vol (mm^3)	Peak t	change-point onset	change-point offset	comorbid (~,>,<) pure depression[1]
				Depression > No Depression					
Instructions									
r. Insula	38	8	−2	71	1917	7.09	74	82	<
l. Precentral G.*	−50	4	4	54	1458	5.84	99	115	<
l. Precentral G.*	−56	−8	16	15	405	5.83	73	81	<
l. Middle Frontal G.	−40	34	16	14	378	6.88	62	70	~
Medial Frontal G.	4	34	26	88	2376	7.58	62	77	~
l. Inferior Frontal G.	−50	−2	26	19	513	6.79	77	88	
Cingulate G.*	2	4	28	50	1350	6.88	62	81	<
Cingulate G.	−14	−4	26	26	702	5.9	71	81	
Cingulate G.	10	−10	28	24	648	6.11	65	83	<
Early Speech Prep									
l. Precentral G.	−56	−4	8	36	972	5.97	100	114	~
l. Prefrontal G.	−50	4	16	20	540	5.54	104	112	~
Cingulate G.	16	−28	38	16	432	6.35	103	111	~
Late Speech Prep									
l. Insula	−34	−16	14	14	378	5.56	152	160	
r. Insula	34	−8	22	76	2052	6.01	148	162	
l. Postcentral G.	−52	−22	22	24	648	6.54	157	163	~
r. Caudate	14	2	20	33	891	5.97	151	161	
Cingulate G.	10	34	20	15	405	6.69	144	152	
l. Sub-gyral	−34	−20	34	31	837	5.88	148	162	~
l. Sub-gyral*	−16	−40	34	17	459	6.33	154	161	<
Recovery									
r. Cerebellum: Culmen	26	−44	−20	22	594	6.08	164	170	~
Lingual G.*	8	−62	−4	176	4752	7.52	163	171	<
Lingual G.	−8	−82	−2	20	540	6.84	164	169	~
				No Depression > Depression					
Instructions									
Posterior Cingulate	−4	−44	10	16	432	−6.47	70	74	~
Cuneus	−8	−76	20	18	486	−6.64	69	95	~
r. Cuneus	16	−74	16	34	918	−5.66	85	97	~
Early Speech Prep									
l. Caudate	−14	−22	26	16	432	−5.87	116	123	
Late Speech Prep									
l. Lentiform Nucleus	−26	8	8	31	837	−6.67	132	142	
Recovery									
Posterior Cingulate G.*	14	−56	14	55	1485	−6.53	176	190	>
l. Precentral G.	−44	−10	40	16	432	−5.89	165	173	~

Note. These clusters were masked with the clusters that exhibited group average activation differences during the social evaluative threat task. vol = volume; G. = Gyrus. [1] Post-hoc group contrasts that test whether comorbid participants exhibited similar (~; not significantly different from each other, but both groups are different than control participants), greater (>), or less (<) activation than participants with pure depression ($p < .05$). The lack of a symbol means that comorbid participants did not exhibit significantly different activation than control participants and participants with pure depression.
* Those regions for which comorbid participants' activation significantly differed from both pure depression and pure social anxiety groups.

Table 5 Change-point analysis of the BOLD responses to the social evaluative threat task of participants with and without social anxiety disorder

Region	x	y	z	voxels	vol (mm^3)	Peak t	change-point onset	change-point offset	comorbid (~,>,<) social anxiety
				Social Anxiety > No Social Anxiety					
Instructions									
Cerebellum: Declive*	8	−58	−14	325	8775	12.52	66	102	<
r. Lingual G.*	26	−74	−2	15	405	5.34	69	79	<
r. Superior Temporal G.	56	−38	4	31	837	7.68	66	83	~
Early Speech Prep									
No suprathreshold voxels									
Late Speech Prep									
No suprathreshold voxels									
Recovery									
r. Cerebellum: Declive*	26	−56	−20	142	3834	9.03	164	174	<
l. Cerebellum: Declive	−20	−62	−20	83	2241	7.45	163	171	~
				No Social Anxiety > Social Anxiety					
Instructions									
l. Insula	−32	8	−4	54	1458	−7.21	68	80	
r. Precentral G.	50	−8	22	151	4077	−6.6	67	81	~
l. Inferior Frontal G.*	−52	8	10	66	1782	−6.62	68	86	>
r. Middle Frontal G.	34	52	8	19	513	−7.21	68	82	~
Cingulate G.	4	−8	34	237	6399	−7.91	66	91	
l. Cingulate/Supramarginal G.	−26	−26	38	159	4293	−6.94	66	81	~
Early Speech Prep									
No suprathreshold voxels									
Late Speech Prep									
No suprathreshold voxels									
Recovery									
r. Insula	44	−2	−2	103	2781	−6.67	164	184	~
l. Insula	−40	4	2	124	3348	−7.4	164	184	~
l. Postcentral G.	−38	−20	38	29	783	−6.89	166	177	~

Note. These clusters were masked with the clusters that exhibited group average activation differences during the social evaluative threat task. vol = volume; G. = Gyrus. [1] Post-hoc group contrasts that test whether comorbid participants exhibited similar (~; not significantly different from each other, but both groups are different than control participants), greater (>), or less (<) activation than participants with pure social anxiety ($p < .05$). The lack of a symbol means that comorbid participants did not exhibit significantly different activation than control participants and participants with pure social anxiety.
* Those regions for which comorbid participants' activation significantly differed from both pure depression and pure social anxiety groups.

due to depressed participants re-exerting the effort they anticipated it would take to perform the upcoming speech. Future investigations that explicitly assess ruminative thoughts as well as motivation/anticipated effort in depression are necessary to test the veracity of these formulations.

The vigilance-avoidance hypothesis for participants with social anxiety was only partially supported. Participants without depression (i.e., those with either social anxiety or no disorder) exhibited decreased activation in the medial frontal cortex during the instructions period. Consistent with the vigilance hypothesis, deactivation in this region co-occurs with cognitive engagement to external stimuli, [45] suggesting that participants with pure social anxiety were paying relatively more attention to external stimuli (the speech instructions) than were participants with depression. Further supporting this formulation, participants with both pure social anxiety and comorbid social anxiety/depression exhibited greater activation in other regions associated with attending to external stimuli, including the occipital cortex and superior temporal gyrus [46], than did

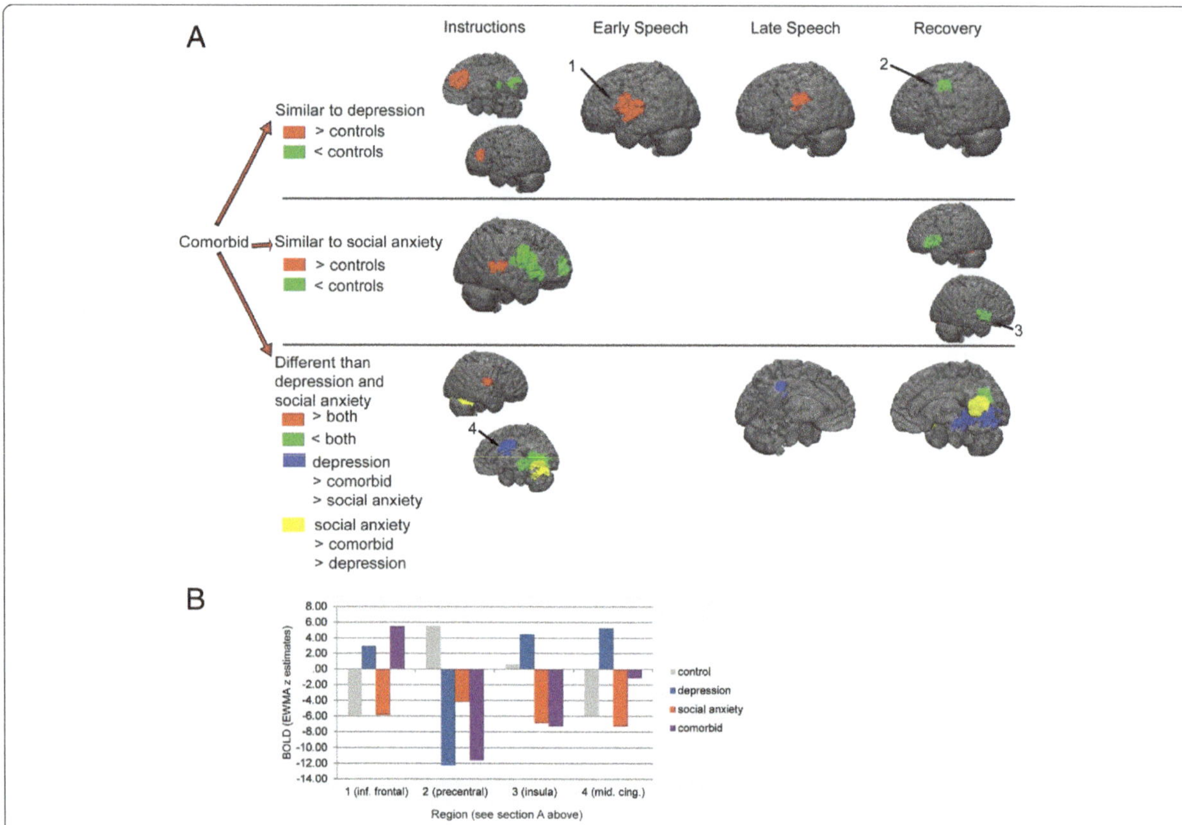

Figure 3 Post-hoc group contrasts that compare the activation of the comorbid group with that of the pure depression and social anxiety groups. A. To have demonstrated similar activation as one of the two pure diagnostic groups, the comorbid group must have exhibited activation that was not significantly different from the pure diagnostic group, and the activation of both the comorbid and pure diagnostic groups must have been significantly different than controls. To have demonstrated different activation than the two pure diagnostic groups, the comorbid group must have exhibited significantly different activation from both the pure depression and social anxiety groups. **B**. Each group's beta estimates of the EWMA z statistic for selected regions. BOLD = blood oxygenation level dependent. EWMA z = exponentially weighted moving average z-statistic (temporally smoothed deviations from baseline period).

participants without social anxiety. Consistent with the avoidance hypothesis, during recovery, social anxiety and comorbid participants exhibited decreased activation in the insula, a region associated with monitoring internal states [47], especially those associated with threat [48]. Together, this pattern of findings suggest that participants with social anxiety exhibited heightened engagement with the stressor when first learning about it (during instructions period) and significant disengagement from the stressor when learning that they would not have to give a speech after all. In addition, we found evidence that this vigilance-avoidance pattern of brain activation may have been adaptive. Across socially anxious participants, the tendency to exhibit greater lingual gyrus activation during the instructions period and decreased insula activation during recovery predicted participants' tendency to perceive the speech task as less demanding. Contrary to predictions, however, having social anxiety did not predict greater medial frontal cortex activation during the early part of the stressor. One possibility that should be tested in future investigations is that the preparation of the speech was too threatening for participants. Indeed, individual differences in social anxiety have been found to be better predictors of differential responses to mildly threatening social situations than to highly threatening social situations [49].

As predicted, the comorbid participants responded similarly to the participants with pure depression and pure social anxiety in a majority of the suprathreshold voxels. Notably, however, during the speech period, the comorbid participants exhibited activation patterns that more closely matched the participants with pure depression than the participants with pure social anxiety (Figure 3). In future studies, investigators should examine whether this asymmetrical influence of these two diagnoses on brain responses to social threat extend to other

Table 6 Change-point analysis of the interaction of depression and social anxiety in BOLD responses to the social evaluative threat task

Region	x	y	z	voxels	vol (mm³)	Peak t	change-point onset	change-point offset	Control	Depression	Social Anxiety	Co-morbid
					Comorbid and/or Control > Depression and/or Social Anxiety							
Instructions												
l. Parahippocampal G	−40	−38	−2	34	918	7.3	65	82	2.52^{b}	-6.09^{a}	-8.17^{a}	-1.43^{ab}
l. Insula	−40	4	−2	28	756	6.84	64	69	7.10^{c}	-8.56^{a}	-5.08^{ab}	-0.16^{b}
l. Insula	−38	−16	8	15	405	5.77	70	78	3.26^{b}	-6.15^{a}	-6.46^{a}	-2.08^{ab}
l. Insula	−40	−8	20	195	5265	8.47	64	79	2.25^{b}	-9.35^{a}	-9.24^{a}	-4.41^{a}
r. Insula*	50	−14	14	30	810	5.78	65	71	2.56^{b}	-7.62^{a}	-7.50^{a}	1.00^{b}
l. Precentral G.	−38	8	22	15	405	5.99	65	75	0.03^{b}	-4.14^{ab}	-6.87^{a}	0.26^{b}
Early Speech Prep												
l. Insula	−50	−34	22	36	972	5.89	115	121	9.46^{c}	-11.72^{a}	-1.47^{b}	2.00^{b}
Late Speech Prep												
l. Lentiform Nucleus	−32	4	−2	15	405	5.58	148	157	3.51^{b}	-3.26^{a}	-3.48^{a}	1.39^{ab}
Recovery												
l. Middle Temporal G.*	−44	−38	2	36	972	7.3	160	170	4.01^{b}	-7.12^{a}	-6.40^{a}	2.08^{b}
l. Precentral G.	−38	−14	32	23	621	7.07	164	177	4.36^{b}	-8.80^{a}	-4.96^{a}	-3.08^{a}
					Depression and/or Social Anxiety > Comorbid and/or Control							
Instructions												
Cerebellum: Declive*	8	−62	−20	14	378	−5.38	90	95	-7.42^{a}	10.43^{c}	26.22^{d}	2.94^{b}
Cuneus*	−8	−68	4	446	12042	−7.94	65	84	3.28^{a}	27.79^{c}	29.39^{c}	12.44^{b}
r. Inferior Frontal G.	40	20	−10	15	405	−6.07	69	81	-11.20^{a}	7.13^{c}	-4.78^{b}	-8.58^{ab}
r. Insula	40	4	−4	23	621	−6.57	71	84	-11.09^{a}	8.04^{b}	-7.03^{a}	-7.09^{a}
r. Cuneus*	22	−76	8	37	999	−6.06	67	79	-1.70^{a}	15.35^{b}	21.56^{c}	3.66^{a}
Early Speech Prep												
No suprathreshold voxels												
Late Speech Prep												
No suprathreshold voxels												
Recovery												
Lingual G.	8	−56	−4	448	12096	−7.4	161	172	-3.95^{a}	27.24^{c}	18.43^{bc}	16.44^{b}
Precuneus*	−2	−68	26	21	567	−6.21	164	171	-6.24^{a}	24.31^{c}	23.38^{c}	12.11^{b}

Note. These clusters were masked with the clusters that exhibited group average activation differences during the social evaluative threat task. vol = volume; G. = Gyrus. Different subscripts represent significantly differences between the groups, calculated using simple slopes analyses on the beta coefficients (presented here) from the multiple regression models.
* Those regions for which comorbid participants' activation significantly differed from both pure depression and pure social anxiety groups.

facets of neural and behavioral functioning. In the few brain regions in which the comorbid participants exhibited different activations than did the participants with pure diagnoses, two patterns emerged. First, the comorbid participants exhibited intermediate activation levels in the middle cingulate cortex, precentral gyrus, and posterior cingulate. This finding raises the intriguing possibility that in these regions the psychological and neural effects of having both depression and social anxiety interact. Second, compared with the pure diagnostic groups, the comorbid group and never-disordered control participants exhibited more tempered responses in the insula (less deactivation) and cuneus (less activation). Future investigations should target these regions as possible sites of dysregulation for individuals with comorbid depression and social anxiety in which neural reactivity to stress is dampened despite heightened self-reported reactivity.

In addition to unpacking the psychological mechanisms that underlie these differences in activation among the diagnostic groups, future studies that replicate and extend this work should address other elements of the current design. For example, investigators should recruit larger samples of both male and female medication-free participants to replicate and extend the present findings to determine whether they generalize to males and to ensure that they are not influenced by medication status. Also, although the speech stressor we used induced similar levels of neural activation during the early-stress period in the depressed and socially anxious participants, the social threat inherent in this task is theoretically more relevant to social anxiety than to depression. Indeed, the participants with social anxiety did report a slightly higher increase in negative affect in response to the social threat stressor than did the participants with depression. By exploring more depression-relevant stressors, future studies should be able to distinguish activation patterns that generalize to other types of stressors from patterns that are specific to the speech stressor.

Conclusions

In sum, the present study is among the first to delineate the neural functioning of comorbidity, and is the first to examine specifically the neural functioning of comorbid depression and social anxiety. We used innovative statistical and methodological techniques to probe temporal aspects of stress-induced neural responding and demonstrated that change-point analyses are more sensitive to temporal differences in activation than standard GLM analyses. This change-point approach allowed us to identify both when and where neural activation differences occurred as a function of diagnosis and yielded several intriguing patterns of activation. Future investigations should assess more explicitly the psychological mechanisms that might underlie these neural activation patterns, as well as possible diagnosis-related differences in functional connectivity among these regions [50] during exposure to stress. Elucidating these unique and shared neural responses to social evaluative threat in individuals with pure depression, pure social anxiety, and comorbid depression/social anxiety may facilitate the selection or development of effective interventions for these debilitating disorders.

Additional file

Additional file 1: Supplementary information and tables.

Competing interests

The authors declare that, except for income received from our primary employer, no financial support or compensation has been received from any individual or corporate entity over the past three years for research or professional service and there are no personal financial holdings that could be perceived as constituting a potential conflict of interest.

Acknowledgments

The authors declare that, except for income received from our primary employer, no financial support or compensation has been received from any individual or corporate entity over the past three years for research or professional service and there are no personal financial holdings that could be perceived as constituting a potential conflict of interest.

The authors thank Juliana Gonzales, Kalpa Bhattacharjee, Arkadiy Maksimovskiy, and Maria Lemus for their help in data collection and preparation. This research was funded by NIMH Grant MH080683 awarded to Ian H. Gotlib. Dr. Waugh had full access to all of the data in the study and takes responsibility for the integrity of the data and the accuracy of the data analysis.

Author details

[1]Department of Psychology, Wake Forest University, P.O. Box 7778, Winston Salem, NC 27109, USA. [2]Department of Psychology, Stanford University, Stanford, CA, USA. [3]Department of Psychology, University of Miami, Coral Gables, FL, USA.

Authors' contributions

CW helped conceive of the design of the study, conducted the data analyses, and took the lead on writing the manuscript. JPH and MCC helped conceive of the design of the study, conducted the fMRI sessions, consulted on data analyses, and contributed to writing the manuscript. JJ helped conceive of the design of the study and contributed to writing the manuscript. IHG helped conceive of the design of the study, consulted on data analyses, and contributed to writing the manuscript. All authors have read and approve of this manuscript.

References

1. Kessler RC, Berglund P, Demler O, Jin R, Walters EE: **Lifetime prevalence and age-of-onset distributions of DSM-IV disorders in the national comorbidity survey replication.** *Arch Gen Psychiatry* 2005, **62**(6):593–602.
2. Brown TA, Campbell LA, Lehman CL, Grisham JR, Mancill RB: **Current and lifetime comorbidity of the DSM-IV anxiety and mood disorders in a large clinical sample.** *J Abnorm Psychol* 2001, **110**(4):585–599.
3. Gilboa-Schechtman E, Presburger G, Marom S, Hermesh H: **The effects of social anxiety and depression on the evaluation of facial crowds.** *Behav Res Ther* 2005, **43**:467–474.
4. Stein MB, Fuetsch M, Muller N, Hofler M, Lieb R, Wittchen H-U: **Social anxiety disorder and the risk of depression.** *Arch Gen Psychiatry* 2001, **58**:251–256.
5. Gotlib IH, Hamilton JP: **Neuroimaging and depression: Current status and unresolved issues.** *Curr Dir Psychol Sci* 2008, **17**(2):159–163.
6. Phan KL, Fitzgerald DA, Nathan PJ, Tancer ME: **Association between amygdala hyperactivity to harsh faces and severity of social anxiety in generalized social phobia.** *Biol Psychiatry* 2006, **59**:424–429.
7. Sheline YI, Barch DM, Donnelly JM, Ollinger JM, Snyder AZ, Mintun MA: **Increased amygdala response to masked emotional faces in depressed subjects resolves with antidepressant treatment: An fMRI study.** *Biol Psychiatry* 2001, **50**:651–658.
8. Gotlib IH, Sivers H, Gabrieli JDE, *et al*: **Subgenual anterior cingulate activation to valenced emotional stimuli in major depression.** *Neuroreport* 2005, **16**:1731–1734.
9. Siegle GJ, Thompson W, Carter CS, Steinhauer SR, Thase ME: **Increased amygdala and decreased dorsolateral prefrontal BOLD responses in unipolar depression: Related and independent features.** *Biol Psychiatry* 2007, **61**:198–209.
10. Blair K, Shaywitz J, Smith BW, *et al*: **Response to emotional expressions in generalized social phobia and generalized anxiety disorder: Evidence for separate disorders.** *Am J Psychiatry* 2008, **165**(9):1193–1202.
11. Lorberbaum JP, Kose S, Johnson MR, *et al*: **Neural correlates of speech anticipatory anxiety in generalized social phobia.** *Neuroreport* 2004, **15**(18):2701–2705.
12. Andreescu C, Butters M, Lenze EJ, *et al*: **fMRI activation in late-life anxious depression: A potential biomarker.** *Int J Geriatr Psychiatry* 2009, **24**(8):820–828.
13. Etkin A, Schatzberg AF: **Common abnormalities and disorder-specific compensation during implicit regulation of emotional processing in Generalized Anxiety and Major Depressive Disorders.** *Am J Psychiatry* 2011, **168**(9):968–978.
14. Monroe SM, Simons AD: **Diathesis-stress theories in the context of life stress research: Implications for the depressive disorders.** *Psychol Bull* 1991, **110**(3):406–425.

15. Allen JL, Rapee RM, Sandberg S: **Severe life events and chronic adversities as antecedents to anxiety in children: A matched control study.** *J Abnorm Child Psychol* 2008, **36**:1047–1056.
16. Young EA, Abelson JL, Cameron OG: **Effect of comorbid anxiety disorders on the Hypothalamic-Pituitary-Adrenal Axis response to a social stressor in major depression.** *Biol Psychiatry* 2004, **56**:113–120.
17. Amir N, Foa EB, Coles ME: **Automatic activation and strategic avoidance of threat-relevant information in social phobia.** *J Abnorm Psychol* 1998, **107**(2):285–290.
18. Koster EHW, Verschuere B, Crombez G, Van Damme S: **Time-course of attention for threatening pictures in high and low trait anxiety.** *Behav Res Ther* 2005, **43**(8):1087–1098.
19. Mogg K, Bradley B, Miles F, Dixon R: **Time course of attentional bias for threat scenes: Testing the vigilance-avoidance hypothesis.** *Cognition & Emotion* 2004, **18**(5):689–700.
20. Amir N, Elias J, Klumpp H, Przeworski A: **Attentional bias to threat in social phobia: facilitated processing of threat or difficulty disengaging attention from threat?** *Behav Res Ther* 2003, **41**(11):1325–1335.
21. McCullough ME, Orsulak P, Brandon A, Akers L: **Rumination, fear, and cortisol: An in vivo study of interpersonal transgressions.** *Health Psychol* 2007, **26**(1):126–132.
22. Nolen-Hoeksema S: **The Role of Rumination in Depressive Disorders and Mixed Anxiety/Depressive Symptoms.** *J Abnorm Psychol* 2000, **109**(3):504–511.
23. Young EA, Lopez JF, Murphy-Weinberg V, Watson SJ, Akil H: **Hormonal evidence for altered responsiveness to social stress in major depression.** *Neuropsychopharmacology* 2000, **23**(4):411–418.
24. Mikolajczak M, Roy E, Luminet O, de Timary P: **Resilience and hypothalamic-pituitary-adrenal axis reactivity under acute stress in young men.** *Stress* 2008, **11**(6):477–482.
25. Waugh CE, Panage S, Mendes WB, Gotlib IH: **Cardiovascular and affective recovery from anticipatory threat.** *Biol Psychol* 2010, **84**:169–175.
26. Wager TD, Waugh CE, Lindquist M, Noll DC, Fredrickson BL, Taylor SF: **Brain mediators of cardiovascular responses to social threat, Part I: Reciprocal dorsal and ventral sub-regions of the medial prefrontal cortex and heart-rate reactivity.** *NeuroImage* 2009, **47**:821–835.
27. Lindquist M, Waugh C, Wager TD: **Modeling state-related fMRI activity using change-point theory.** *NeuroImage* 2007, **35**:1125–1141.
28. *User's guide for the structured clinical interview for DSM-IV Axis 1 disorders [computer program].* Version 20th edition.: ; 1995.
29. Turner SM, Beidel DC, Dancu CV, Stanley MA: **An empirically derived inventory to measure social fears and anxiety: The Social Phobia and Anxiety Inventory.** *Psychological Assessment: A Journal of Consulting and Clinical Psychology* 1989, **1**(1):35–40.
30. Beck AT, Steer RA, Brown GK: *Manual for the Beck Depression Inventory-II.* San Antonio, TX: Psychological Corporation; 1996.
31. Fredrickson BL, Mancuso RA, Branigan C, Tugade MM: **The undoing effect of positive emotions.** *Motiv Emotion* 2000, **24**(4):237–258.
32. Glover GH, Law CS: **Spiral-in/out BOLD fMRI for increased SNR and reduced susceptibility artifacts.** *Magn Reson Med* 2001, **46**(3):515–522.
33. Cox RW: **AFNI: Software for analysis and visualization of functional magnetic resonance neuroimages.** *Comput Biomed Res* 1996, **29**:162–173.
34. Talairach J, Tournoux P: *Co-Planar Stereotaxic Atlas of the Human Brain.* Stuttgart, Germany: Thieme; 1988.
35. Sackheim HA: **The definition and meaning of treatment-resistant depression.** *J Clin Psychiatry* 2001, **62**:10–17.
36. Ward BD: **Simultaneous inference for fMRI data.** *Accessed August* 2007, **()**. http://afni.nimh.nih.gov/afni/docpdf/AlphaSim.pdf.
37. Jaccard J, Turrisi R: **Interaction effects in multiple regression**. In *Thousand Oaks*. Vol 07–072 2nd edition. CA: Sage University Press; 2003.
38. Mendes WB, Gray HM, Mendoza-Denton R, Major B, Epel ES: **Why egalitarianism might be good for your health: Physiologial thriving during stressful intergroup encounters.** *Psychol Sci* 2007, **18**(11):991–998.
39. Tomaka J, Blascovich J, Kelsey RM, Leitten CL: **Subjective, physiological, and behavioral effects of threat and challenge appraisal.** *J Pers Soc Psychol* 1993, **65**(2):248–260.
40. Watson D, Clark LA, Tellegen A: **Development and validation of brief measures of positive and negative affect: The PANAS scales.** *J Pers Soc Psychol* 1988, **54**(6):1063–1070.
41. Amodio DM, Frith CD: **Meeting of minds: The medial frontal cortex and social cognition.** *Nat Rev Neurosci* 2006, **7**:268–277.
42. Sturm VE, Sollberger M, Seeley WW, *et al*: **Role of right pregenual anterior cingulate cortex in self-conscious emotional reactivity.** *Social Cognitive and Affective Neuroscience.* 2012; doi:10.1093/scan/nss023.
43. Waugh CE, Hamilton JP, Gotlib IH: **The neural temporal dynamics of the intensity of emotional experience.** *NeuroImage* 2010, **49**:1699–1707.
44. Critchley HD, Mathias CJ, Josephs O, *et al*: **Human cingulate cortex and autonomic control: Converging neuroimaging and clinical evidence.** *Brain* 2003, **126**(10):2139–2152.
45. Shulman GL, Fiez JA, Corbetta M, *et al*: **Common blood flow changes across visual tasks: II decreases in cerebral cortex.** *J Cogn Neurosci* 1997, **9**(5):648–663.
46. Fiez JA, Peterson SE: **Neuroimaging studies of word reading.** *Proc Natl Acad Sci U S A* 1998, **95**(3):914–921.
47. Craig AD: **Opinion: How do you feel? Interoception: the sense of the physiological condition of the body.** *Nat Rev Neurosci* 2002, **3**(8):655–666.
48. Nitschke JB, Sarinopoulos I, Mackiewicz KL, Schaefer HS, Davidson RJ: **Functional neuroanatomy of aversion and its anticipation.** *NeuroImage* 2006, **29**(1):106–116.
49. Gramer M, Saria K: **Effects of social anxiety and evaluative threat on cardiovascular responses to active performance situations.** *Biol Psychol* 2007, **74**(1):67–74.
50. Carballedo A, Scheuerecker J, Meisenzahl E, *et al*: **Functional connectivity of emotional processing in depression.** *J Affect Disord* 2011, **134**(1–3):272–279.

4

Sleep quality and neural circuit function supporting emotion regulation

Jared D Minkel[1*], Kristin McNealy[1], Peter J Gianaros[2], Emily M Drabant[3], James J Gross[3], Stephen B Manuck[2] and Ahmad R Hariri[1,4]

Abstract

Background: Recent laboratory studies employing an extended sleep deprivation model have mapped sleep-related changes in behavior onto functional alterations in specific brain regions supporting emotion, suggesting possible biological mechanisms for an association between sleep difficulties and deficits in emotion regulation. However, it is not yet known if similar behavioral and neural changes are associated with the more modest variability in sleep observed in daily life.

Methods: We examined relationships between sleep and neural circuitry of emotion using the Pittsburgh Sleep Quality Index and fMRI data from a widely used emotion regulation task focusing on cognitive reappraisal of negative emotional stimuli in an unselected sample of 97 adult volunteers (48 women; mean age 42.78±7.37 years, range 30–54 years old).

Results: Emotion regulation was associated with greater activation in clusters located in the dorsomedial prefrontal cortex (dmPFC), left dorsolateral prefrontal cortex (dlPFC), and inferior parietal cortex. Only one subscale from the Pittsburgh Sleep Quality Index, use of sleep medications, was related to BOLD responses in the dmPFC and dlPFC during cognitive reappraisal. Use of sleep medications predicted lesser BOLD responses during reappraisal, but other aspects of sleep, including sleep duration and subjective sleep quality, were not related to neural activation in this paradigm.

Conclusions: The relatively modest variability in sleep that is common in the general community is unlikely to cause significant disruption in neural circuits supporting reactivity or regulation by cognitive reappraisal of negative emotion. Use of sleep medication however, may influence emotion regulation circuitry, but additional studies are necessary to determine if such use plays a causal role in altering emotional responses.

Keywords: Emotion, Emotion regulation, Sleep, Sleep quality, FMRI

Background

Sleep problems are highly comorbid with psychiatric disorders [1,2] and have been found to predict the onset of both depressive episodes [3] and mania [4]. Although available data suggest a causal link between sleep and psychiatric symptoms, a compelling biological mechanism has not yet been reported. One hypothesis is that poor sleep compromises neural systems supporting emotion regulation [5]. Although this hypothesis was first based on clinical experience and anecdote, it has more recently been supported by independent lines of research that have established key neural and behavioral correlates of sleep deprivation in controlled laboratory experiments [6,7].

In general, these experiments have identified the prefrontal cortex, which plays a key role in the cognitive control of emotion [8], as particularly sensitive to sleep loss [9]. Experimental sleep deprivation studies have reported subjective [10], physiological [11], and neural [7] changes consistent with exaggerated responsiveness to negative emotional stimuli. The strongest support for this position comes from a study reporting decreased functional connectivity between the medial prefrontal cortex (mPFC) and amygdala in sleep deprived subjects

* Correspondence: jared.minkel@duke.edu
[1]Laboratory of NeuroGenetics, Department of Psychology & Neuroscience, Duke University, 417 Chapel Dr., Durham, NC 27708, USA
Full list of author information is available at the end of the article

viewing intense negative (i.e., disgusting and disturbing) photographs [7]. Although this emotion elicitation paradigm did not directly assess emotion regulation, the pathway involved shares considerable overlap with canonical emotion regulation circuitry [12], indicating that sleep deprivation results in deficient capacity to regulate strong emotional arousal. However, a serious limitation of studies to date is that they have used experimental paradigms with relatively long periods of sustained wakefulness that are very rare in real world settings.

In the present study, we extend the literature on the influence of sleep on neural substrates of emotion in three important ways. First, a well-characterized emotion regulation paradigm was administered during BOLD fMRI. This paradigm allows for the robust engagement of neural circuits, including the amygdala and mPFC, involved in emotional reactivity as well as cognitive reappraisal [13]. Cognitive reappraisal may be a particularly important process because it is one of the primary ways people can voluntarily alter their own emotional experiences [14] and is believed to represent a psychological mechanism by which people with psychiatric disorders improve mood and prevent relapse during cognitive behavior therapy [15,16]. To our knowledge, this is the first study to investigate relationships between sleep and emotion regulation per se. Second, self-reported sleep variables were collected using a widely utilized measure [17], allowing for the mapping of relationships between neural function associated with emotional regulation and individual differences in sleep variables commonly encountered in real-world settings. Third, our relatively large (N = 97), community-based sample allows greater generalizability than previous studies that have used smaller samples (less than 30), extreme levels of sleep deprivation rarely encountered in real-world settings, and young adult samples. Based on the existing literature, we hypothesized that sleep problems, particularly short sleep-duration, would predict deficits in neural activation supporting emotion regulation. Specifically, we predicted sleep problems would be associated with greater amygdala activation in response to negative emotional stimuli and lower activation in the mPFC during regulation of negative emotional stimuli.

Methods

Participants

Participants were recruited from Phase II of the Adult Health and Behavior project (AHAB II), which assesses a wide range of behavioral and biological traits among middle-aged community volunteers. All participants had completed both the emotion regulation fMRI task and the Pittsburgh Sleep Quality Index (PSQI) and were in good general health. The University of Pittsburgh Institutional Review Board approved the study and all participants provided informed consent in accordance with its regulations. Participants were evaluated for current *DSM-IV* Axis I disorders using the Mini-International Neuropsychiatric Interview (MINI [18]) and excluded only for history of psychosis. The participants were free of medical diagnoses of cancer, stroke, diabetes requiring insulin treatment, and chronic kidney or liver disease. Additional exclusion criteria included use of psychotropic, glucocorticoid, hypolipidemic, antiarrhythmic, antihypertensive, and prescription weight loss medication. Sleep medications were allowed if they were not taken more than 7 of 14 days prior to eligibility determination.

Our initial sample included 106 unselected participants, but 8 were removed for amygdala coverage less than 90%. One additional participant was removed for abnormally high motion artifact, leaving a final sample of 97 participants (48 women; mean age 42.78 ± 7.37 years, range 30–54 years old).

Measures

Pittsburgh Sleep Quality Index (PSQI)

All participants completed the PSQI, a 19-item self-rated questionnaire for evaluating general sleep patterns over the previous month [17]. The questionnaire is scored to produce seven clinically-derived component scores, each of which is converted to a 0–3 scale where higher numbers indicate more problematic sleep. Many of the component scores are based on a single item or reflect a single calculation based on two or more items. The component scores are subjective sleep quality, sleep latency, sleep duration, habitual sleep efficiency (a measure of time spent asleep to total time spent in bed), sleep disturbances, use of sleeping medication, and daytime dysfunction. The combined score is reported as Global Sleep Quality. Global scores greater than 5 indicate clinically meaningful sleep disturbance.

Center for Epidemiologic Studies Depression Scale (CES-D)

To ensure that observed relationships were not better accounted for by co-occurring symptoms of mood disorders, depression symptoms were also evaluated using the CES-D [19]. The CES-D is a 20-item measure of depression symptoms that has been evaluated and used in many studies of psychiatric symptoms and disorders. A cutoff score of 16 has been used to differentiate those who are likely to have clinically meaningful levels of depressive symptoms from those who are not [20].

Emotion regulation paradigm

The emotion regulation task in this experiment was adapted from a previously validated paradigm [8,13]. The task consisted of 30 negative photographs and 15 neutral photographs selected from the International Affective Picture System (IAPS) database based on published norms [21]. Negative photographs depicted bodily illness and injury (21 photographs), acts of aggression (3 photographs), members of hate groups (2 photographs), transportation accidents (2 photographs) and human waste (2 photographs). Neutral photographs depicted inanimate objects (10 photographs) or neutral scenes (5 photographs).

Prior to completing the task, subjects were instructed that when cued to "look," they were to maintain attention on the stimulus and allow their emotional reaction to occur without attempting to change it. When cued to "decrease," they were to attempt to reduce their emotional response through cognitive reappraisal (i.e., by thinking of something that makes the photograph seem less negative). Subjects were given examples of reappraisal strategies for specific photographs and then practiced the skill outside the MRI scanner. During the MRI scan each trial consisted of a 2 second cue to either "look" or "decrease" one's emotional response, then a 7 second presentation of either a negative or neutral picture, then a 4 second opportunity to rate the picture, followed by a 1–3 second rest period before the next cue. During the "rate picture" phase, subjects were instructed to report their emotional reaction to each photograph on a scale of 1 to 5, where 1 indicated neutral and 5 indicated feeling strongly negative. The ratings were made using a button response pad in the participant's right hand and recorded in E-Prime software.

Fifteen negative photographs were presented with the "look" cue and 15 were presented with the "decrease" cue. All 15 neutral photographs were presented with the "look" cue (because there is nothing to regulate in response to a neutral photograph). The stimuli were presented in pseudo-random order such that no more than 2 of the same instruction (look vs. regulate) could be presented consecutively and no more than 4 negative stimuli could be presented consecutively. Total time for the task was 11:28 minutes. This design allows for an assessment of neural activation related to the emotional valence of the stimuli (look negative > look neutral) as well as activation related to reappraisal (regulate negative > look negative).

BOLD fMRI data acquisition

Each participant was scanned using a Siemens 3 T Allegra scanner (Siemens AG, Medical Solutions, Erlangen, Germany) developed specifically for advanced brain imaging applications and characterized by increased T2* sensitivity and fast gradients that minimize echo spacing, thereby reducing echo-planar imaging (EPI) geometric distortions and improving image quality. An autoshimming procedure was conducted to minimize field inhomogeneities. A series of 34 interleaved axial slices aligned with the AC-PC plane were acquired with a gradient-echo echo planar imaging sequence (TR/TE = 2000 ms/25 ms; FOV = 200 mm, matrix size 64 × 64; 3.125 × 3.125 × 3 mm voxels; interslice skip = 0). Two initial RF excitations were performed (and discarded) to achieve steady-state equilibrium. However, the first two acquired volumes were discarded during preprocessing to further ensure steady-state equilibrium. All scanning parameters were selected to optimize the quality of the BOLD signal while maintaining a sufficient number of slices to acquire whole brain data. Before the collection of fMRI data for each participant, we acquired a reference EPI scan that we visually inspected for artifacts (e.g., ghosting) as well as good signal across the entire volume of acquisition.

BOLD fMRI data analysis

Whole-brain image analysis of all fMRI data was conducted at the Laboratory of NeuroGenetics at Duke University using the general linear model (GLM) of SPM8 (http://www.fil.ion.ucl.ac.uk/spm). Images for each participant were realigned to the first volume in the time series to correct for head motion, spatially normalized into a standard stereotactic space (Montreal Neurological Institute template) using a 12-parameter affine model (final resolution of functional images = 2 mm isotropic voxels), and smoothed to minimize noise and residual difference in gyral anatomy with a Gaussian filter, set at 6-mm full-width at half-maximum. Preprocessed data sets were analyzed using second-level random-effects models that account for both scan-to-scan and participant-to-participant variability to determine task-specific regional responses.

Variability in single-subject whole-brain functional volumes was determined using the Artifact Recognition Toolbox (http://www.nitrc.org/projects/artifact_detect). Individual whole-brain BOLD fMRI volumes meeting at least one of the following two criteria were identified as artifacts during the determination of task-specific effects: 1) significant mean-volume signal intensity variation 2 (i.e., within volume mean signal greater or less than 4 standard deviations of mean signal of all volumes in time series), and 2) individual volumes where scan-to-scan movement exceeded 2 mm translation or 2° rotation in any direction. Artifacts were then treated as regressors of no interest in subsequent preprocessing steps. One participant was removed from further analyses due to abnormally high artifact (37% of whole-brain BOLD fMRI volumes). The remaining participants had, on average, 2.64% of all volumes identified as artifacts, thus we believe this approach enhanced our capacity to determine task-specific effects by minimizing the influence of volumes with substantial variability without compromising our power to detect task-specific effects by excluding a large number of volumes.

Following preprocessing, linear contrasts employing canonical hemodynamic response functions were used to estimate condition-specific (i.e. negative > neutral and regulate > look) BOLD responses for each individual. Individual contrast images (i.e., weighted sum of the beta images) were then used in second-level random effects models accounting for scan-to-scan and participant-to-participant variability to determine mean condition-specific regional responses using one-sample t-tests. A voxel-level statistical threshold of $p < 0.05$, FWE corrected for multiple comparisons (across the anatomical amygdala ROIs for negative > neutral, and across whole brain for regulate > look) was applied. An additional extent threshold of 10 contiguous voxels was applied to both ROI and whole brain analyses.

Based on previous findings [7,13,22] we selected the amygdala as a region of interest (ROI) where we expected to find effects of emotional reactivity (negative > neutral contrast). A bilateral amygdala ROI mask was created from the Automated Anatomical Labeling (AAL) atlas [23]. Because of the potential for signal loss and noise often observed in the amygdala and adjacent regions, single-subject BOLD fMRI data were included in subsequent analyses only if there was a minimum of 90% signal coverage in the amygdala masks bilaterally. Although we anticipated finding main effects of task in regions previously identified [8,13], these analyses were completed using whole brain analyses. No additional ROI masks were created.

BOLD parameter estimates from clusters exhibiting condition-effects (negative > neutral; regulate > look) were extracted using the VOI tool in SPM8 and exported for analyses in R and SPSS (v.18). Extracting parameter estimates from functional clusters activated by our fMRI paradigm, rather than clusters specifically correlated with our independent variables of interest, precludes the possibility of any correlation coefficient inflation that may result when an explanatory covariate is used to select a region of interest [24]. We have used this more conservative and rigorous analytic strategy in recent studies [25,26].

Statistical analyses

The influence of sleep duration on emotional reactivity and emotion regulation was investigated using regression analyses. Because sleep duration was measured prior to the emotion regulation task and because it is believed to play a causal role in influencing subjective responses and neural responses during emotional reactivity and regulation, it was treated as an independent variable in all regression analyses. Dependent variables included subjective emotional responses to photographs as well as extracted BOLD parameter estimates from max voxels of clusters showing significant condition-effects and ratings of emotional reactions during each condition. Dependent variables were analyzed to ensure they were approximately normally distributed prior to entry into regression analyses. Relationships among subjective emotional reactions and extracted BOLD parameter estimates were investigated using Pearson correlations. Because we made a priori predictions that poorer sleep would predict less brain activation during emotion regulation and less subjective regulatory success, one-tailed significance tests were used in these analyses. For all other analyses, two-tailed significance tests were used.

Results

Negative emotion induction and regulation manipulation checks

Emotional reactivity

Subjective responses to photographs were compared using paired samples t-tests. Two subjects were excluded based on abnormal or missing self-report data. These analyses confirmed that negative photographs elicited significantly greater negative emotion than neutral photographs ($t(95) = 37.02, p < .001$).

Based on previous findings [7,22], we focused our analyses of neural responses associated with emotional reactivity (negative > neutral contrast) on amygdala activation. A significant condition-effect was found in both the left (89 voxels, $t = 5.73$, $p < .001$; -20, -6, -14) and right (39 voxels, $t = 4.70$, $p < .001$; 20, -4, -16) amygdala (Figure 1).

Emotion regulation

Cognitive reappraisal was associated with significantly less intense subjective negative emotion than simply viewing negative photographs ($t(95) = 9.65$, $p < .001$). These results confirmed that the emotion regulation paradigm produced the intended subjective effects and that participants were able to regulate their emotional responses through reappraisal.

Analyses of neural responses associated with cognitive reappraisal (regulate > look contrast) revealed significant main effects of task in three clusters located within the medial prefrontal cortex (mPFC), left dorsolateral prefrontal cortex (dlPFC), and inferior parietal cortex (IPC, Figure 2). Regulatory success (computed as the difference between subjective responses in the regulate negative and look negative conditions) was significantly correlated with activation in the mPFC ($r = .206$, $p = .044$) and IPC ($r = .213$, $p = .037$) and trended toward a significant relationship with activation in the left dlPFC cluster ($r = .184$, $p = .073$), indicating that greater activation in these clusters was associated with more effective use of reappraisal, as indexed by lower overall subjective emotional responses to the negative stimuli.

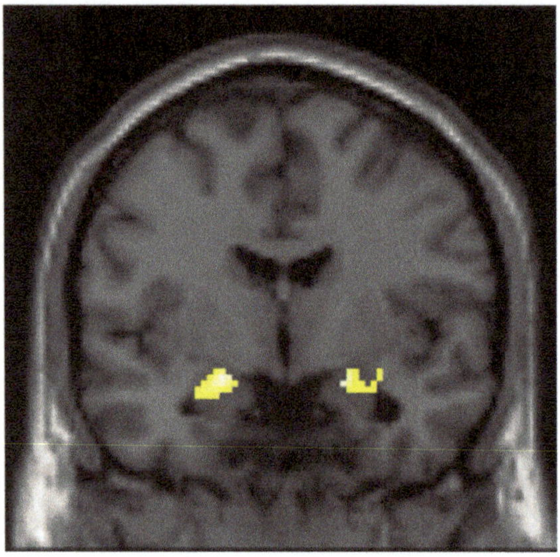

Figure 1 Statistical parametric map illustrating amygdala activation associated with viewing IAPS photographs (look negative > look neutral). Maximal voxel MNI coordinates for left amygdala activation: -20, -6, -14; 89 voxels, t=5.73, p<.001. Maximal voxel MNI coordinates for right amygdala activation: 20, -4, 16; 39 voxels, t=5.00, p<.001.

Sleep quality analyses

Sleep and emotional reactivity

Sleep was measured using the Pittsburgh Sleep Quality Index (see Table 1 for frequency and severity of sleep problems). Global Sleep Quality, i.e., the composite score reflecting the sum of all subscales) was analyzed to determine overall relationships among sleep and emotional reactivity (see Table 1 for PSQI score descriptive statistics). Global Sleep Quality scores did not predict left (b = –.135, p = .19) or right (b = –.044, p = .67) amygdala activation during the negative > neutral contrast. Global PSQI scores were also unrelated to subjective responses to negative vs. neutral photographs (b = –.134, p = .193). Neither sleep duration nor sleep quality predicted left (ps > .59) or right (ps > .41) amygdala activation in the negative > neutral contrast. Similarly, there was no relationship between PSQI subscales and subjective emotional responses to negative vs. neutral photographs in the "look" condition (ps > .29), except for a trend toward poorer subjective sleep quality predicting *less* intense subjective emotional responses (b = –.189, p = .066).

Sleep and emotion regulation

Global PSQI scores predicted activation in the mPFC cluster, (b = –.190, p = .03) such that worse sleep was associated with less mPFC activity (Figure 3). Global PSQI scores were not significantly related to activation in the dlPFC cluster (b = –.052, p = .31) or the IPC cluster (r = .003, p = .49). Similarly, Global PSQI scores were not significantly related to self-reported regulatory success (r = .008, p = .47). Analyses of PSQI subscales revealed a significant relationship between use of sleep medication and activation in the mPFC cluster (b = –.23, p = .02), left dlPFC cluster (b = –.22, p = .02) and IPC cluster (b = –.196, p = .03). Use of sleep medication did not predict self-reported regulatory success however (b = 0.017, p = .44). Use of sleep medication was relatively rare with 12 subjects (6 women) reporting such use in the last month. Of these, 7 reported using sleep medication less than once per week and 5 reported using sleep medications 1–2 times per week. Due to these small groups, they were combined and compared to those who did not use sleep medications (n = 85, 42 women). Independent samples t-tests confirmed that those who used sleep

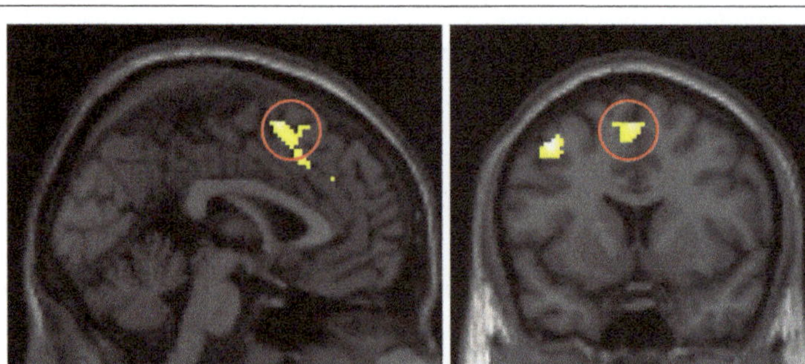

Figure 2 Statistical parametric map illustrating whole brain activation associated with reappraisal of emotional responses to negative IAPS photographs (regulate negative > look negative). The cluster in the dorsal medial prefrontal cortex (mPFC; within the red circle) showed a significant relationship with regulatory success based on subjective responses to IAPS photographs (r=.21, p=.04). Maximal voxel MNI coordinates for medial prefrontal cluster: 0, 10, 60; 241 voxels, t=6.32, p<.001. The cluster in the left dorsolateral prefrontal cortex (dlPFC), maximal voxel MNI coordinates for dlPFC cluster: -42, 8, 52; 198 voxels, t=7.11, p<.001, showed a marginally significant relationship with regulatory success (r=.18, p=.07). A third cluster (not visible here) was located in the inferior parietal cortex and had maximal voxel MNI coordinates -50, -58, 46; 481 voxels, t=6.98, p<.001.

Table 1 Pittsburgh Sleep Quality Index Component Scores

		Frequency (N=97)			
Subscale	**M (SD)**	**Normal 0**	**Mild 1**	**Moderate 2**	**Severe 3**
Subjective Sleep Quality	.94 (.67)	24	56	16	1
Sleep Latency	.85 (.73)	31	53	10	3
Sleep Duration	.87 (.64)	26	59	11	1
Habitual Sleep Efficiency	.30 (.64)	76	14	6	1
Sleep Disturbances	1.31 (.53)	1	67	27	2
Use of Sleeping Medication	.18 (.50)	85	7	5	0
Daytime Dysfunction	.71 (.56)	33	59	5	0

medication demonstrated less activation in the mPFC cluster ($t(23.1) = 3.85, p < .001$) and dlPFC cluster ($t(23.2) = 3.17$, p = .002) than those who did not use sleep medications, but differences in activation in the IPC cluster showed a non-significant trend ($t(95) = 1.56, p = .06$; Figure 4). All other PSQI subscales failed to predict activation in the dlPFC cluster (all $b < .12, ps > .26$), mPFC cluster (all $b < .11, ps > .16$), or IPC cluster (all $b < .10, ps > .20$). Furthermore, controlling for all other PSQI subscales had no effect on relationships between use of sleep medications and neural activation supporting emotion regulation (mPFC cluster: $b = -.20, p = .04$, dlPFC: $b = -.24, p = .02$, IPC cluster: $b = -.24, p = .02$). Removing participants who reported using sleep medication from the analyses resulted in a non-significant relationship between Global Sleep Quality and activation in the mPFC ($b = -0.75, p = .50$).

One final analysis we conducted was to create a composite score of all PSQI subscales except medication use. Here we included all participants, including those who reported using sleep medication, but did not allow this medication use to affect their Global PSQI score. The relationship between mPFC activation and this composite sleep score was nearly significant (b = 0.16, p = .06) suggesting that it may have not been the use of sleep medication per se that accounted for this relationship.

Control analyses

Additional analyses were completed in order to ensure that our findings related to sleep and emotion were not

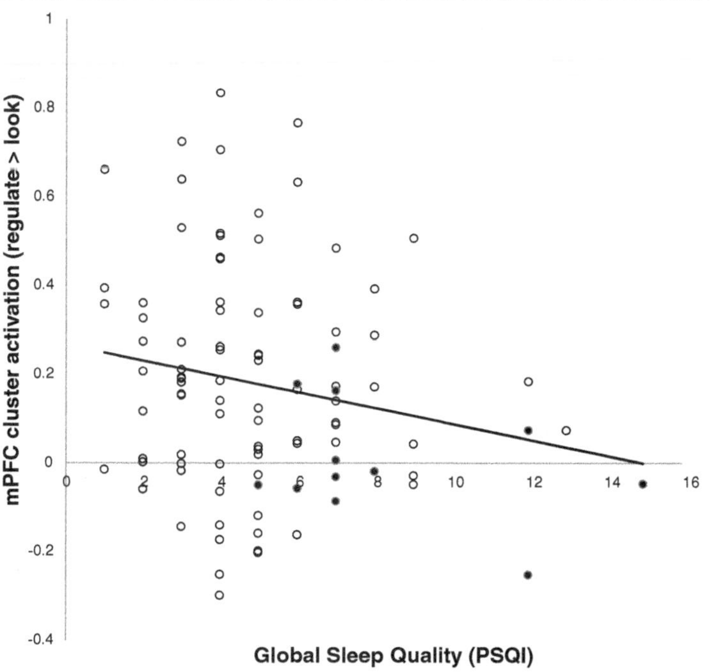

Figure 3 Scatter plot showing individual differences in activation in the medial prefrontal cortex (mPFC) for the regulate negative > look negative contrast based on global sleep quality scores for the PSQI. Worse sleep predicted less mPFC cluster activation (b = -.190, $p = .03$). Filled circles indicate participants who reported using sleep medication within the last month.

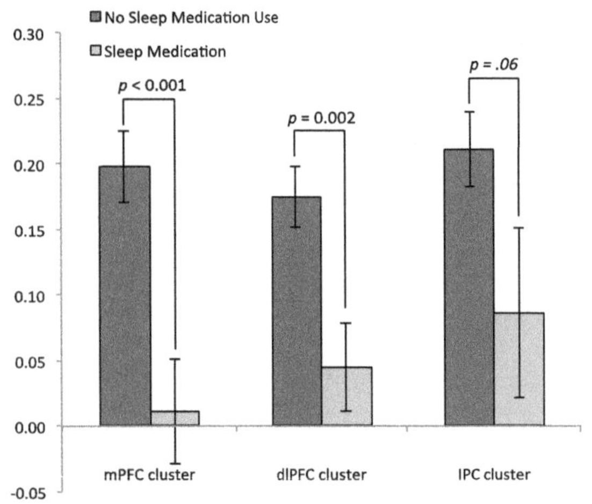

Figure 4 Activation during the regulate negative > look negative condition was greater for those who denied use of sleep medication in the last 30 days (dark gray bars, n = 85) than for those who endorsed it (light gray bars, n = 12). Differences were significant in the medial prefrontal cluster (mPFC, $p = .001$) and left dorsolateral prefrontal cluster (dlPFC, $p = .004$) and there was a non-significant trend in the inferior parietal cortex cluster (IPC, $p = .06$).

better accounted for by mood problems. Depression symptoms, measured by the CES-D, were highly correlated with PSQI Global scores ($r = .56$, $p < .001$), but were not significantly correlated with activation in the clusters identified above ($ps > .20$). Similarly, subjects scoring above the CES-D cutoff score of 16 (n = 14) did not show significantly different activation relative to those scoring below the cutoff score in any of the clusters identified above ($ps > .62$). There was a non-significant trend toward greater depression symptoms predicting less self-reported regulatory success ($b = -.177$, $p = 0.09$).

Discussion

Inadequate sleep is thought to produce exaggerated emotional responses by compromising the top-down inhibitory control of the prefrontal cortex over amygdala driven emotional arousal [5-7]. If true, this could be a promising mechanism that contributes to relatively high rates of depression in industrialized and developing nations. Our findings suggest however, that findings from experimental settings, where wakefulness can be extended for long durations, were not replicated in our sample where more modest variability in sleep was observed. Because this was a large, unselected sample from the community, we believe the findings are more relevant for public policy than smaller self-selected samples typical of experimental studies. Although there was a significant relationship between the composite PSQI score Global Sleep Quality and neural activation in the mPFC, analyses of subscales showed that most aspects of sleep were unrelated to emotional functioning. Perhaps most important was the finding that there were no significant relationships between emotional responses to negative photographs and either how much participants slept (sleep duration) or their reports of how well they slept (subjective sleep quality). We interpret these findings as evidence that the human nervous system can preserve regulatory efficiency of negative emotion within the variability in sleep observed in the general population. Because our paradigm measured emotional reactivity with and without voluntary regulation strategies, we believe these findings are particularly robust. It is important to emphasize, however, that these findings cannot necessarily be extended to clinical populations. There is substantial evidence that relationships between sleep and emotion may be very different in people with psychiatric diagnoses such as Bipolar Disorder and Major Depression [4,27] and additional investigations of underlying biological mechanisms to explain those differences are needed. One final caveat is that in an unselected sample, people are free to choose their own sleep schedule and those who are most sensitive to sleep loss may choose to sleep more than those who are more resilient. The emotional consequences of sleep loss may be more profound in subgroups that cannot choose their own sleep schedules, such as emergency personnel and shift workers. Additional studies are needed to investigate possible emotional consequences of abnormal sleep in these populations.

Our secondary analyses suggested that the relationship between the composite PSQI score Global Sleep Quality and neural activation during cognitive reappraisal was primarily driven by the PSQI subscale related to sleep medications. Use of sleep medication was associated with reduced activation in both the dorsolateral prefrontal and medial prefrontal clusters. This finding, if replicated, would suggest that sleep medication should be used with caution, especially in people with a predisposition for mood problems. We would like to emphasize, however, that this was an unexpected finding from a correlational study that cannot establish a causal relationship between sleep medication use and the abnormalities identified. In addition, data were not available on the class of sleep medications these participants used, so additional studies are needed to investigate what influence, if any, different classes of sleep medication have on emotion regulation circuitry. It is also possible that a third variable can explain both sleep medication use and abnormal neural responses during the emotion regulation task. Perhaps the most likely such variable, namely depressive symptoms, was ruled out by our analyses. There was no relationship between depression and neural substrates of emotion regulation in this community sample. Future studies could extend these findings considerably by evaluating emotion regulation before and after the administration of sleep medications. Because the participants who used sleep medication also reported greater sleep disturbances overall, it is further possible that this relationship more generally reflects a negative impact of moderate to severe sleep disturbance on the engagement of prefrontal regions during cognitive reappraisal of emotional stimuli.

The analyses reported above have several important limitations we would like to emphasize. First, we estimated average sleep duration using self-report, where objective methods such as actigraphy or polysomnography would have been more accurate, suggesting that we may have failed to detect a true correlation. Our relatively large sample size partially attenuates this concern, but future studies might be able to detect small, but statistically significant effects through actigraphy or polysomnography. Second, our sample consisted of adults in the age range of 30 to 54 years. There is reason to believe that sleep may have different effects on emotion throughout the lifespan [5,10] and additional studies of different age groups are needed to better understand these relationships in children, adolescents, and the elderly. Finally, although depression symptoms were measured and could therefore be evaluated as possible confounds, there were many other potential confounds, such as stress or anxiety, that we could not evaluate in this study.

Conclusions

We believe that the analyses presented above demonstrated two important findings. First, they suggest that healthy normal adults can cope with mild to moderate sleep problems without showing large changes in neural or subjective emotional functioning, at least in response to passive experiences of negative stimuli. Nevertheless, only a handful of studies have investigated the neurobiological bases of emotional changes associated with sleep and more research is needed to understand main effects and individual differences in affective responses to sleep loss. Second, we found evidence suggesting that taking sleep medications may result in altered neural function supporting emotion regulation, and that these alterations may more broadly reflect the negative impact of moderate to severe sleep disturbances. Although preliminary, we believe this finding justifies additional studies designed to evaluate the impact of sleep medications on emotion regulation.

Competing interests

The authors report no biomedical financial interests or potential conflicts of interest.

Authors' contributions

JDM conceived of the analyses reported here, completed statistical analyses and drafted the manuscript. KM completed first level MRI analyses and consulted on additional analyses. PJG participated in the design of the emotion regulation task and helped to draft the manuscript. JJG provided expertise in designing the emotion regulation task and helped to draft the manuscript. SBM participated in the design of the experiment and coordinated data exchange between sites. ARH participated in the design of the experiment, co-wrote the manuscript, and provided mentorship for all analyses completed. All authors read and approved the final manuscript.

Acknowledgments

This work was supported by the National Institutes of Health grant PO1 HL040962 (SBM). JDM was supported by National Institute on Drug Abuse (NIDA) Grant P30 DA023026. PJG was supported by National Heart Lung and Blood Institute Grants R01-HL089850 and R01-HL101421.

Author details

[1]Laboratory of NeuroGenetics, Department of Psychology & Neuroscience, Duke University, 417 Chapel Dr., Durham, NC 27708, USA. [2]Department of Psychology, University of Pittsburgh, Pittsburgh, Pennsylvania, USA. [3]Department of Psychology, Stanford University, Stanford, CA, USA. [4]Institute for Genome Sciences & Policy, Duke University, Durham, NC 27708, USA.

References

1. Wulff K, Gatti S, Wettstein JG, Foster RG: **Sleep and circadian rhythm disruption in psychiatric and neurodegenerative disease.** *Nat Rev Neurosci* 2010, **11**:589–599.
2. Benca RM, Obermeyer WH, Thisted RA, Gillin JC: **Sleep and psychiatric disorders: a meta-analysis.** *Arch Gen Psychiatry* 1992, **49**:651.
3. Chang PP, Ford DE, Mead LA, Cooper-Patrick L, Klag MJ: **Insomnia in young men and subsequent depression.** *Am J Epidemiol* 1997, **146**:105.
4. Plante DT, Winkelman JW: **Sleep disturbance in bipolar disorder: therapeutic implications.** *Am J Psychiatry* 2008, **165**:830.
5. Dahl RE, Lewin DS: **Pathways to adolescent health sleep regulation and behavior.** *J Adolesc Health* 2002, **31**:175–184.
6. Gujar N, Yoo SS, Hu P, Walker MP: **Sleep deprivation amplifies reactivity of brain reward networks, biasing the appraisal of positive emotional experiences.** *J Neurosci* 2011, **31**:4466.
7. Yoo SS, Gujar N, Hu P, Jolesz FA, Walker MP: **The human emotional brain without sleep–a prefrontal amygdala disconnect.** *Curr Biol* 2007, **17**:R877–R878.
8. Ochsner KN, Ray RD, Cooper JC, Robertson ER, Chopra S, Gabrieli JD, Gross JJ: **For better or for worse: neural systems supporting the cognitive down-and up-regulation of negative emotion.** *Neuroimage* 2004, **23**:483–499.
9. Durmer JS, Dinges DF: **Neurocognitive consequences of sleep deprivation.** *Semin Neurol* 2005, **25**:117–129.
10. Talbot LS, McGlinchey EL, Kaplan KA, Dahl RE, Harvey AG: **Sleep deprivation in adolescents and adults: Changes in affect.** *Emotion* 2010, **10**:831.
11. Franzen PL, Buysse DJ, Dahl RE, Thompson W, Siegle GJ: **Sleep deprivation alters pupillary reactivity to emotional stimuli in healthy young adults.** *Biol Psychol* 2009, **80**:300–305.
12. Davidson RJ, Pizzagalli D, Nitschke JB, Kalin NH: **Parsing the subcomponents of emotion and disorders of emotion: Perspectives from affective neuroscience.** In *Handbook of Affective Sciences*. Edited by Davidson RJ, Scherer KR, Goldsmith HH. New York: Oxford Press; 2003:8–24.
13. Ochsner KN, Bunge SA, Gross JJ, Gabrieli JD: **Rethinking feelings: An fMRI study of the cognitive regulation of emotion.** *J Cogn Neurosci* 2002, **14**:1215–1229.
14. Ochsner KN, Gross JJ: **Cognitive emotion regulation.** *Curr Dir Psychol Sci* 2008, **17**:153.
15. Clark DA, Beck AT: **Cognitive theory and therapy of anxiety and depression: Convergence with neurobiological findings.** *Trends Cogn Sci* 2010, **14**:418–424.
16. Strunk DR, DeRubeis RJ, Chiu AW, Alvarez J: **Patients' competence in and performance of cognitive therapy skills: Relation to the reduction of**

relapse risk following treatment for depression. *J Consult Clin Psychol* 2007, **75:**523.

17. Buysse DJ, Reynolds CF, Monk TH, Berman SR, Kupfer DJ: The Pittsburgh Sleep Quality Index: a new instrument for psychiatric practice and research. *Psychiatry Res* 1989, **28:**193–213.
18. Lecrubier Y, Sheehan DV, Weiller E, Amorim P, Bonora I, Harnett Sheehan K, Janavs J, Dunbar GC: The Mini International Neuropsychiatric Interview (MINI). A short diagnostic structured interview: reliability and validity according to the CIDI. *Eur Psychiatry* 1997, **12:**224–231.
19. Radloff LS: The CES-D Scale: A Self Report Depression Scale for Research in the General Population. *Applied Psychol Measurement* 1977, **1:**385–401.
20. Boyd JH, Weissman MM, Thompson WD, Myers JK: Screening for depression in a community sample: Understanding the discrepancies between depression symptom and diagnostic scales. *Arch Gen Psychiatry* 1982, **39:**1195.
21. Lang PJ, Bradley MM, Cuthbert BN: International affective picture system (IAPS): Affective ratings of pictures and instruction manual. *Technical Report A-8* 2008.
22. Hariri AR, Mattay VS, Tessitore A, Fera F, Weinberger DR: Neocortical modulation of the amygdala response to fearful stimuli. *Biol Psychiatry* 2003, **53:**494–501.
23. Tzourio-Mazoyer N, Landeau B, Papathanassiou D, Crivello F, Etard O, Delcroix N, Mazoyer B, Joliot M: Automated anatomical labeling of activations in SPM using a macroscopic anatomical parcellation of the MNI MRI single-subject brain. *Neuroimage* 2002, **15:**273–289.
24. Viviani R: Unbiased ROI selection in neuroimaging studies of individual differences. *Neuroimage* 2010, **50:**184–189.
25. Hyde LW, Gorka A, Manuck SB, Hariri AR: Perceived social support moderates the link between threat-related amygdala reactivity and trait anxiety. *Neuropsychologia* 2011, **49:**651–656.
26. Carré JM, Fisher PM, Manuck SB, Hariri AR: Interaction between trait anxiety and trait anger predict amygdala reactivity to angry facial expressions in men but not women. *Soc Cogn Affect Neurosci* 2010.
27. Wu JC, Bunney WE: The biological basis of an antidepressant response to sleep deprivation and relapse: review and hypothesis. *Am J Psychiatry* 1990, **147:**14.

Anterior cingulate cortex and insula response during indirect and direct processing of emotional faces in generalized social anxiety disorder

Heide Klumpp[1*], David Post[1], Mike Angstadt[2], Daniel A Fitzgerald[1] and K Luan Phan[1,2,3]

Abstract

Background: Generalized social anxiety disorder (gSAD) is associated with a heightened neural sensitivity to signals that convey threat, as evidenced by exaggerated amygdala and/or insula activation when processing face stimuli that express negative emotions. Less clear in the brain pathophysiology of gSAD are cortical top down control mechanisms that moderate reactivity in these subcortical emotion processing regions. This study evaluated amygdala, insula, and anterior cingulate cortex (ACC) activity in gSAD with a novel "Emotional Faces Shifting Attention Task" (EFSAT), an adaptation of perceptual assessment tasks well-known to elicit amygdala response. In healthy volunteers, the task has been shown to engage the amygdala when attention is directed to emotional faces and the ACC when attention is directed to shapes, away from emotional faces.

Methods: During functional MRI, 29 participants with gSAD and 27 healthy controls viewed images comprising a trio of faces (angry, fear, or happy) alongside a trio of geometric shapes (circles, rectangles, or triangles) within the same field of view. Participants were instructed to match faces or match shapes, effectively directing attention towards or away from emotional information, respectively.

Results: Participants with gSAD exhibited greater insula, but not amygdala, activation compared to controls when attending to emotional faces. In contrast, when attention was directed away from faces, controls exhibited ACC recruitment, which was not evident in gSAD. Across participants, greater ACC activation was associated with less insula activation.

Conclusions: Evidence that individuals with gSAD exhibited exaggerated insula reactivity when attending to emotional faces in EFSAT is consistent with other studies suggesting that the neural basis of gSAD may involve insula hyper-reactivity. Furthermore, greater ACC response in controls than gSAD when sustained goal-directed attention is required to shift attention away from social signals, together with a negative relationship between ACC and bilateral insula activity, indicate the ACC may have served a regulatory role when the focus of attention was directed to shapes amidst emotional faces.

Keywords: Social anxiety, fMRI, Emotional faces, Threat processing, Brain imaging

* Correspondence: hklumpp@psych.uic.edu
[1]Mood and Anxiety Disorders Research Program, Department of Psychiatry (HK, DP, DAF, KLP), University of Illinois at Chicago, 1747 W. Roosevelt Rd, Chicago, IL 60608, USA
Full list of author information is available at the end of the article

Background

Generalized social anxiety disorder (gSAD) is characterized by extreme fears of potential scrutiny encompassing most social situations [1,2] and, therefore, can lead to impaired functioning in educational, occupational, and interpersonal domains [1,3,4]. Clinical manifestations of gSAD reflect a heightened threat processing system. These include excessive attention to negative social-signals (e.g., angry, fearful facial expressions [5]); fear-based physiological responses (autonomic changes) in anticipation of [6,7], or during [8], anxiety-evoking situations; and negative predictions about social events [9].

Thus far, models of the neural pathophysiology of gSAD have focused on an enhanced threat processing system that have fundamentally evolved from amygdala-centric 'functional' brain activation paradigms. In light of the central role amygdala plays in mediating fear and threat-related processing [7,10-12], its response to emotional information has been a predominant focus in affective neuroscience. As one example, when coupled with functional neuroimaging, perceptual matching tasks are designed to isolate the influence of emotional face content by contrasting a matching face condition with a sensorimotor control condition (i.e., matching shapes) and to robustly elicit amygdala response in healthy volunteers [13-16]. Building on this paradigm, studies of gSAD have shown amygdala reactivity to threat exceeds that of healthy individuals [17,18] and the extent of this reactivity has been shown to reflect symptom severity [19].

There is increasing evidence that the neural substrates of gSAD extend beyond the amygdala. In addition, there is a growing realization that functional neuroimaging paradigms should move beyond perceptual assessment tasks that primarily probe subcortical reactivity in key emotion processing regions. First, accumulating data point to insula hyper-reactivity in regard to processing negative emotional information in gSAD [20-27], and evidence of a correlation between anterior insula (aINS) reactivity to threat-relevant cues and symptom severity [24] also supports the notion that exaggerated aINS reactivity underlies anxiety disorders [28,29]. It has been posited that negative beliefs are mediated by feeling states, a core function of the aINS [30,31]. That is, aberrant insula activiation in anxiety is thought to be driven by sensitivity to aversive interoceptive signals and/or inaccurate interpretations of ordinary changes in bodily state [28,29]. Second, the prefrontal cortex (PFC) has reciprocal connections with the amygdala [32-34] and aINS [30,35-39], yet less is known about prefrontal mechanisms in gSAD. The relative gap in knowledge may relate to the interest in aberrant amygdala activation in anxiety and use of perceptual matching tasks, which are not well-validated to probe PFC regions.

Several functional neuroimaging tasks exist that are known to robustly recruit PFC areas by engaging cognitive functions such as 'top down' attentional control—that is, the ability to effectively resolve the type of conflict that occurs when cognitive goals compete with salient distractors for limited processing resources [40-48]. For example, to reflect the competition for processing resources imposed by distractors, tasks such as the emotional counting Stroop [48-50], modified dot probe detection [51,52], and "faces/houses" [40,53] have in common the rapid and simultaneous presentation of non-emotional, task-relevant stimuli and salient distractors (e.g., 500 ms or less; [40,51-54]). Studies using such tasks have shown that anxiety-prone [40,41,55,56] and clinically anxious patients [49,50,57], including those with gSAD [49], exhibit deficiencies in the recruitment of the anterior cingulate cortex (ACC) and other emotion regulation areas (e.g., dorsolateral PFC) in the presence of threat distractors. Excessive attention to threat appears to encompass impoverished top-down control at least when the window of information processing is markedly restricted (i.e., when visual processing is fast).

Current models propose that there is a balance between attending to the task at hand and to the emotional salience that surround the given task. Resolving emotional conflict must occur in the context that salient emotional cues not only capture but sustain visual attention [58]. Consequently, prefrontal areas should engage during the maintenance of goal-directed attention even when the window of information processing is extended to that of direct emotion processing.

In order to capture this balance, we adapted the face matching task into a relatively slow, easy-to-perform blocked perceptual matching task known as the "Emotional Faces Shifting Attention Task" (EFSAT), which requires subjects to shift their attention towards and away from emotional faces. In contrast to the traditional faces-only and shapes-only images, in EFSAT both image types were configured to be in the same field of view (Figure 1). Therefore, the instruction to "Match Shapes"

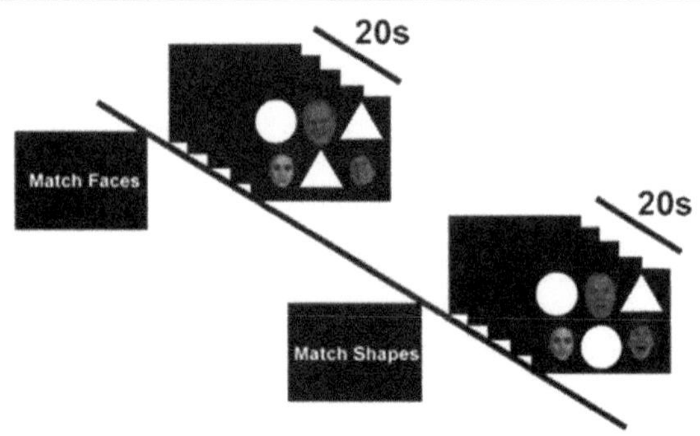

Figure 1 Schematic of an exemplar Match Faces and Match Shapes blocks in the Emotional Faces Shifting Attention Task (EFSAT).

directed attention *away* from emotional faces whereas "Match Faces" directed attention *towards* emotional faces. Analogous to traditional perceptual assessment tasks, each matching trial was presented for 4 sec in back-to-back blocks. In a recent study [59], we demonstrated the modification was successful as healthy volunteers engaged the amygdala to "Match Faces" and the rostral ACC to "Match Shapes" indicating the ACC effectively impeded the processing of task-irrelevant emotional faces presented alongside shapes. Thus, EFSAT complements traditional attentional control paradigms shown to recruit PFC areas.

In an effort to assess neural correlates of sustained attentional control in gSAD, participants performed the EFSAT during functional MRI. Our predictions for emotion processing (Match Faces > Match Shapes) were individuals with gSAD compared to demographically matched healthy controls (HC) would demonstrate: 1) exaggerated amygdala and anterior insula reactivity, 2) a positive relationship between activation in these regions and symptom severity, and 3) subcortical effects would be most pronounced when the faces constituted social signals of threat (angry and fear). Regarding attentional control (Match Shapes > Match Faces), we predicted gSAD compared to HC would exhibit: 1) reduced ACC activation, and 2) deficient ACC response would be most pronounced in the presence of distracting threat faces. Lastly, given reciprocal subcortical-ACC associations, we hypothesized insula activation to emotion processing would negatively correlate with ACC response during attentional control across participants.

Methods

Participants

Twenty-seven matched HC were recruited through community advertisements. The current HC group incorporates six new participants to the cohort in the previous EFSAT study involving only healthy volunteers [59], which previously served as a validation of this novel task and prompted pursuing the current study and informed the stated hypotheses. Twenty-nine individuals diagnosed with gSAD were identified through community advertisement and an outpatient psychiatric clinic. Participants completed the Structured Clinical Interview for DSM-IV [60] conducted by a licensed psychologist in addition to measures of symptoms and negative mood, such as the Liebowitz Social Anxiety Scale "LSAS" [61] and Beck Depression Inventory "BDI" [62]. All of the subjects were free of psychotropic medications except for two individuals with gSAD who were taking a selective serotonin reuptake inhibitor. None of the participants with gSAD had a current major depressive episode or severe depression symptoms (i.e., BDI score of 30 or greater; [62]). Furthermore, none of the participants with gSAD had recent substance abuse/dependence (within 6 months of study) or a lifetime history of major psychiatric illness (e.g., bipolar, psychotic disorder). All participants were between 18 and 55 years of age, right-handed, and free of current and past major medical or neurologic illness, as confirmed by a Board Certified physician. None of the participants tested positive for alcohol or illegal substances. GSAD and HC groups were matched for age ($t(54) = 0.02$, $p = 0.99$), gender ($\chi^2(1, N = 56) = 0.25$, $p = 0.62$), and race/ethnicity ($\chi^2(3, N = 56) = 4.54$, $p = 0.21$). All participants provided written informed consent, as approved by the Institutional Review Boards (ethics committee) of the University of Michigan Medical School in compliance with the Helsinki Declaration. See Table 1 for group characteristics.

Emotional faces shifting attention task

During fMRI scanning, participants performed the EFSAT, which consisted of trials depicting a trio of geometric shapes (circles, rectangles, triangles) presented

Table 1 Group characteristics (Mean ± SD)

	gSAD (n = 29)	HC (n = 27)	t (*df* = 56)	*p*
Age (years)	24.9 ± 6.3	24.9 ± 5.9	0.02	0.99
Gender	18 F/11 M	15 F/12 M		
Race/Ethnicity	6Asa/3AA/2H/18C	3Asa/1AA/0H/23C		
Social Anxiety Severity	77.3 ± 15.4	7.8 ± 6.3	21.69	<0.001
State Anxiety Level	42.9 ± 8.6	24.0 ± 5.4	9.72	<0.001
Trait Anxiety Level	49.1 ± 8.4	26.6 ± 4.0	12.69	<0.001
Depression Level	12.0 ± 7.9	0.67 ± 1.0	7.41	<0.001

gSAD, Generalized Social Anxiety Disorder participants.
HC, Healthy Control participants.
F, Female.
M, Male.
Asa, Asian American; AA, African American; H, Hispanic; C, Caucasian.
Social anxiety severity measured with the Liebowitz Social Anxiety Scale.
State and trait anxiety levels measured with the Spielberger State-Trait Anxiety Inventory.
Depression level measured with the Beck Depression Inventory.

alongside a trio of faces within the same field of view (Figure 1). During the "Match Faces" condition, participants had to select from one of two bottom faces (one emotional vs. one neutral) which matched the emotional expression of the top target face, whereas in the "Match Shapes" condition, participants selected from the two top shapes the one matching the bottom target shape. The faces were chosen from a validated stimulus set [63], were presented without repetition, and equally represented both genders.

The task comprised 36 back-to-back blocks: 18 blocks of matching shapes interleaved with 18 blocks of matching emotional faces, counterbalanced across two runs. Each target emotional face condition (angry, fear, happy) was presented in six 20-second blocks; these were presented pseudo-randomly, without subsequent repetition of individual faces. Each block began with a 4 second cue to either "Match Faces" (attend *to* faces) or "Match Shapes" (attend *away* from faces) followed by the four sequential matching trials, each lasting 4 seconds. Participant responses were recorded via button press.

Functional imaging: acquisition and analysis

Functional imaging was performed with blood-oxygen-level-dependent (BOLD) sensitive whole-brain fMRI on a 3.0 Tesla GE Signa System (General Electric; Milwaukee, WI) using a standard radio frequency coil. Images were acquired with 30 axial, 5-mm-thick slices using a standard T2*-sensitive gradient echo reverse spiral acquisition sequence (2 s repetition time; 25 ms echo time; 64 × 64 matrix; 24 cm field of view; flip angle 77°; 3.75 × 3.75 × 5 mm final voxel size). A high-resolution, T1-weighted volumetric anatomical scan was also acquired for anatomical localization. Data from all participants met the criteria for quality with minimal motion correction (movements were less than 2 mm in any one direction across each functional run) and the first 4 volumes from each run were discarded to allow for T1 equilibration effects. Conventional preprocessing steps were used in Statistical Parametric Mapping (SPM8) software package (Wellcome Trust Centre for Neuroimaging, London www.fil.ion.ucl.ac.uk/spm). Briefly, images were temporally corrected to account for differences in slice time collection, spatially realigned to the first image of the first run, normalized to a Montreal Neurological Institute (MNI) template, and smoothed with an 8 mm isotropic Gaussian kernel.

A general linear model was applied to the time series, convolved with the canonical hemodynamic response function and with a 128 s high-pass filter. Blocks of Match Faces (shapes in 'background') and Match Shapes (faces in 'background') were modeled separately based on the target emotion or shape (angry, fearful, or happy / circle, square, or triangle) resulting in six regressors, the effects of which were estimated for each voxel for each participant and taken to the second level for random effects analysis.

A region of interest (ROI)-based Analysis of Variance (ANOVA) was conducted to test our *a priori* hypotheses—specifically, within the bilateral amygdala, anterior insula, and anterior cingulate cortex (ACC) as defined by atlas-based anatomical ROIs with Automated Anatomical Labeling (AAL) toolbox within SPM, in the context of main effects of Group (gSAD, HC), Emotion (angry, fear, happy), and Group by Emotion interaction. Activations were deemed significant at a p-value of <0.05, corrected for multiple comparisons within the *a priori* anatomically-confined ROI (i.e., a small volume correction [SVC]). For completeness, we also report activation clusters outside *a priori* ROIs at a whole-brain threshold of $p < 0.001$ uncorrected with at least 10 contiguous voxels.

To clarify the direction of activation and to examine correlations, parameter estimates of peak activation (β weights, arbitrary units [a.u.]) were extracted from spherical (10-mm diameter) ROIs from each participant and submitted to *post hoc* t-tests in the Statistical Package for the Social Sciences (SPSS) (Chicago, IL version 18).

Pearson correlational analyses were conducted to evaluate the predicted positive relationship between amygdala and/or insula activation with symptom severity, and the association between subcortical (amygdala, aINS) activation and ACC response.

Behavioral data were submitted to a 2 (Group: gSAD, HC) x 3 (Emotion: fear, angry, happy) ANOVA with repeated measures for the Emotion factor for Match Faces and emotional 'distractor' for Match Shapes. All significant main effects and interactions were followed up with two-tailed t-tests, $p < 0.05$.

Results

Behavioral data: match faces

For accuracy, results revealed a main effect of Emotion [$F(2,108)$ 4.41, $p < 0.016$] but no main effect of Group or Emotion x Group interaction (all $p_s > 0.05$). The main effect of Emotion showed participants were more accurate at matching fearful than angry faces ($p < 0.007$); no differences were evident for fearful versus happy ($p = 0.13$) or angry versus happy faces ($p = 0.12$). Similarly, mean reaction times (RT) for accurate trials showed a main effect of Emotion [$F(2,108)$ 36.0, $p < 0.001$] but no main effect of Group or Emotion x Group interaction (all $p_s > 0.05$). The main effect of Emotion revealed participants were faster at matching happy than angry faces ($p < 0.001$) and faster at matching fearful than angry faces ($p < 0.001$). There was a non-significant trend for matching fearful faster than happy faces ($p = 0.08$). See Table 2 for behavioral descriptives.

Table 2 Accuracy and reaction times (in milliseconds) for accurate trials (Mean ± SD)

Contrast	gSAD (n = 29)	HC (n = 27)	t (*df* = 56)	*p*
Accuracy				
Attend Angry vs. Shapes	85.6 ± 11.8	86.6 ± 10.9	0.31	0.76
Attend Fear vs. Shapes	92.7 ± 9.1	90.7 ± 10.1	0.75	0.46
Attend Happy vs. Shapes	90.8 ± 11.0	86.3 ± 14.2	1.34	0.19
Attend Shapes vs. Angry (distractor)	94.1 ± 8.1	93.7 ± 8.0	0.20	0.84
Attend Shapes vs. Fear (distractor)	90.1 ± 14.4	95.5 ± 7.6	1.75	0.09
Attend Shapes vs. Happy (distractor)	91.2 ± 11.5	93.4 ± 7.5	0.81	0.42
Reaction Times				
Attend Angry vs. Shapes	1479.6 ± 405.8	1419.9 ± 219.5	0.68	0.50
Attend Fear vs. Shapes	1337.9 ± 371.9	1285.7 ± 218.5	0.63	0.53
Attend Happy vs. Shapes	1303.7 ± 340.4	1231.0 ± 207.4	0.96	0.34
Attend Shapes vs. Angry (distractor)	1021.1 ± 273.5	957.8 ± 122.4	1.11	0.27
Attend Shapes vs. Fear (distractor)	985.4 ± 239.9	946.2 ± 144.4	0.74	0.47
Attend Shapes vs. Happy (distractor)	975.6 ± 236.4	944.3 ± 157.7	0.58	0.57

Behavioral data: match shapes

Regarding accuracy, there were no main effects for (distractor) Emotion or Group and no evidence of a (distractor) Emotion x Group interaction (all $p_s > 0.05$). All participants exhibited similar accuracy when matching shapes alongside angry, fearful, and happy distractor faces. Results for RT were analogous as there were no main effects for (distractor) Emotion or Group and no (distractor) Emotion x Group interaction (all $p_s > 0.05$). Participants showed comparable RT among each distractor emotion: shapes-angry, shapes-fearful, and shapes-happy (all $p_s > 0.05$). See Table 2 for behavioral descriptives.

Functional MRI

An ANOVA revealed a main effect of Group for anterior insula and ACC (Table 3). *Post hoc* t-tests showed greater bilateral anterior insula activity for gSAD versus HC [left (−32, 22, 8), F-score = 12.02, volume = 560 mm^3, $_{svc}$corrected $p < 0.01$; right (32, 26, 4), F-score = 8.03, volume = 440 mm^3, $_{svc}$corrected $p < 0.03$] when attending to emotional faces (vs. shapes) (Figure 2). Conversely, gSAD showed less activation in left rostral ACC (rACC) compared to HC [(-6, 30, -6), F-score = 6.72, volume = 368 mm^3, $_{svc}$corrected $p < 0.05$] when attending to shapes (vs. emotional faces) (Figure 3). The main effect of Emotion and the Group x Emotion interaction were non-significant in *a priori* regions.

Correlational analyses

Extent of anterior insula (aINS) reactivity in gSAD corresponded with the intensity of social anxiety symptoms (LSAS-total score) though significance was evident in the left aINS (r = 0.32, $p < 0.04$, one-tailed) but not right aINS (r = 0.20, $p = 0.1$, one-tailed). No correlations emerged for aINS reactivity and general anxiety (i.e., trait anxiety; [64] or depression level [62] (all $p_s > 0.05$) in the gSAD group.

We observed a negative relationship between both left aINS and rostral ACC (r = −0.35, $p < 0.009$, two-tailed) and right aINS and rostral ACC (r = −0.45, $p < 0.001$, two-tailed) (Figure 4). Of note, these correlations remained significant even after the removal of the HC and gSAD outliers.

Table 3 Whole-brain voxel-wise analysis of variance

Region	MNI Coordinates			Volume	*F* statistic
Main Effect of Group					
Anterior insula	**-32**	**22**	**8**	**560**	**12.02**
	32	**26**	**4**	**440**	**8.03**
Anterior cingulate cortex	**-6**	**30**	**-6**	**368**	**6.72**
Middle occipital gyrus	-30	-98	-4	104	16.03
	28	-86	4	248	13.44
Supramarginal gyrus	-64	-42	32	224	14.15
Supplementary motor area	8	-16	52	128	12.43
Main Effect of Emotion					
Hippocampus	-34	-14	-12	104	9.30
Inferior frontal operculum	-36	10	26	112	8.73
Group x Emotion Interaction					
Superior frontal gyrus	-18	32	54	1080	12.01
Caudate	16	-16	24	184	9.91
	22	0	24	152	8.72
Middle frontal gyrus	40	-2	62	104	8.48

A priori areas within the atlas-based anatomical regions of interest are shown in bold.
MNI, Montreal Neurological Institute.

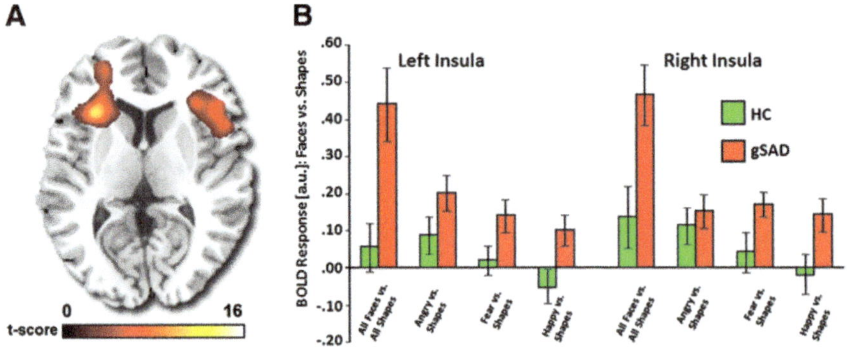

Figure 2 A priori region of interest: Anterior insula. A) Voxel-wise main effect of group for the contrast Match Faces > Match Shapes, along with Match Angry > Match Shapes, Match Fear > Match Shapes, and Match Happy > Match Shapes, showing bilateral anterior insula (aINS) displayed on statistical F-map at $p < 0.05$; cluster size >10 contiguous voxels (family-wise error corrected for multiple comparisons across small volumes of interest). Color scale reflects *F*-score. **B**) Bar graphs depicting extracted parameter estimates of activation from the aINS ROI within each group showing Generalized Social Anxiety Disorder exhibited greater bilateral anterior insula activation than Healthy Controls ($p < 0.05$).

Discussion

In this functional MRI study, we examined amygdala, anterior insula (aINS), and anterior cingulate cortex (ACC) activation in patients with generalized social anxiety disorder (gSAD) and demographically matched healthy controls (HC) with a novel "Emotional Faces Shifting Attention Task" (EFSAT). The paradigm is an adaptation of widely used emotional faces matching tasks known to evoke exaggerated amygdala and/or insula reactivity in gSAD [17,18]. By spatially combining the traditionally separate faces-only and shapes-only image trials into one trial within one field of view, attention was modulated by having it directed towards or away from emotional faces in order to complete the matching task.

The primary objective in this study was to evaluate attentional modulation with EFSAT in patients with gSAD. When attending to emotional content (Match Faces > Match Shapes), we hypothesized individuals with gSAD relative to HC would exhibit exaggerated amygdala and aINS reactivity particularly to threat expressions (angry, fearful). Our prediction was partially supported. Though no group effects emerged for amygdala, participants with gSAD compared to HC showed bilateral aINS hyper-reactivity when attending to faces, regardless of emotional valence. We also expected a positive correlation between subcortical reactivity and symptom intensity in gSAD. In support, greater left aINS reactivity to emotional faces corresponded with greater symptom severity in gSAD but not with general anxiety or depression

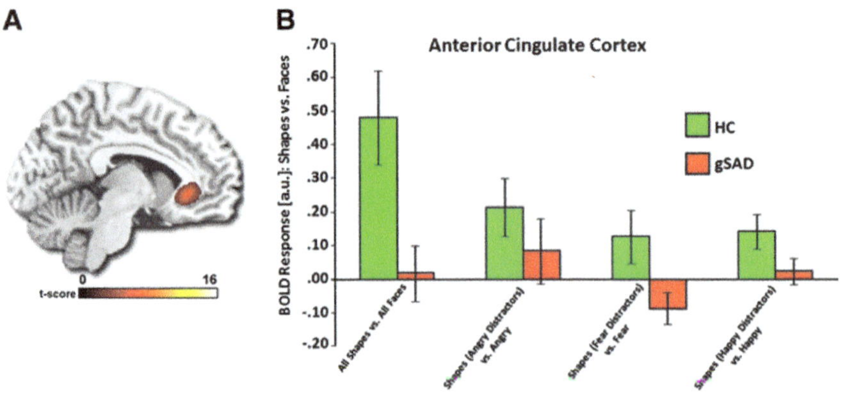

Figure 3 A priori region of interest: Anterior cingulate cortex. A) Voxel-wise main effect of group for the contrast Match Shapes > Match Faces, along with Match Shapes (Angry distractor) > Match Angry, Match Shapes (Fear distractor) > Match Fear, and Match Shapes (Happy distractor) > Match Happy, showing anterior cingulate cortex (ACC) displayed on statistical F-map at $p < 0.05$; cluster size >10 contiguous voxels (family-wise error corrected for multiple comparisons across small volumes of interest). Color scale reflects *F*-score. **B**) Bar graphs depicting extracted parameter estimates of activation from the ACC ROI activation within each group showing Healthy Controls exhibited ACC activation, whereas, Generalized Social Anxiety Disorder showed no 'activation'.

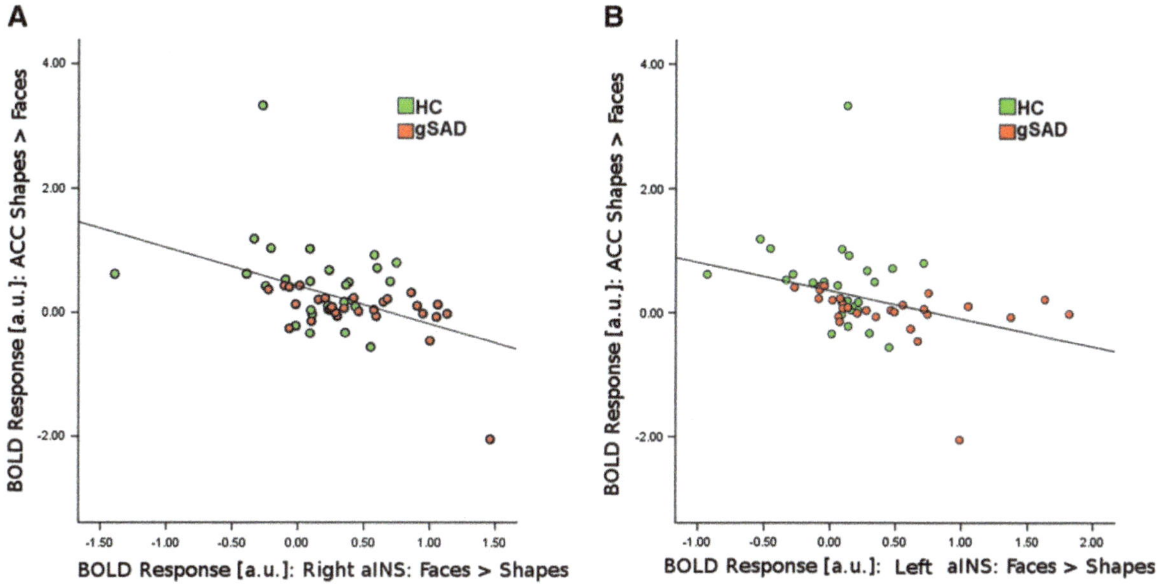

Figure 4 Correlation between extent of activation from the anterior cingulate cortex (ACC) ROI and extent of activation in A) right anterior insula and B) left anterior insula ROIs across all subjects. Generalized Social Anxiety Disorder subjects are coded in red; Healthy Controls are coded in green.

level; however, results were weak (i.e., only revealed with one-tailed t-test). Nevertheless, overall findings substantiate the proposal that interoception, a function of aINS that aids in bringing bodily state to awareness [30,31], underlies anxiety by means of negative beliefs that facilitate, or are the result of, exaggerated interoceptive signals [28,29].

When attending away from emotional faces (Match Shapes > Match Faces), we hypothesized gSAD relative to HC would exhibit reduced ACC engagement and that deficient ACC response would be most pronounced in the presence of distracting threat faces. Evidence of enhanced rostral ACC in our HC group is consistent with its role in regulatory control [40,46,65,66]. Specifically, its recruitment when attention was shifted to shapes indicates it served a gating function in modulating the processing of face distractors. We did not find evidence of group effects for dorsal ACC, another region involved in the inhibition of emotional processing [45,66] suggesting EFSAT may not tap into regulatory regions associated with conflict resolution or stimulus appraisal [66]. Again, our hypothesis was partially supported in that gSAD showed a lack of rostral ACC response; however, there was no interaction with the emotional valence of task-irrelevant faces. To our knowledge, the only other study of implicit attentional control in gSAD comprised an event-related emotional conflict task, an emotional counting Stroop paradigm. Results showed patients with gSAD or generalized anxiety disorder lacked dorsal ACC recruitment to congruent and incongruent negative pictures compared to healthy volunteers [49]. Methodological differences do not premit direct comparison with our study, however, evidence of deficient ACC activation during conflict resolution or sustained goal-directed attention suggests impoverished ACC plays a role in excessive attention to emotional information in gSAD and potentially other disorders of emotion dysregulation.

Across participants, we hypothesized a negative relationship between ACC response during attentional control and subcortical (amygdala and/or aINS) reactivity to emotional faces. The prediction was supported, but only in aINS and not amygdala. In a previous study, we showed greater aINS reactivity to threat faces in gSAD than controls, with reduced functional connectivity between aINS and dorsal ACC activity in gSAD indicating exaggerated aINS reactivity was due to a deficiency in 'top down' control or appraisal [23]. Here, we observe a negative aINS-ACC relationship across subjects based on direct and indirect emotion processing, respectively, along with evidence of enhanced rostral ACC and reduced bilateral aINS activation in the HC group. Given that the ACC is thought to interact with and/or modulate aINS response to salient signals, we interpret that individuals who exhibit deficient ACC engagement when attentional control is required are those who are likely to exhibit enhanced aINS reactivity when their attention is directed towards emotional stimuli.

Conclusions

Findings should be considered in the context of several important limitations. Due to the lack of a baseline (e.g., fixation) condition, findings cannot be interpreted in relation to a change from a non-cognitive and non-emotional task. The lack of 'neutral' target expressions does not permit dissociation between face and emotion-processing influences. Additionally, the paradigm failed to elicit differential amygdala response between gSAD and controls and insula hyper-reactivity in gSAD was not specific to threat. Together, the task may, in these aspects, not be as sensitive as traditional perceptual matching paradigms. Interestingly, subjects with gSAD have been shown to judge happy faces as less approachable than controls [67]. Although we did not measure potential interpretation bias, we cannot rule out the possibility that insula activation in gSAD involved a less positive judgment of happy faces. Lastly, the gSAD group exhibited greater levels of depression and general anxiety (i.e., trait anxiety) than controls; therefore, we cannot rule out potential influences of depression and general anxiety on results.

Despite limitations, these findings suggest a simple, volitional shift in attention to and away from emotional faces differentiates patients with gSAD from healthy controls in terms of engagement of regions integral to emotion processing and attentional control. During direct and indirect processing of emotional faces, gSAD patients exhibit exaggerated insula reactivity and deficient ACC recruitment, respectively, and different valences, both positive and negative, of socio-emotional information.

Competing interests

The authors declare that they have no competing interests.

Authors' contributions

HK conceived and designed the study, conducted data analyses and interpretation, and wrote the manuscript. DP and DAF conducted data analyses and interpretation, and participated in drafting the manuscript. MA helped design the study, collected the data, and participated in drafting the manuscript. KLP conceived and designed the study, conducted data interpretation, and participated in drafting the manuscript. All authors read and approved the final manuscript.

Acknowledgements

This work was supported by grants from the National Institutes of Health, National Institute of Mental Health (MH076198 to KLP and MH093679 to HK).

Author details

[1]Mood and Anxiety Disorders Research Program, Department of Psychiatry (HK, DP, DAF, KLP), University of Illinois at Chicago, 1747 W. Roosevelt Rd, Chicago, IL 60608, USA. [2]Department of Psychiatry (MA, KLP), University of Michigan, Ann Arbor, MI, USA. [3]Neuropsychiatric Research Program (KLP), Mental Health Service, Jesse Brown VA Medical Center, Chicago, IL, USA.

References

1. Kessler RC, Chiu WT, Demler O, Merikangas KR, Walters EE: **Prevalence, severity, and comorbidity of 12-month DSM-IV disorders in the National Comorbidity Survey Replication.** *Arch Gen Psychiatry* 2005, **62:**617–627.
2. Stein MB, Stein DJ: **Social anxiety disorder.** *Lancet* 2008, **371:**1115–1125.
3. Kessler RC, McGonagle KA, Zhao S, Nelson CB, Hughes M, Eshleman S, Wittchen H-U, Kendler KS: **Lifetime and 12-month prevalence of DSM-III-R psychiatric disorders in the United States: results from the national comorbidity survey.** *Arch Gen Psychiatry* 1994, **51:**8–19.
4. Ruscio AM, Brown TA, Chiu WT, Sareen J, Stein MB, Kessler RC: **Social fears and social phobia in the USA: results from the National Comorbidity Survey Replication.** *Psychol Med* 2008, **38:**15–28.
5. Bögels SM, Mansell W: **Attention processes in the maintenance and treatment of social phobia: hypervigilance, avoidance and self-focused attention.** *Clin Psychol Rev* 2004, **24:**827–856.
6. Cornwell BR, Johnson L, Berardi L, Grillon C: **Anticipation of public speaking in virtual reality reveals a relationship between trait social anxiety and startle reactivity.** *Biol Psychiatry* 2006, **59:**664–666.
7. Davidson RJ: **Affective style, psychopathology, and resilience: brain mechanisms and plasticity.** *Am Psychol* 2000, **55:**1196–1214.
8. McTeague LM, Lang PJ, Laplante M-C, Cuthbert BN, Strauss CC, Bradley MM: **Fearful imagery in social phobia: generalization, comorbidity, and physiological reactivity.** *Biol Psychiatry* 2009, **65:**374–382.
9. Heimberg RG: **Cognitive assessment strategies and the measurement of outcome of treatment for social phobia.** *Behav Res Ther* 1994, **32:**269–280.
10. Adolphs R, Tranel D, Damasio H, Damasio AR: **Fear and the human amygdala.** *J Neurosci* 1995, **15:**5879–5891.
11. Davis M, Whalen PJ: **The amygdala: vigilance and emotion.** *Mol Psychiatry* 2001, **6:**13–34.
12. Phan KL, Wager T, Taylor SF, Liberzon I: **Functional neuroanatomy of emotion: a meta-analysis of emotion activation studies in PET and fMRI.** *NeuroImage* 2002, **16:**331–348.
13. Hariri AR, Whalen PJ: **The amygdala: inside and out.** *F1000 Biol Rep* 2011, **3:**2.
14. Hariri AR, Tessitore A, Mattay VS, Fera F, Weinberger DR: **The amygdala response to emotional stimuli: a comparison of faces and scenes.** *NeuroImage* 2002, **17:**317–323.
15. Hariri AR, Drabant EM, Munoz KE, Kolachana BS, Mattay VS, Egan MF, Weinberger DR: **A susceptibility gene for affective disorders and the response of the human amygdala.** *Arch Gen Psychiatry* 2005, **62:**146–152.
16. Sergerie K, Chochol C, Armony JL: **The role of the amygdala in emotional processing: a quantitative meta-analysis of functional neuroimaging studies.** *Neurosci Biobehav Rev* 2008, **32:**811–830.
17. Etkin A, Wager TD: **Functional neuroimaging of anxiety: a meta-analysis of emotional processing in PTSD, Social Anxiety Disorder, and Specific Phobia.** *Am J Psychiatry* 2007, **164:**1476–1488.
18. Freitas-Ferrari MC, Hallak JEC, Trzesniak C, Filho AS, Machado-de-Sousa JP, Chagas MHN, Nardi AE, Crippa JAS: **Neuroimaging in social anxiety disorder: a systematic review of the literature.** *Prog Neuropsychopharmacol Biol Psychiatry* 2010, **34:**565–580.
19. Phan KL, Fitzgerald DA, Nathan PJ, Tancer ME: **Association between amygdala hyperactivity to harsh faces and severity of social anxiety in generalized social phobia.** *Biol Psychiatry* 2006, **59:**424–429.
20. Amir N, Klumpp H, Elias J, Bedwell JS, Yanasak N, Miller LS: **Increased activation of the anterior cingulate cortex during processing of disgust faces in individuals with social phobia.** *Biol Psychiatry* 2005, **57:**975–981.
21. Ball TM, Sullivan S, Flagan T, Hitchcock CA, Simmons A, Paulus MP, Stein MB: **Selective effects of social anxiety, anxiety sensitivity, and negative affectivity on the neural bases of emotional face processing.** *NeuroImage* 2012, **59:**1879–1887.
22. Evans KC, Wright CI, Wedig MM, Gold AL, Pollack MH, Rauch SL: **A functional MRI study of amygdala responses to angry schematic faces in social anxiety disorder.** *Depress Anxiety* 2008, **25:**496–505.
23. Klumpp H, Angstadt M, Phan KL: **Insula reactivity and connectivity to anterior cingulate cortex when processing threat in generalized social anxiety disorder.** *Biol Psychol* 2012, **89:**273–276.
24. Schmidt S, Mohr A, Miltner WHR, Straube T: **Task-dependent neural correlates of the processing of verbal threat-related stimuli in social phobia.** *Biol Psychol* 2010, **84:**304–312.
25. Shah SG, Klumpp H, Angstadt M, Nathan PJ, Phan KL: **Amygdala and insula response to emotional images in patients with generalized social anxiety disorder.** *J Psychiatry Neurosci* 2009, **34:**296–302.
26. Straube T, Kolassa I-T, Glauer M, Mentzel H-J, Miltner WHR: **Effect of task conditions on brain responses to threatening faces in social phobics: an event-related functional magnetic resonance imaging study.** *Biol Psychiatry* 2004, **56:**921–930.

27. Straube T, Mentzel H-J, Miltner WHR: **Common and distinct brain activation to threat and safety signals in social phobia.** *Neuropsychobiology* 2005, **52:**163–168.
28. Paulus MP, Stein MB: **An insular view of anxiety.** *Biol Psychiatry* 2006, **60:**383–387.
29. Paulus MP, Stein MB: **Interoception in anxiety and depression.** *Brain Struct Funct* 2010, **214:**451–463.
30. Craig ADB: **How do you feel–now? The anterior insula and human awareness.** *Nat Rev Neurosci* 2009, **10:**59–70.
31. Jones CL, Ward J, Critchley HD: **The neuropsychological impact of insular cortex lesions.** *J Neurol Neurosurg Psychiatr* 2010, **81:**611–618.
32. Amaral DG, Price JL: **Amygdalo-cortical projections in the monkey (Macaca fascicularis).** *J Comp Neurol* 1984, **230:**465–496.
33. Ghashghaei HT, Barbas H: **Pathways for emotion: interactions of prefrontal and anterior temporal pathways in the amygdala of the rhesus monkey.** *Neuroscience* 2002, **115:**1261–1279.
34. Ghashghaei HT, Hilgetag CC, Barbas H: **Sequence of information processing for emotions based on the anatomic dialogue between prefrontal cortex and amygdala.** *NeuroImage* 2007, **34:**905–923.
35. Augustine JR: **Circuitry and functional aspects of the insular lobe in primates including humans.** *Brain Res Brain Res Rev* 1996, **22:**229–244.
36. Craig AD: **How do you feel? interoception: the sense of the physiological condition of the body.** *Nat Rev Neurosci* 2002, **3:**655–666.
37. Mesulam MM, Mufson EJ: **Insula of the old world monkey. III: efferent cortical output and comments on function.** *J Comp Neurol* 1982, **212:**38–52.
38. Nelson SM, Dosenbach NUF, Cohen AL, Wheeler ME, Schlaggar BL, Petersen SE: **Role of the anterior insula in task-level control and focal attention.** *Brain Struct Funct* 2010, **214:**669–680.
39. Seeley WW, Menon V, Schatzberg AF, Keller J, Glover GH, Kenna H, Reiss AL, Greicius MD: **Dissociable intrinsic connectivity networks for salience processing and executive control.** *J Neurosci* 2007, **27:**2349–2356.
40. Bishop S, Duncan J, Brett M, Lawrence AD: **Prefrontal cortical function and anxiety: controlling attention to threat-related stimuli.** *Nat Neurosci* 2004, **7:**184–188.
41. Bishop SJ, Jenkins R, Lawrence AD: **Neural processing of fearful faces: effects of anxiety are gated by perceptual capacity limitations.** *Cereb Cortex* 2007, **17:**1595–1603.
42. Botvinick MM, Braver TS, Barch DM, Carter CS, Cohen JD: **Conflict monitoring and cognitive control.** *Psychol Rev* 2001, **108:**624–652.
43. Carter CS, Braver TS, Barch DM, Botvinick MM, Noll D, Cohen JD: **Anterior cingulate cortex, error detection, and the online monitoring of performance.** *Science* 1998, **280:**747–749.
44. Duncan J, Owen AM: **Common regions of the human frontal lobe recruited by diverse cognitive demands.** *Trends Neurosci* 2000, **23:**475–483.
45. Etkin A, Egner T, Peraza DM, Kandel ER, Hirsch J: **Resolving emotional conflict: a role for the rostral anterior cingulate cortex in modulating activity in the amygdala.** *Neuron* 2006, **51:**871–882.
46. Kanske P, Kotz SA: **Emotion speeds up conflict resolution: a new role for the ventral anterior cingulate cortex?** *Cereb Cortex* 2011, **21:**911–919.
47. MacDonald AW III, Cohen JD, Stenger VA, Carter CS: **Dissociating the role of the dorsolateral prefrontal and anterior cingulate cortex in cognitive control.** *Science* 2000, **288:**1835–1838.
48. Whalen PJ, Bush G, Shin LM, Rauch SL: **The emotional counting Stroop: a task for assessing emotional interference during brain imaging.** *Nat Protoc* 2006, **1:**293–296.
49. Blair KS, Geraci M, Smith BW, Hollon N, Devido J, Otero M, Blair JR, Pine DS: **Reduced dorsal anterior cingulate cortical activity during emotional regulation and top-down attentional control in generalized social phobia, generalized anxiety disorder, and comorbid generalized social phobia/generalized anxiety disorder.** *Biol Psychiatry* 2012, **72:**476–482.
50. Shin LM, Whalen PJ, Pitman RK, Bush G, Macklin ML, Lasko NB, Orr SP, McInerney SC, Rauch SL: **An fMRI study of anterior cingulate function in posttraumatic stress disorder.** *Biol Psychiatry* 2001, **50:**932–942.
51. Carlson JM, Reinke KS, Habib R: **A left amygdala mediated network for rapid orienting to masked fearful faces.** *Neuropsychologia* 2009, **47:**1386–1389.
52. Pourtois G, Schwartz S, Seghier ML, Lazeyras F, Vuilleumier P: **Neural systems for orienting attention to the location of threat signals: an event-related fMRI study.** *NeuroImage* 2006, **31:**920–933.
53. Vuilleumier P, Armony JL, Driver J, Dolan RJ: **Effects of attention and emotion on face processing in the human brain: an event-related fMRI study.** *Neuron* 2001, **30:**829–841.
54. Pessoa L, Kastner S, Ungerleider LG: **Attentional control of the processing of neutral and emotional stimuli.** *Brain Res Cogn Brain Res* 2002, **15:**31–45.
55. Klumpp H, Ho SS, Taylor SF, Phan KL, Abelson JL, Liberzon I: **Trait anxiety modulates anterior cingulate activation to threat interference.** *Depress Anxiety* 2011, **28:**194–201.
56. Krug MK, Carter CS: **Adding fear to conflict: a general purpose cognitive control network is modulated by trait anxiety.** *Cogn Affect Behav Neurosci* 2010, **10:**357–371.
57. Price RB, Eldreth DA, Mohlman J: **Deficient prefrontal attentional control in late-life generalized anxiety disorder: an fMRI investigation.** *Transl Psychiatry* 2011, **1:**e46.
58. Hajcak G, Olvet DM: **The persistence of attention to emotion: brain potentials during and after picture presentation.** *Emotion* 2008, **8:**250–255.
59. Klumpp H, Angstadt M, Phan KL: **Shifting the focus of attention modulates amygdala and anterior cingulate cortex reactivity to emotional faces.** *Neurosci Lett* 2012, **514:**210–213.
60. First MB, Spitzer RL, Gibbon M, Williams JBW: *Structured Clinical Interview for the DSM-IV Axis I Disorders: SCID-I/P, Version 2.0.*: Biometrics Research Department, New York State Psychiatric Institute; 1997.
61. Liebowitz MR: **Social phobia.** *Mod Probl Pharmacopsychiatry* 1987, **22:**141–173.
62. Beck AT, Steer RA, Brown GK: *Manual for the Beck Depression Inventory-II.* San Antonio, TX: Psychological Corp; 1996.
63. Gur RC, Schroeder L, Turner T, McGrath C, Chan RM, Turetsky BI, Alsop D, Maldjian J, Gur RE: **Brain activation during facial emotion processing.** *NeuroImage* 2002, **16:**651–662.
64. Spielberger CD, Gorsuch RL, Lushene R, Vagg PR, Jacobs GA: *Manual for the State-Trait Anxiety Inventory.* Palo Alto, CA: Consulting Psychologists Press; 1983.
65. Bush G, Luu P, Posner MI: **Cognitive and emotional influences in anterior cingulate cortex.** *Trends Cogn Sci* 2000, **4:**215–222.
66. Etkin A, Egner T, Kalisch R: **Emotional processing in anterior cingulate and medial prefrontal cortex.** *Trends Cogn Sci* 2011, **15:**85–93.
67. Campbell DW, Sareen J, Stein MB, Kravetsky LB, Paulus MP, Hassard ST, Reiss JP: **Happy but not so approachable: the social judgments of individuals with generalized social phobia.** *Depress Anxiety* 2009, **26:**419–424.

6

An fMRI study of unconditioned responses in post-traumatic stress disorder

Clas Linnman[1*], Thomas A Zeffiro[2], Roger K Pitman[1] and Mohammed R Milad[1]

Abstract

Background: Both fear and pain processing are altered in post-traumatic stress disorder (PTSD), as evidenced by functional neuroimaging studies showing increased amygdala responses to threats, and increased insula, putamen and caudate activity in response to heat pain. Using psychophysiology and functional magnetic resonance imaging, we studied conditioned and unconditioned autonomic and neuronal responses in subjects with PTSD versus trauma-exposed non-PTSD control (TENC) subjects. A design using an electric shock selected by subjects to be 'highly annoying but not painful' as an unconditioned stimulus (US) with partially reinforced cues allowed us to partly disentangle the expectancy- and prediction-error components from sensory components of the unconditioned response.

Results: Whereas responses to the conditioned stimulus (CS) were similar in PTSD and TENC, the former displayed higher putamen, insula, caudate and amygdala responses to the US. Reactivity to the US in the anterior insula correlated with PTSD symptom severity. Functional connectivity analyses using the putamen as a seed region indicated that TENC subjects had increased amygdala-putamen connectivity during US delivery; this connection was disengaged in PTSD.

Conclusions: Our results indicate that although neural processing of fear learning in people with PTSD seems to be comparable with controls, neural responses to unconditioned aversive stimuli in PTSD seem to be increased.

Background

In classic fear conditioning, an initially neutral, and later conditioned stimulus (CS+) is paired with an aversive unconditioned stimulus (US) such as an electric shock. After pairing, the neutral stimulus is able to elicit fear on its own. Much has been learned about the neural responses induced by the CS+ presentation. In healthy people, conditioned stimuli activate the amygdala, brainstem, insula and parts of anterior cingulate cortex (ACC) [1]. Less is known about changes occurring in response to the presentation of the more biologically relevant US [2]. Responses to a US in healthy subjects are accompanied by increased activity in the brainstem, thalamus, and cingulate, sensory and insular cortices [3-5], structures also known to respond to noxious stimuli [6].

Understanding the neural mechanisms that mediate aversive unconditioned responses may be clinically relevant. Brain regions involved in fear learning, such as the amygdala and the ACC, are implicated in the pathophysiology of several anxiety disorders such as post-traumatic stress disorder (PTSD). Other intrinsically aversive stimuli such as trauma reminders, aversive images and fearful faces also elicit increased responses in several brain regions in PTSD, such as the amygdala and the ACC [7]. The unconditioned response represents a specific exemplar of a more general class of aversive stimuli to which people with PTSD may be more sensitive. In addition, understanding how aversive somatosensory stimuli are processed in PTSD may help to explain why pain processing is altered in this disorder [8], and clarify the high comorbidity between PTSD and chronic pain [9,10]. Recent functional magnetic resonance imaging (fMRI) studies of pain processing in PTSD reported increased insular and putamen reactivity to painful heat [11,12]. However, it is unknown whether such alterations in pain processing are driven by

* Correspondence: linnman@nmr.mgh.harvard.edu
[1]Department of Psychiatry, Harvard Medical School & Massachusetts General Hospital, 149 13th street, Charlestown, MA, USA
Full list of author information is available at the end of the article

anticipatory or perceptual properties of noxious stimulation, and whether aversive but not overtly painful somatosensory stimuli are also processed differently in PTSD.

In the present study, we examined the neural correlates of responses to electrical shock stimuli in subjects with PTSD and in trauma-exposed non-PTSD (TENC) control subjects. Within an fMRI fear-conditioning paradigm, we examined neuronal and autonomic responses to CS+ and US presentations in a partial-reinforcement paradigm [13]. The US was a 'highly annoying but not painful' electric shock delivered after 62.5% of the CS+ presentations. This experimental design allowed us to compare neural responses to both the CS+ and US, and to the anticipation and unexpected omission of the US (unreinforced CS+ trials). By contrasting time intervals representing delivered versus non-delivered US, the sensory component of a US response may be in part be isolated from its expectancy- and prediction-error related components. Moreover, we related alterations in brain responses elicited by the US to PTSD symptom severity. Lastly, in a *post hoc* analysis, we explored inter-regional functional connectivity differences in US-elicited responses in the regions in which the subjects with PTSD were found to differ significantly from the TENC subjects.

Methods

The Partners Healthcare System Human Research Committee approved the study, and all subjects gave informed consent.

Subjects

In total, 23 right-handed people with PTSD and 28 right-handed healthy TENC subjects were recruited from the community. All were administered the Structured Clinical Interview for the *Diagnostic and Statistical Manual*, fourth edition (DSM-IV) [14] to determine PTSD diagnostic status and possible comorbid axis I disorders.

For the TENC group, participants with any current mental disorder were excluded. Subjects with PTSD who had current substance dependence were also excluded, as were subjects who had used any psychotropic medication within 4 weeks before participation (1 year for neuroleptics). Data from four PTSD and four TENC subjects were excluded because of excessive head movement while in the scanner, leaving a total sample size of 19 PTSD and 24 TENC subjects. Data from a subset of these participants have already been reported in studies examining fear extinction [15,16]; however, their responses to the US have not previously been reported.

Rating scales

The Clinician-Administered PTSD Scale (CAPS) [17], Neuroticism-Extroversion-Openness Personality Inventory-Revised (NEO PI-R) [18], Spielberger State Trait Anxiety Inventory [19], Beck Anxiety Inventory (BAI) [20] and Beck Depression Inventory (BDI) [21] were administered to all participants. These results, along with demographic data, type of trauma, age at first trauma exposure, and current comorbid disorders are shown in Table 1.

Fear-conditioning procedure

We used a partial-reinforcement classic conditioning paradigm that has previously been described in detail [13]. In the fMRI scanner, each trial began with an image of a room (context) containing an unlit lamp, which was presented for 3 seconds. The lamp was then switched on to show one of three colors (blue, red or yellow). Two of the colors (CS+) were followed by an electric shock (US) in 62.5% of the cases. The third color was never followed by a shock (CS-). The illuminated lamp was presented 32 times, giving a total of 16 safe trials (CS-), 10 CS+ trials followed by the shock, and 6 CS+ trials in which the shock was omitted. Each CS presentation lasted for 6 seconds. Between trials, a black screen was displayed for 12 to 18 seconds. The lamp color sequence was counterbalanced across subjects in pseudo-random order (see Additional file 1 Figure S1).

Electric shock

The US consisted of a 500 ms train of 1 ms spikes at 50 Hz delivered to the second and third fingers of the right hand, with currents ranging from 0.2 to 4.0 mA. Before the experiment, the shock current was individually adjusted so that it would be perceived as 'highly annoying but not painful' by the individual patient. Administration of the US immediately followed CS offset.

Skin conductance

Skin-conductance responses (SCRs) were measured using a skin-conductance coupler (S71-23; Coulbourn Modular Instruments, Allentown, PA, USA) with 8 mm (sensor diameter) radiolucent Ag/AgCl electrodes (BioPac Systems Inc., Goleta, CA, USA). Electrodes were filled with isotonic paste, and placed on the palm of the subject's left hand. The skin-conductance electrodes were separated by 14 mm. The SCR for each CS trial was calculated by subtracting the mean skin-conductance level 2 seconds before CS onset from the highest skin-conductance level recorded during the following CS duration of 6 seconds. SCR responses during the interval after the US, the omitted (non-delivered) US or the CS- offset were calculated by subtracting the mean skin-conductance level recorded during the first 2 seconds of this interval from the highest skin-conductance level during the ensuing 3 seconds. Because autonomic responses are delayed with respect to their antecedent neural activity [22], this 2-second baseline was more or

Table 1 Demographics, comorbidities and type of trauma exposure in the cohort[a] (significant *P* values in bold).

	PTSD[b]	TENC[c]	*P*
Demographics			
Gender, M/F	9/10 (n = 19)	11/13 (n = 24)	0.5[d]
Age, ± SD	36 ± 12 (n = 19)	30 ± 12 (n = 24)	0.16
Years of education	15 ± 2 (n = 19)	17 ± 6 (n = 19)	0.1
Personality[e]			
NEO neuroticism	27 ± 8 (n = 16)	17 ± 9 (n = 22)	**0.001**
NEO extraversion	22 ± 8 (n = 16)	30 ± 6 (n = 22)	**<0.001**
NEO openness	28 ± 6 (n = 16)	32 ± 5 (n = 22)	**0.04**
NEO agreeableness	29 ± 6 (n = 16)	31 ± 6 (n = 22)	0.3
NEO conscientiousness	33 ± 7 (n = 16)	34 ± 7 (n = 22)	0.66
Clinical measures			
CAPS[f] score	67 ± 24 (n = 19)	8 ± 9 (n = 24)	**< 0.001**
BDI[g]score	21 ± 12 (n = 19)	2 ± 3 (n = 24)	**< 0.001**
BAI[h] score	19 ± 13 (n = 17)	5 ± 8 (n = 22)	**< 0.001**
Spielberger Trait anxiety	54 ± 12 (n = 18)	35 ± 9 (n = 21)	**< 0.001**
Spielberger State anxiety	44 ± 12 (n = 18)	34 ± 12 (n = 22)	**< 0.001**
Age at trauma, years	24 ± 15 (n = 19)	19 ± 12 (n = 19)	0.23
Time since trauma, years	11 ± 15 (n = 19)	12 ± 12 (n = 19)	0.95
Subjects with childhood[i] trauma n	9	5	0.10*[d]
Type of trauma exposure, n			
Motor vehicle accidents	3	4	1.0[d]
Sexual assaults	8	3	**0.04[d]**
Physical assaults	5	7	1.0[d]
Childhood abuse	6	3	0.15[d]
Combat	3	0	0.07[d]
Witness to trauma	3	7	0.47[d]
Current comorbidities, n			
Major depression	5	0	**0.01[d]**
Panic disorder	3	0	0.07[d]
Alcohol abuse	1	0	0.44[d]
Other substance abuse	2	0	0.19[d]
Eating disorders	2	0	0.19[d]

[a]Not all ratings were available for all participants; numbers are given in brackets. Participants might also have had more than one type of traumatic event or comorbid disorder.
[b]Post-traumatic stress disorder.
[c]Trauma-exposed normal control.
[d]Fisher's exact probability test. All other data were analyzed with Student's *t*-test, two-tailed.
[e]As measured by the Neuroticism-Extroversion-Openness (NEO) Inventory
[f]CAPS, Clinician-Administered PTSD Scale.
[g]BDI, Beck Depression Inventory.
[h]BAI Beck Anxiety Index.
[i]Before the age of 16 years.

less uncontaminated by the response to the shock. A representative example of SCR is provided (see Additional file 1 Figure S2).

Image Acquisition

MRI data were collected using a 3.0 Tesla whole-body MRI system (Trio; Siemens Medical Systems, Iselin, NJ, USA) equipped for echo planar imaging with a 12-channel head coil. Subjects were instructed to lie as still as possible, and head movement was restricted with foam cushions. After an automated scout image was obtained and automated shimming procedures performed, a high-resolution, T1-weighted, three-dimensional, magnetization-prepared rapid acquisition gradient echo (MPRAGE) volume was collected to facilitate spatial normalization and positioning of the subsequent scans. Functional MRI images, sensitive to blood oxygenation level-dependent (BOLD) contrast, were acquired with an interleaved gradient echo T2*-weighted sequence (TR = 3000 ms, TE = 30, flip angle = 90°), collected in 45 coronal oblique slices tilted 30° down from the anterior-posterior commissural line. The voxel size was 3 ± 3 ± 3 mm.

fMRI data analysis

Preprocessing

SPM8 (Wellcome Trust Center for Neuroimaging, http://www.fil.ion.ucl.ac.uk) was used to process all MRI data. Structural images were segmented and spatially normalized to the Montreal Neurological Institute (MNI) 305 T1 template. Functional images were realigned, corrected for slice timing, coregistered with the structural volume, resampled to 2 ± 2 ± 2 mm, normalized into MNI space using parameters obtained from the structural normalization process, and finally smoothed with an 8 mm full width half-maximum Gaussian kernel to reduce spatial noise and to compensate for residual misregistration in the spatial normalization process. High-pass temporal filtering with a cutoff of 128 seconds was included in the first-level statistical model to remove the effects of low-frequency physiological noise. Serial correlations in the fMRI time series caused by aliased biorhythms were estimated using an autoregressive AR(1) model.

First-level model

After preprocessing, each subject's functional time series was modeled using a general linear model, with six regressors signifying the condition onsets and durations: the context, onsets of the CS+ and the CS-, the US, the omitted US, and the CS- offset. Movement parameters derived from the realignment step for *x*, *y*, *z* and roll, pitch, and yaw were included in the model to reduce the effects of residual motion-related noise. The experimental effects of interest were identified using a statistical model containing boxcar functions representing each of the six experimental conditions, convolved with the SPM8 canonical hemodynamic response function.

We focused our analysis on the responses to three of the experimental events: 1) the CS+, 2) the US and 3) the omitted US. The CS- cue and the interval following its offset were used as control contrasts. This design allowed us to investigate not only fear-conditioned responses but to also directly contrast brain responses induced by the actual delivery of the US with brain responses induced by the immediate expectancy and then the unexpected omission of the US. Because both the US and omitted US intervals occurred immediately after the offset of the CS+, a combination of anticipatory- and prediction-error components influencing the shock response could be identified in the omitted US contrast, as limited by the temporal resolution of the present fMRI paradigm. Multi-collinearity between regressors may lead to instability of parameter estimation and a consequent reduction in sensitivity. In the present design, the inherent multiple collinearity of the classic conditioning design (a cue followed by a shock) was not problematic for these three contrasts, as the correlations between the regressors were very low ($r^2 < 0.01$). However, because of multiple collinearity between regressors identifying cue-induced activations and activity immediately after the termination of the cue ($r^2 = 0.36$), we did not examine this effect.

Second-level model

First-level contrast images representing the effects of CS +, CS-, US, omitted US and CS- offset were obtained for each subject, and modeled at the second level using a mixed-effects linear model with subject, group and task factors. At the second level, voxel-wise contrasts compared the PTSD group with the TENC group for CS+ versus implicit baseline, CS+ versus CS-, US versus implicit baseline, omitted US versus implicit baseline, and US versus omitted US.

Recent studies of pain responses in PTSD have reported alterations in activity in the putamen, amygdala, hippocampus, cingulate, insula and caudate nucleus [11,12,23]. Based on these studies, we also performed restricted voxel-wise analyses within these regions defined from the Anatomical Automatic Labeling (AAL) library [24,25]. Whole-brain and *a priori* regional activations of more than 10 contiguous voxels, adjusted for multiple comparisons within the search volume thresholded at $P < 0.05$ family-wise error (FEW), corrected for multiple comparisons, are reported.

Symptom correlations

First-level contrast images representing the effects of CS + and US were obtained for all subjects with PTSD, and modeled at the second level using a linear regression model with CAPS scores. Correlated clusters of more than 10 contiguous voxels adjusted for multiple comparisons at $P < 0.05$ FWE are reported. Correlation models such as these have been criticized for overinflated correlation coefficients [26], so we therefore did not plot correlations or report *r* values.

Post hoc functional connectivity analysis

To further understand alterations in US responses in PTSD, we performed a psychophysiological interaction (PPI) analysis, a technique allowing estimation of how inter-regional BOLD signal correlations vary with respect to an experimental psychological context. Based on the univariate results, we investigated whether the delivery of the US (versus omitted US) modulated the inter-regional functional connectivity between seed regions and targets elsewhere in the brain differently in PTSD and TENC subjects. Four seed regions (the left and right putamen, the left middle frontal gyrus, and the left parahippocampal gyrus) were chosen based on the peak observed hyperactivation to the US of these regions in the PTSD group. We contrasted inter-regional influences of the seeds during the US interval with those during the omitted US interval to elucidate how the delivery of the US modulated seed functional connectivity to other brain regions. The corresponding PPI design matrix had three columns: the interaction between the experimental manipulation and seed time series, the main effect of experimental manipulation (US or omitted US), and the physiological effect (hemodynamically deconvolved seed region time series). In accordance with the task-related univariate analysis, we also included six estimated movement parameters to account for any residual effects due to inter-scan head motion. The voxel-wise regression of voxel time series from the entire brain on the three predictor variables resulted in a first-level PPI contrast for each seed region in every subject. Subsequently, these PPI contrast images were modeled in a second-level group analysis using a mixed-effects repeated-measures linear model with subjects, diagnosis and seed region as factors. This second-level analysis resulted in a statistical parametrical map of regions that displayed differences between TENC and PTSD subjects in alterations of seed functional connectivity depending on the presence or absence of the US. Clusters of more than 10 contiguous voxels adjusted for multiple comparisons at $P < 0.05$ FWE are reported.

Results

Shock levels and skin-conductance responses

PTSD and TENC subjects chose similar shock levels and displayed similar levels of autonomic skin-conductance responses to the CS+ and the US. Subjects with PTSD displayed slightly higher skin-conductance responses to the non-reinforced CS- cue, but the magnitude of responses to the CS- was generally low (Table 2; see Additional file 1 Figure S3. Figure S4). There were no significant differences between PTSD and TENC subjects in brain activations to the CS+, the CS- or to the contrast CS+ versus CS-.

Table 2 Shock levels and skin-conductance responses (in square root microSiemens, $\mu S^{1/2}$) to the conditioned stimulus, the unconditioned stimulus (US) and the omitted US ± standard error (significant *P* values in bold).

	PTSD[a]	TENC[b]	*P*
Shock level, mA	2.13 ± 0.16	2.20 ± 0.18	0.77
CS[c]+ response, $\mu S^{1/2}$	0.27 ± 0.08	0.17 ± 0.04	0.24
CS- response, $\mu S^{1/2}$	0.08 ± 0.04	-0.01 ± 0.04	**0.04**
Unconditioned response, $\mu S^{1/2}$	0.79 ± 0.11	0.71 ± 0.07	0.56
Omitted US response, $\mu S^{1/2}$	0.26 ± 0.05	0.21 ± 0.03	0.36

[a]Post-traumatic stress disorder.
[b]Trauma-exposed normal control.
[c]CS, conditional stimulus (positive or negative).

Brain responses to the unconditioned stimuli

For all subjects, the delivery of the US-elicited responses in the primary and secondary somatosensory cortices, insula, cingulate gyrus, thalamus and brainstem (Figure 1). In the whole-brain between-group contrast, people with PTSD exhibited higher BOLD reactivity to the US in the bilateral putamen, left middle frontal gyrus and left parahippocampal gyrus. Within the *a priori* regions of interest (ROI), subjects with PTSD displayed additional significant hyper-reactivity in the bilateral amygdala, left hippocampus, right dorsal ACC, bilateral posterior insula, left anterior insula, and bilateral caudate and putamen. No regions displayed lower reactivity in the PTSD group (Table 3; Figure 2).

Brain responses to the omitted US

During those trials in which the shock was unexpectedly omitted, at a time point when immediate anticipation, prediction error and relief from not getting shocked are intermingled in the hemodynamic response measurable in the current fMRI experiment, subjects with PTSD displayed significantly greater activity in hippocampus. This difference was driven by a lack of deactivation of the hippocampus to the omitted US in the PTSD group. No other significant between-group differences were noted in this analysis (Table 3).

Brain responses to US versus the omitted US

To partially separate sensory components of the US from anticipatory, prediction error and relief components, we contrasted US versus omitted US in PTSD versus TENC subjects (two-way ANOVA). Within the *a priori* ROI, this contrast showed significantly greater reactivity of the putamen and the anterior insula in the PTSD group (Table 3).

Symptom correlations

We found a significant correlation between PTSD symptoms (CAPS scores) and US-induced BOLD activation in the right inferior frontal gyrus/anterior insula (MNI_{xyz} = 28, 34, 0, cluster size = 329 voxels, $Z = 7.93$, $P_{FWE\ corrected} = 0.002$) (Figure 3).

Functional connectivity of hyperactivated regions

To further elucidate the findings from the univariate analysis, we performed *post hoc* functional connectivity analyses on the regions displaying higher BOLD response to the US in PTSD versus TENC subjects. We chose the US and the omitted US as the conditions possibly inducing altered functional connectivity. In other words, we investigated how the functional connectivity of the seed regions was different during the delivery of the US compared with the omitted delivery of the US.

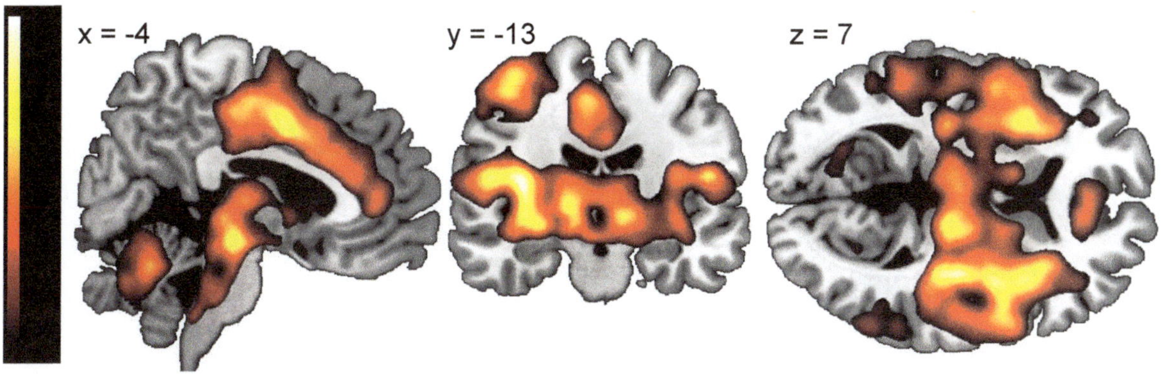

Figure 1 Main effect of unconditioned responses. Unconditioned stimulus (US) versus negative conditioned stimulus (CS)- offset in subjects with post-traumatic stress disorder (PTSD) and trauma-exposed non-PTSD control (TENC) subjects. Although the US was 'highly annoying' rather than painful, it elicited massive neuronal responses in classic pain regions including the brainstem, the thalamus, the contralateral sensory cortices, the insula and the middle cingulate. Activations are displayed at a threshold of T > 4 on a template magnetic resonance imaging (MRI) scan.

Individual seeds of the putamen, middle frontal gyrus and parahippocampal gyrus were extracted and used in a psychophysiological interaction (PPI), that is, connectivity, analysis.

Left putamen

The left putamen displayed the most prominent hyperactivation in the PTSD group, consistent with previous studies using painful levels of heat [11,12], but its role in PTSD is less well described. We thus chose the putamen region *post hoc* to perform a functional connectivity analysis. The seed consisted of a 6 mm sphere centrered at the peak location (MNI_{xyz} = -22, 0, -6). When comparing PPI effects of the left putamen between PTSD and TENC subjects, there were significant differences in functional connectivity shifts. The TENC group showed a a more positive PPI effect between the left putamen and the left temporal lobe including the amygdala. In other words, the shock delivery led to a larger increase in functional connectivity between the putamen and the amygdala in the TENC group as compared to connectivity shifts in the PTSD group (Table 4; Figure 4a).

Right putamen

The right putamen seed (a 6 mm sphere) was centred at the peak location (MNI_{xyz} = 18, 10, -12). Contrasting PPI effects of the right putamen between PTSD and TENC subjects showed differences in functional connectivity shifts similar to the left putamen seed, with a more positive PPI effect in the TENC group between the right putamen and the left temporal lobe including the amygdala, that is, indicating a larger increase in functional connectivity between these two regions at the shock delivery in the TENC group compared with the PTSD group (Table 4).

Left middle frontal gyrus

The left middle frontal gyrus seed (a 6 mm sphere) was centred at the peak location (MNI_{xyz} = -22, -4, 48). Contrasting PPI effects of the left middle frontal gyrus between PTSD and TENC subjects showed no significant differences in PPI effects.

Left parahippocampal gyrus

The left parahippocampal gyrus seed (a 6 mm sphere) was centred at the peak location (MNI_{xyz} = -18, -38, -4). Contrasting PPI effects of the left parahippocampal gyrus between PTSD and TENC subjects showed differences in functional connectivity shifts, with a more positive PPI effect in the TENC group between the left parahippocampal gyrus and right inferior parietal lobule, and the left medial frontal gyrus and the right precentral gyrus, that is, indicating a larger increase in functional connectivity between the seed and these three regions at the delivery of the shock in the TENC group compared with the PTSD group (Table 4 and Figure 4b).

Discussion

The predictable and 'annoying' shock (the unconditioned stimuli (US)) elicited activation in several brain regions associated with pain processing [6], suggesting that stimuli may not need to be perceived as overtly painful to activate the so called 'pain matrix'. Subjects with PTSD had significantly higher BOLD reactivity in the putamen, middle frontal gyrus and parahippocampal gyrus compared with the TENC subjects. The ROI analysis further revealed the amygdala, hippocampus, dorsal ACC, insula and caudate nucleus to be hyperactive in the PTSD US response. These findings are consistent with previous studies indicating higher putamen and insula reactivity to heat pain in PTSD [11,12], and

Table 3 Univariate analysis results

Contrast / ROI[a]	MNI[b], peak *x, y, z*	*Z*-score	Size, voxels	Cluster *P* value, FWE[c]	Region
US[d]					
PTSD[e] > TENC[f]					
Whole brain	**-22, 0, -6**	**5.51**	**111**	**< 0.0001**	**Left putamen**
	(-24, 10, -14)	-5.47			
	(-32, 2, -4)	-4.93			
	18, 10 -12	**5.47**	**90**	**< 0.0001**	**Right putamen**
	(20, 10, -4)	-5.13			
	-22, -4, 48	**5.25**	**19**	**0.003**	**Left middle frontal gyrus**
	-18, -38, -4	**5.07**	**11**	**0.007**	**Left parahippocampal gyrus**
Putamen	**16, 12, -10**	**5.34**	**359**	**< 0.0001**	**Right ventral putamen**
	(30, -20, 6)	-3.79			
	(28, -2, -6)	-3.73			
	-26, 2, -4	**5.11**	**840**	**< 0.0001**	**Left putamen**
	(-22, 8, -10)	-4.88			
	(-32, -12, -6)	-4.75			
Amygdala	**-22, 6, -16**	**4.3**	**48**	**0.01**	**Left amygdala**
	24, 2, -16	**4.27**	**81**	**0.005**	**Right amygdala**
Hippocampus	**-18, -32, 4**	**4.43**	**36**	**0.029**	**Left hippocampus**
	(-22, -24, -8)	-3.74			
	-26, -34, 8	**3.79**	**18**	**0.028**	**Left hippocampus**
	(-14, -32, 10)	-3.52			
	-26, -12, -12	**3.69**	**25**	**0.042**	**Left hippocampus**
	(-20, -4, 12)	-3.62			
Cingulate	**8, 12, 42**	**3.8**	**19**	**0.013**	**Right dorsal acc**
Insula	**34, -20, 4**	**4.97**	**36**	**0.006**	**Right posterior insula**
	-26, 14, -16	**5.05**	**28**	**0.008**	**Left piriform insula**
	-34, -6, 16	**4.14**	**13**	**0.017**	**Left middle insula**
	-36, -22, 4	**4.08**	**17**	**0.014**	**Left posterior insula**
Caudate	**-14, 16, -8**	**4.2**	**67**	**0.006**	**Right caudate**
	(16, 18, 0)	-3.81			
	16, 0, 16	**3.86**	**24**	**0.021**	**Right caudate**
	-12, 10, 14	**4.41**	**297**	**0.001**	**Left caudate body**
	(-18, -2, 22)	-4.16			
TENC > PTSD	No significant differences in whole brain or ROI				
Omitted US					
PTSD > TENC					
Whole brain	No significant differences in whole brain				
Hippocampus	**22, -10, -20**	**3.77**	**54**	**0.009**	**Right anterior hippocampus**
	(30, -10, -18)	-3.46			
TENC > PTSD	No significant differences in whole brain or ROI				
US minus omitted US					
PTSD > TENC					
Whole brain	No significant differences in whole brain				
Putamen	**20, 12, -10**	**3.89**	**69**	**0.003**	**Right ventral putamen**
	20, 0, 12	**3.48**	**13**	**0.032**	
Insula	**-28, 16, -18**	**4.05**	**52**	**0.016**	**Left orbital insula**

Clusters are in bold, with sub-peaks in brackets.

[a]Region of interest

[b]Montreal Neurological Institute.

[c]Family-wise error.

[d]US, unconditioned stimulus

[e]Post-traumatic stress disorder.

[f]Trauma-exposed normal control.

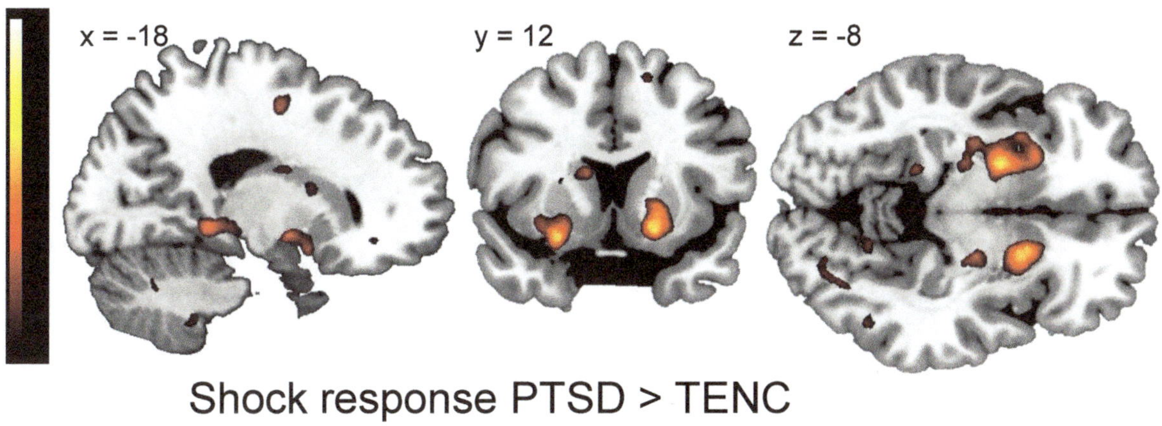

Figure 2 Increased putamen unconditioned stimulus (US) responses in subjects with post-traumatic stress disorder (PTSD). US responses in PTSD minus trauma-exposed non-PTSD control (TENC) displayed at T > 4 on a template magnetic resonance imaging (MRI) scan. The bilateral putamen displayed the most prominent hyperactivation in PTSD, no region displayed hypoactivation in PTSD.

increased caudate signaling to heat pain after traumatic memory induction [23]. Subjects with PTSD displayed hyperactivation of the amygdala and dorsal ACC to the US, findings that are consistent with several previous studies suggesting amygdala and cingulate involvement in processing aversive stimuli [5,27-29] and hyperactivation in PTSD [30]. Thus, a highly annoying but not overtly painful electrical shock can be used to replicate previous studies indicating alterations in PTSD pain processing. The benefits of using experimental stimuli that are not overtly painful are obvious.

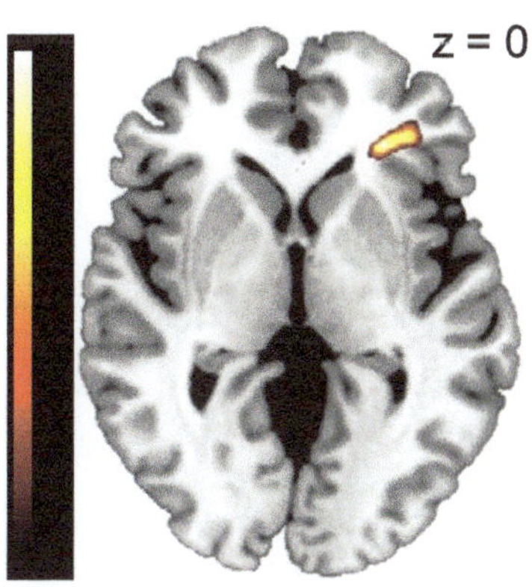

Figure 3 Post-traumatic stress disorder (PTSD) symptom severity correlates with the magnitude of unconditioned stimulus (US) reactivity. Positive correlations between blood oxygenation level-dependent (BOLD) US signal in the right anterior insula/inferior frontal gyrus and Clinician-Administered PTSD Scale (CAPS) score in the 19 subjects with PTSD investigated. The correlation map is displayed at a threshold of T > 4 on a template magnetic resonance imaging (MRI) scan.

The CS+ led to comparable increases in skin conductance in both the PTSD and the TENC group, suggesting no differences in the fear induced by the conditioned cues. Moreover, there were no differences in the neural response to the CS+, replicating behavioral studies that suggested intact fear learning in PTSD [31-35], but other studies have disagreed [36-38]. Autonomic responses to the US were of comparable magnitude in PTSD and TENC subjects, as has been previously reported [34,36].

Subjects with PTSD displayed increased putamen reactivity to the US, an effect that was not observed after the omitted US. Moreover, the putamen hyperactivation to the US in the PTSD group remained significant when controlling for responses to the omitted US, (PTSD (US vs. omitted US) vs. TENC (US vs. omitted US); Table 3). We therefore interpret the putamen reactivity as driven mostly by sensation rather than alterations in anticipation of the aversive stimulus or a signal of error prediction. It has been shown that learning of the CS-US relationship allows healthy people to engage in endogenous pain inhibition [39-41]. When endogenous opioid neurotransmission is blocked with naloxone in healthy subjects, a moderately painful US leads to increased putamen and insular responses [42], similar to the present findings. There is evidence that people with PTSD have an altered opioidergic system [43-45], and the findings in the present study seem to support this.

With regard to the functional connectivity results, two major effects were seen when comparing connectivity at the omitted US and the delivered US: TENC subjects (compared with subjects with PTSD), displayed a larger increase in putamen to temporal lobe/amygdala connectivity at the delivered US compared with the omitted

Table 4 Psychophysiological interaction analysis

Seed	MNI[a], peak x, y, z	Z-score	Size, voxels	Cluster P value, FWE[b]	Region[c]
Left putamen					
TENC[d] > PTSD[e]	**-44, -12, -16**	**4.65**	**295**	**0.01**	**Left temporal lobe**
	(-32, 0, -30)	4.01			Left parahippocampal lobe/amygdala
	(-30, -10, -22)	3.72			Left parahippocampal gyrus
PTSD > TENC	No significant differences				
Right putamen					
TENC > PTSD	**-30, 0, -32**	**4.54**	**248**	**0.019**	**Left temporal lobe wm/amygdala**
	(-48, 8, -30)	3.97			Left middle temporal gyrus
	(-56, 4, -26)	3.44			Left middle temporal gyrus
PTSD > TENC	No significant differences				
Left middle frontal gyrus					
TENC > PTSD	No significant differences				
PTSD > TENC	No significant differences				
Left parahippocampal gyrus					
TENC > PTSD	**44, -34, 42**	**4.45**	**449**	**0.001**	**Right inferior parietal lobule**
	48, -38, 50	-4.27			Right inferior parietal lobule
	52, -26, 50	-3.77			Right postcentral gyrus
	-10, 66, 10	**4.42**	**263**	**0.017**	**Left medial frontal gyrus**
	(-14, 62, 0)	-4.06			Left medial frontal gyrus
	(-8, 62, 18)	-3.45			Left medial frontal gyrus
	34, -20, 68	**4.37**	**487**	**0.001**	**Right precentral gyrus**
	(34, -16, 46)	-4.14			Right precentral gyrus
	(22, -16, 74)	-4.12			Right precentral gyrus
PTSD > TENC	No significant differences				

[a]Montreal Neurological Institute.
[b]Family-wise error.
[c]Regions were identified based on nearest gray matter.
[d]Post-traumatic stress disorder.
[e]Trauma-exposed normal control.

US. Moreover, TENC subjects (compared with subjects with PTSD) displayed an increase in parahippocampal gyrus connectivity to the inferior parietal lobule, the precentral gyrus and the medial frontal gyrus (Figure 4a, b). We speculate that the PPI results may be indicative of an altered network processing of aversive stimuli PTSD, but further studies are needed to elucidate how the observed network connectivity changes might relate to the emotional and functional response to aversive stimuli in PTSD.

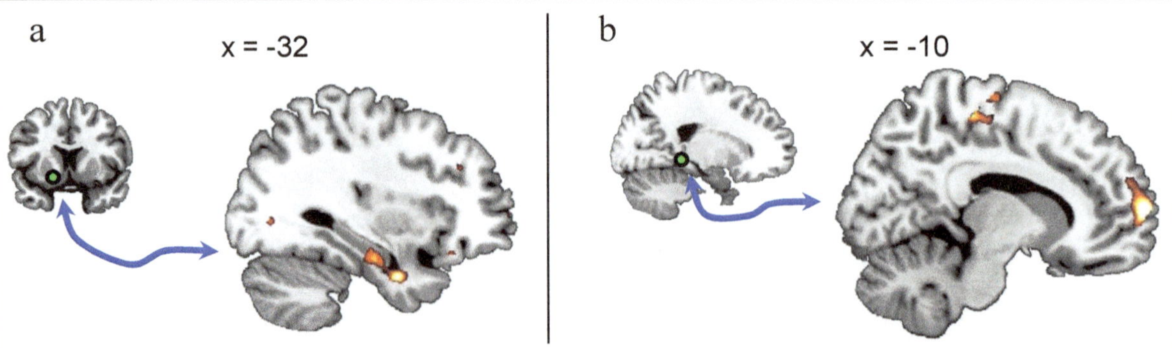

Figure 4 Psychophysiological interaction (PPI) analysis. The PPI analysis contrasted the unconditioned stimulus (US) versus omitted US, modeling the change in regional coupling between the seed induced by the delivery of the US. The green sphere indicates the location of **(A)** the putamen seed and **(B)** the parahippocampal seed. Group differences (trauma-exposed non-PTSD control (TENC) > PTSD) in psychophysiological interaction effects are displayed at a threshold of T > 3 on a template magnetic resonance imaging (MRI) scan.

Higher right anterior insula US reactivity was correlated with higher PTSD symptom severity on the CAPS. This result is consistent with findings of Mickleborough and colleagues [23], who reported a positive correlation between CAPS scores and insula signaling during heat pain after traumatic memory activation. Dickie and colleagues [46] reported a positive CAPS-insula correlation with remembered fearful faces. Felmingham and colleagues [47] reported a positive correlation between CAPS and insula activation to masked fear faces. Thus, this relationship seems to be consistent whether the stimuli are perceived as painful, highly annoying but not painful, encoded as aversive, or subliminally aversive. However, Strigo and colleagues [12] found the rostral anterior insula reactivity to painful stimulation to be negatively correlated to CAPS avoidance scores. One possible explanation for this discrepancy is that in the Strigo experiment, pain stimulation was delivered without a predictive cue, whereas the study of Mickleborough and the present study entailed a predictive cue.

The putamen is best known as a motor output region [48], but both nociception [49,50] and emotion [51] are processed in the putamen and the adjacent nucleus accumbens [52,53]. Moreover, the putamen is structurally and functionally connected to the medial orbitofrontal cortex and the amygdala [54], two regions implicated in PTSD. The observed increased putamen activation in PTSD corresponds to regions known to receive projections from the dorsal anterior cingulate and orbital cortex [55]. Altered basal ganglia function has previously been reported in PTSD for other paradigms: putamen blood flow and reactivity after script-driven imagery in PTSD has been correlated to aspects of flashback intensity and dissociative states [23,56], caudate and putamen volume are decreased in people with PTSD with headaches [57], and people with PTSD display diminished caudate and putamen signal to reward [58]. Thus, future studies could be aimed at elucidating PTSD alterations in both approach and avoidance behaviors involving corticostriatal circuitry [55,59].

Limitations and alternate interpretations

We have interpreted the neuronal responses and connectivity modulations related to the omitted US as reflecting immediate expectancy ('I am going to get shocked right now'). It could be argued, however, that these results also represent a prediction error and relief signal ('Oh, I guess I did not get shocked'). Our experimental design did not allow us to distinguish between these two responses, thus further studies with higher temporal resolution should be designed and conducted to further examine this point.

Conclusions

Previous studies have implicated the putamen and insula in altered pain processing in PTSD. The present study extends to this literature by showing that the functional activation of these brain regions is also altered in response to highly annoying but not overtly painful stimuli, and that such alterations are likely to be driven by sensory aspects of the aversive stimulus rather than by expectancy- and prediction-error components.

Additional material

Additional file 1: Figure S1 Paradigm design and timing. Figure S2 Skin conductance responses within three different trials in one representative subject. Figure S3 Skin conductance responses to the conditioned stimulus. Figure S4 Skin conductance responses to the unconditioned stimulus. Figure S5 Skin conductance responses to the omitted unconditioned stimulus.

List of abbreviations

ACC: anterior cingulate cortex; BAI: Beck Anxiety Inventory; BDI: Beck Depression Inventory; CAPS: Clinician-Given PTSD Scale; CS conditioned stimulus; fMRI functional magnetic resonance imaging; FWE: family-wise error corrected for multiple comparisons; PPI: psychophysiological interaction; PTSD: post-traumatic stress disorder; SCR: skin-conductance response; STAI: Spielberger State Trait Anxiety Inventory; TENC: trauma-exposed non-PTSD controls; US: unconditioned stimulus.

Acknowledgements

This work was supported by the National Institutes of Health grant to MRM (Grant # 1R01MH081975). CL received support from the Swedish Society for Medical Research (SSMF).

Author details

[1]Department of Psychiatry, Harvard Medical School & Massachusetts General Hospital, 149 13th street, Charlestown, MA, USA. [2]Neural Systems Group, Massachusetts General Hospital, 149 13th street, Charlestown, MA, USA.

Authors' contributions

CL collected and analyzed the data, and wrote the manuscript. TAZ contributed to data analysis and to the final version of the manuscript. RKP participated in experimental design and the final version of the manuscript. MRM designed the study, collected data and contributed to the final version of the manuscript. All authors read and approved the final manuscript.

Competing interests

The authors declare that they have no competing interests.

References

1. Sehlmeyer C, Schoning S, Zwitserlood P, Pfleiderer B, Kircher T, Arolt V, Konrad C: **Human fear conditioning and extinction in neuroimaging: a systematic review.** *PloS one* 2009, **4(6)**:e5865.
2. Domjan M: **Pavlovian conditioning: a functional perspective.** *Annual review of psychology* 2005, **56**:179-206.
3. Knight DC, Waters NS, King MK, Bandettini PA: **Learning-related diminution of unconditioned SCR and fMRI signal responses.** *Neuroimage* 2010, **49(1)**:843-848.
4. Dunsmoor JE, Bandettini PA, Knight DC: **Impact of continuous versus intermittent CS-UCS pairing on human brain activation during Pavlovian fear conditioning.** *Behavioral neuroscience* 2007, **121(4)**:635-642.

5. Dunsmoor JE, Bandettini PA, Knight DC: **Neural correlates of unconditioned response diminution during Pavlovian conditioning.** *Neuroimage* 2008, **40(2)**:811-817.
6. Apkarian AV, Bushnell MC, Treede RD, Zubieta JK: **Human brain mechanisms of pain perception and regulation in health and disease.** *Eur J Pain* 2005, **9(4)**:463-484.
7. Liberzon I, King AP, Britton JC, Phan KL, Abelson JL, Taylor SF: **Paralimbic and medial prefrontal cortical involvement in neuroendocrine responses to traumatic stimuli.** *Am J Psychiatry* 2007, **164(8)**:1250-1258.
8. Asmundson GJ, Katz J: **Understanding the co-occurrence of anxiety disorders and chronic pain: state-of-the-art.** *Depression and anxiety* 2009, **26(10)**:888-901.
9. Beckham JC, Crawford AL, Feldman ME, Kirby AC, Hertzberg MA, Davidson JR, Moore SD: **Chronic posttraumatic stress disorder and chronic pain in Vietnam combat veterans.** *Journal of psychosomatic research* 1997, **43(4)**:379-389.
10. Otis JD, Keane TM, Kerns RD: **An examination of the relationship between chronic pain and post-traumatic stress disorder.** *Journal of rehabilitation research and development* 2003, **40(5)**:397-405.
11. Geuze E, Westenberg HG, Jochims A, de Kloet CS, Bohus M, Vermetten E, Schmahl C: **Altered pain processing in veterans with posttraumatic stress disorder.** *Archives of general psychiatry* 2007, **64(1)**:76-85.
12. Strigo IA, Simmons AN, Matthews SC, Grimes EM, Allard CB, Reinhardt LE, Paulus MP, Stein MB: **Neural correlates of altered pain response in women with posttraumatic stress disorder from intimate partner violence.** *Biol Psychiatry* 2010, **68(5)**:442-450.
13. Milad MR, Wright CI, Orr SP, Pitman RK, Quirk GJ, Rauch SL: **Recall of fear extinction in humans activates the ventromedial prefrontal cortex and hippocampus in concert.** *Biol Psychiatry* 2007, **62(5)**:446-454.
14. First M, Spitzer RL, Gibbon M, Williams JBW: **Structured Clinical Interview for DSM-Iv Axis I Disorders - Patient Edition (SCID-I/P, Version 2.0).** New York: Biometrics Reserach Depatment New York State Psychiatric Institute; 1995.
15. Milad MR, Pitman RK, Ellis CB, Gold AL, Shin LM, Lasko NB, Zeidan MA, Handwerger K, Orr SP, Rauch SL: **Neurobiological basis of failure to recall extinction memory in posttraumatic stress disorder.** *Biol Psychiatry* 2009, **66(12)**:1075-1082.
16. Rougemont-Bucking A, Linnman C, Zeffiro TA, Zeidan MA, Lebron-Milad K, Rodriguez-Romaguera J, Rauch SL, Pitman RK, Milad MR: **Altered processing of contextual information during fear extinction in PTSD: an fMRI study.** *CNS neuroscience & therapeutics* 2010.
17. Blake DD, Weathers FW, Nagy LM, Kaloupek DG, Gusman FD, Charney DS, Keane TM: **The development of a clinician-administered PTSD Scale.** *Journal of traumatic stress* 1995, **8(1)**:75-90.
18. Costa P, McCrae R: **Revised NEO Personality Inventory (NEO-PI-R) and NEO Five-Factor Inventory (NEO-FFI) professional manual.** Odessa, FL: Psychological Assessment Resources; 1992.
19. Spielberger C, Gorsuch R, Lushene R: **Manual for the State-Trait Anxiety Inventory.** Palo Alto, CA: Consulting Psychologists Press; 1970.
20. Beck AT, Epstein N, Brown G, Steer RA: **An inventory for measuring clinical anxiety: psychometric properties.** *Journal of consulting and clinical psychology* 1988, **56(6)**:893-897.
21. Beck AT, Ward CH, Mendelson M, Mock J, Erbaugh J: **An inventory for measuring depression.** *Archives of general psychiatry* 1961, **4**:561-571.
22. Boucsein W: **Electrodermal activity.** New York: Plenum Press; 1992.
23. Mickleborough MJ, Daniels JK, Coupland NJ, Kao R, Williamson PC, Lanius UF, Hegadoren K, Schore A, Densmore M, Stevens T, *et al*: **Effects of trauma-related cues on pain processing in posttraumatic stress disorder: an fMRI investigation.** *J Psychiatry Neurosci* 2010.
24. Maldjian JA, Laurienti PJ, Kraft RA, Burdette JH: **An automated method for neuroanatomic and cytoarchitectonic atlas-based interrogation of fMRI data sets.** *Neuroimage* 2003, **19(3)**:1233-1239.
25. Tzourio-Mazoyer N, Landeau B, Papathanassiou D, Crivello F, Etard O, Delcroix N, Mazoyer B, Joliot M: **Automated anatomical labeling of activations in SPM using a macroscopic anatomical parcellation of the MNI MRI single-subject brain.** *Neuroimage* 2002, **15(1)**:273-289.
26. Vul E, Harris C, Winkielman P, Pashler H: **Puzzlingly high correlations in fMRI studies of emotion, personality, and social cognition.** *Perspectives on Psychological Science* 2009, **4(3)**:274-290.
27. Shackman AJ, Salomons TV, Slagter HA, Fox AS, Winter JJ, Davidson RJ: **The integration of negative affect, pain and cognitive control in the cingulate cortex.** *Nat Rev Neurosci* 2011, **12(3)**:154-167.
28. Milad MR, Quirk GJ, Pitman RK, Orr SP, Fischl B, Rauch SL: **A role for the human dorsal anterior cingulate cortex in fear expression.** *Biol Psychiatry* 2007, **62(10)**:1191-1194.
29. Linnman C, Rougemont-Bucking A, Beucke JC, Zeffiro TA, Milad MR: **Unconditioned responses and functional fear networks in human classical conditioning.** *Behavioural brain research* 2011.
30. Shin LM, Liberzon I: **The neurocircuitry of fear, stress, and anxiety disorders.** *Neuropsychopharmacology: official publication of the American College of Neuropsychopharmacology* 2010, **35(1)**:169-191.
31. Milad MR, Orr SP, Lasko NB, Chang Y, Rauch SL, Pitman RK: **Presence and acquired origin of reduced recall for fear extinction in PTSD: results of a twin study.** *Journal of psychiatric research* 2008, **42(7)**:515-520.
32. Peri T, Ben-Shakhar G, Orr SP, Shalev AY: **Psychophysiologic assessment of aversive conditioning in posttraumatic stress disorder.** *Biol Psychiatry* 2000, **47(6)**:512-519.
33. Grillon C, Morgan CA: **Fear-potentiated startle conditioning to explicit and contextual cues in Gulf War veterans with posttraumatic stress disorder.** *Journal of abnormal psychology* 1999, **108(1)**:134-142.
34. Orr SP, Milad MR, Metzger LJ, Lasko NB, Gilbertson MW, Pitman RK: **Effects of beta blockade, PTSD diagnosis, and explicit threat on the extinction and retention of an aversively conditioned response.** *Biological psychology* 2006, **73(3)**:262-271.
35. Vythilingam M, Lawley M, Collin C, Bonne O, Agarwal R, Hadd K, Charney DS, Grillon C: **Hydrocortisone impairs hippocampal-dependent trace eyeblink conditioning in post-traumatic stress disorder.** *Neuropsychopharmacology* 2006, **31(1)**:182-188.
36. Orr SP, Metzger LJ, Lasko NB, Macklin ML, Peri T, Pitman RK: **De novo conditioning in trauma-exposed individuals with and without posttraumatic stress disorder.** *Journal of abnormal psychology* 2000, **109(2)**:290-298.
37. Blechert J, Michael T, Vriends N, Margraf J, Wilhelm FH: **Fear conditioning in posttraumatic stress disorder: evidence for delayed extinction of autonomic, experiential, and behavioural responses.** *Behav Res Ther* 2007, **45(9)**:2019-2033.
38. Norrholm SD, Jovanovic T, Olin IW, Sands LA, Karapanou I, Bradley B, Ressler KJ: **Fear extinction in traumatized civilians with posttraumatic stress disorder: relation to symptom severity.** *Biol Psychiatry* 2010.
39. Johansen JP, Tarpley JW, LeDoux JE, Blair HT: **Neural substrates for expectation-modulated fear learning in the amygdala and periaqueductal gray.** *Nature neuroscience* 2010, **13(8)**:979-986.
40. Helmstetter FJ, Tershner SA: **Lesions of the periaqueductal gray and rostral ventromedial medulla disrupt antinociceptive but not cardiovascular aversive conditional responses.** *J Neurosci* 1994, **14(11 Pt 2)**:7099-7108.
41. Helmstetter FJ, Tershner SA, Poore LH, Bellgowan PS: **Antinociception following opioid stimulation of the basolateral amygdala is expressed through the periaqueductal gray and rostral ventromedial medulla.** *Brain research* 1998, **779(1-2)**:104-118.
42. Eippert F, Bingel U, Schoell E, Yacubian J, Buchel C: **Blockade of endogenous opioid neurotransmission enhances acquisition of conditioned fear in humans.** *J Neurosci* 2008, **28(21)**:5465-5472.
43. Baker DG, West SA, Orth DN, Hill KK, Nicholson WE, Ekhator NN, Bruce AB, Wortman MD, Keck PE Jr, Geracioti TD Jr: **Cerebrospinal fluid and plasma beta-endorphin in combat veterans with post-traumatic stress disorder.** *Psychoneuroendocrinology* 1997, **22(7)**:517-529.
44. Liberzon I, Taylor SF, Phan KL, Britton JC, Fig LM, Bueller JA, Koeppe RA, Zubieta JK: **Altered central micro-opioid receptor binding after psychological trauma.** *Biol Psychiatry* 2007, **61(9)**:1030-1038.
45. Pitman RK, van der Kolk BA, Orr SP, Greenberg MS: **Naloxone-reversible analgesic response to combat-related stimuli in posttraumatic stress disorder. A pilot study.** *Archives of general psychiatry* 1990, **47(6)**:541-544.
46. Dickie EW, Brunet A, Akerib V, Armony JL: **An fMRI investigation of memory encoding in PTSD: influence of symptom severity.** *Neuropsychologia* 2008, **46(5)**:1522-1531.
47. Felmingham K, Williams LM, Kemp AH, Liddell B, Falconer E, Peduto A, Bryant R: **Neural responses to masked fear faces: sex differences and**

trauma exposure in posttraumatic stress disorder. *Journal of abnormal psychology* 2010, **119(1)**:241-247.
48. Bhatia KP, Marsden CD: **The behavioural and motor consequences of focal lesions of the basal ganglia in man.** *Brain* 1994, **117(Pt 4)**:859-876.
49. Bingel U, Glascher J, Weiller C, Buchel C: **Somatotopic representation of nociceptive information in the putamen: an event-related fMRI study.** *Cereb Cortex* 2004, **14(12)**:1340-1345.
50. Borsook D, Upadhyay J, Chudler EH, Becerra L: **A key role of the basal ganglia in pain and analgesia–insights gained through human functional imaging.** *Molecular pain* 2010, **6**:27.
51. Haber SN: **The primate basal ganglia: parallel and integrative networks.** *Journal of chemical neuroanatomy* 2003, **26(4)**:317-330.
52. Borsook D, Becerra L, Carlezon WA Jr, Shaw M, Renshaw P, Elman I, Levine J: **Reward-aversion circuitry in analgesia and pain: implications for psychiatric disorders.** *European journal of pain* 2007, **11(1)**:7-20.
53. Becerra L, Breiter HC, Wise R, Gonzalez RG, Borsook D: **Reward circuitry activation by noxious thermal stimuli.** *Neuron* 2001, **32(5)**:927-946.
54. Cohen MX, Schoene-Bake JC, Elger CE, Weber B: **Connectivity-based segregation of the human striatum predicts personality characteristics.** *Nature neuroscience* 2009, **12(1)**:32-34.
55. Haber SN, Kim KS, Mailly P, Calzavara R: **Reward-related cortical inputs define a large striatal region in primates that interface with associative cortical connections, providing a substrate for incentive-based learning.** *J Neurosci* 2006, **26(32)**:8368-8376.
56. Osuch EA, Benson B, Geraci M, Podell D, Herscovitch P, McCann UD, Post RM: **Regional cerebral blood flow correlated with flashback intensity in patients with posttraumatic stress disorder.** *Biol Psychiatry* 2001, **50(4)**:246-253.
57. Filipovic BR, Djurovic B, Marinkovic S, Stijak L, Aksic M, Nikolic V, Starcevic A, Radonjic V: **Volume changes of corpus striatum, thalamus, hippocampus and lateral ventricles in posttraumatic stress disorder (PTSD) patients suffering from headaches and without therapy.** *Central European neurosurgery* 2010.
58. Elman I, Lowen S, Frederick BB, Chi W, Becerra L, Pitman RK: **Functional neuroimaging of reward circuitry responsivity to monetary gains and losses in posttraumatic stress disorder.** *Biol Psychiatry* 2009, **66(12)**:1083-1090.
59. Stein MB, Paulus MP: **Imbalance of approach and avoidance: the yin and yang of anxiety disorders.** *Biol Psychiatry* 2009, **66(12)**:1072-1074.

7

Emotion regulation in social anxiety disorder: behavioral and neural responses to three socio-emotional tasks

Michal Ziv*, Philippe R Goldin, Hooria Jazaieri, Kevin S Hahn and James J Gross

Abstract

Background: Social anxiety disorder (SAD) is thought to involve deficits in emotion regulation, and more specifically, deficits in cognitive reappraisal. However, evidence for such deficits is mixed.

Methods: Using functional magnetic resonance imaging (fMRI) of blood oxygen-level dependent (BOLD) signal, we examined reappraisal-related behavioral and neural responses in 27 participants with generalized SAD and 27 healthy controls (HC) during three socio-emotional tasks: (1) looming harsh faces (Faces); (2) videotaped actors delivering social criticism (Criticism); and (3) written autobiographical negative self-beliefs (Beliefs).

Results: Behaviorally, compared to HC, participants with SAD had lesser reappraisal-related reduction in negative emotion in the Beliefs task. Neurally, compared to HC, participants with SAD had lesser BOLD responses in reappraisal-related brain regions when reappraising faces, in visual and attention related regions when reappraising criticism, and in the left superior temporal gyrus when reappraising beliefs. Examination of the temporal dynamics of BOLD responses revealed late reappraisal-related increased responses in HC, compared to SAD. In addition, the dorsomedial prefrontal cortex (DMPFC), which showed reappraisal-related increased activity in both groups, had similar temporal dynamics in SAD and HC during the Faces and Criticism tasks, but greater late response increases in HC, compared to SAD, during the Beliefs task. Reappraisal-related greater late DMPFC responses were associated with greater percent reduction in negative emotion ratings in SAD patients.

Conclusions: These results suggest a dysfunction of cognitive reappraisal in SAD patients, with overall reduced late brain responses in prefrontal regions, particularly when reappraising faces. Decreased late activity in the DMPFC might be associated with deficient reappraisal and greater negative reactivity.

Trial registration: ClinicalTrials.gov identifier: NCT00380731

Keywords: Social anxiety, Emotion regulation, Reappraisal, fMRI, DMPFC, Temporal dynamics

Background

Social anxiety disorder (SAD) is characterized by heightened anxiety in a wide array of social situations [1]. It has been suggested that these elevated levels of anxiety may be due to ineffective emotion regulation [2]. Specifically, it has been suggested that patients with SAD use adaptive emotion regulation strategies, such as cognitive reappraisal, less frequently than non-anxious healthy adults [3]. In healthy individuals, cognitive reappraisal, which involves changing the meaning of a stimulus that gives rise to an emotion, can modify emotional reactions to anxiety-provoking situations, leading to greater psychological flexibility and emotional well being [4]. In SAD, deficits in cognitive reappraisal are thought to be related to difficulty in modifying the negative thoughts that arise before, during, and after social evaluative situations [5].

Neuroimaging findings

One source of evidence regarding reappraisal in SAD comes from neuroimaging studies. To date, three studies have investigated the neural correlates of cognitive reappraisal in SAD. In the first study, Goldin and

* Correspondence: ziv.michal@gmail.com
Department of Psychology, Stanford University, Jordan Hall, Bldg. 420, 94305-2130 Stanford, CA, USA

colleagues examined cognitive reappraisal of social (harsh facial expressions) and physical (violent scenes) threat in SAD patients and healthy controls. Regulation during social threat, but not physical threat, was associated with diminished recruitment of brain systems implicated in cognitive reappraisal (dorsomedial and dorsolateral prefrontal cortex (PFC)), and attention modulation (medial cuneus, posterior cingulate cortex, and parietal cortex) in SAD, compared to healthy controls [5].

In a second study by this group, using negative self-beliefs, the temporal dynamics of the BOLD response, in addition to its signal magnitude, were analyzed [3]. Findings revealed greater early activity in healthy controls during reappraisal of negative self-beliefs in brain networks implicated in reappraisal (dorsomedial, dorsolateral, and ventrolateral PFC), language (left inferior frontal gyrus), and visual (precuneus, inferior parietal) processing, while SAD patients had greater late responses in dorsomedial and ventrolateral PFC, insula, and visual processing regions. Taken together, these two studies suggest a failure to recruit reappraisal-related prefrontal regions in SAD. This differential activity of prefrontal regulatory regions in SAD has been observed in other neuroimaging studies [6-10].

The third study that explicitly addressed the neural correlates of emotion regulation in SAD, by Bruhl and colleagues [11], reported results that are discrepant with the two studies reported above. In this study, patients were instructed either to perform 'reality checking' or to simply anticipate and then look at negative, positive, and neutral pictures. Thus, in contrast to the first two studies, which compared patients to healthy controls, this study compared patients applying cognitive control with patients not using cognitive control. The authors found regulation-related reduced activity in emotion reactivity regions (amygdala, insula, thalamus), and in the dorsolateral PFC and cingulated cortex, with no regions with increased activity due to cognitive control.

Explaining mixed findings

One possible explanation for the mixed findings may be the different contexts that were examined. Each of these studies focused on only one emotional probe: faces, beliefs, or non-socially specific affective pictures. However, in the SAD literature, it has been shown that the choice of emotional probes and experimental paradigms has a much larger effect on the results of fMRI investigations than is typically thought [12].

In addition to using different stimuli, another source of variability in the imaging literature is the different data analytic approaches used in each study. The majority of studies in SAD so far have used BOLD signal magnitude analyses that usually collapse across time. Only a handful of studies examined the temporal dynamics of the BOLD responses [3,13-15]. Of these studies, only one [3] has specifically focused on emotion regulation processes. Analysis of BOLD signal temporal dynamics can reveal information that might be hidden when averaging across time. It can also reveal between-group differences in brain regions that have the same averaged response among two groups, such as a pattern of early brain responses in one group, or delayed responses in the other group. Indeed, the one study examining temporal dynamics of emotion regulation processes in SAD found delayed BOLD signal onset in the dorsomedial and ventrolateral PFC regions in patients, relatively to healthy controls [3].

The present study

The goal of the present study was to examine behavioral and fMRI BOLD responses in patients with SAD compared to healthy controls (HC) when reappraising socio-emotional stimuli. To test whether emotion dysregulation in SAD is related to a specific socio-emotional stimulus, or whether this is a more general core deficit, three contexts were compared: (1) looming harsh faces (Faces); (2) dynamic video clips of actors delivering social criticism (Criticism); and (3) written autobiographical social anxiety-related negative self-beliefs (Beliefs). To our knowledge, no study has directly tested reappraisal-related BOLD responses in patients with SAD across several distinct socio-emotional tasks that vary in both content and form.

Behaviorally, we hypothesized that, compared to HC, patients with SAD would be less successful in down regulating negative emotional reactivity when implementing cognitive reappraisal in each of the three tasks. Neurally, we hypothesized that, compared to HC, patients with SAD would have: (1) lesser BOLD responses in reappraisal-related PFC regions; and (2) delayed (that is, late) BOLD responses in reappraisal-related PFC regions. In addition to analyzing the differential and common BOLD responses separately for each task, we examined BOLD signal temporal dynamics in regions showing similar reappraisal-related increased activity in SAD and HC across all three tasks. The purpose of this analysis was to see whether there are cognitive reappraisal-related brain responses that are stimulus-independent, and whether more refined timing differences in patients and HC could be revealed using analyses of the BOLD signal temporal dynamics.

Methods

Participants

This study was part of a randomized controlled trial (RCT) of cognitive-behavioral therapy (CBT) for SAD, and data from participants in this RCT have been published in other baseline brain papers [3,10]. Participants included 27 (12 women) unmedicated (minimum of three months since stopping pharmacotherapy) adults who met *DSM-IV-TR* [16] criteria for primary generalized SAD and 27 (13 women) HC with no lifetime history of psychiatric disorders (Table 1). As reported in Ziv et al. [10], patients were recruited through clinician referrals and advertisements on community and online bulletin boards. Two PhD-level clinical psychologists assessed each potential participant using the Anxiety Disorders Interview Schedule for *DSM-IV-TR Lifetime version (ADIS-IV-L)* [17]. Only patients who met clinical diagnostic criteria for a principal diagnosis of current generalized SAD (defined as greater than moderate anxiety/fear for five or more distinct social situations) or HC with no current or past history of DSM-IV disorders were eligible for participation.

Patients and HC did not differ significantly in age or years of education (see Table 1). All participants were right-handed as assessed by the Edinburgh Handedness Inventory [18]. Potential patients were excluded if they reported current pharmacotherapy or psychotherapy, history of neurological disorders, and current psychiatric disorders (other than SAD, generalized anxiety disorder, agoraphobia without a history of panic attacks, dysthymia, or specific phobia). HC were not permitted to meet criteria for any current or past psychiatric disorders.

Among patients, current Axis-I co-morbidity included two with panic attacks, two with generalized anxiety disorder, two with dysthymia, and two with specific phobia. Past Axis-I co-morbidity included six with major depression, one with post-traumatic stress disorder, four with substance abuse, and one with eating disorder. Thirteen patients reported past (that is, ended >1 year ago) non-cognitive-behavioral psychotherapy, and seven reported past pharmacotherapy. The study was approved by the Stanford Medical Research Institutional Review Board (Protocol ID #79403). All participants provided informed consent in accordance with Stanford University Human Subjects Committee rules.

Table 1 Demographic and clinical variables

	SAD $n = 27$	HC $n = 27$	t-value	Partial eta^2
Women (n)	12	13		
Age (mean years ± SD)	31.1 ± 7.6	32.6 ± 9.5	0.6	
Education (mean years ± SD)	16.3 ± 2.3	17.5 ± 1.5	2.0	
Ethnicity				
- Caucasian	12	17		
- Asian	5	8		
- Latino	6	2		
- Native American	1	0		
- Native Hawaiian	1	0		
- Filipino	1	0		
- African American	1	0		
LSAS-SR (Mean ± SD)	99.3 ± 11.8	15.3 ± 9.1	29.2[1]	0.94

[1]P <0.0001.
LSAS-SR = Liebowitz Social Anxiety Scale - Self-Report.

Clinical assessment

To assess social anxiety symptom severity, participants completed the Liebowitz Social Anxiety Scale-Self-Report (LSAS-SR) [19]. This questionnaire assesses both fear and behavioral avoidance of social situations, and is widely used in the research of SAD [20].

To provide greater sensitivity, from 67 patients who were eligible for the study, we selected a subgroup of 27 SAD patients with the highest social anxiety symptom severity (range of LSAS-SR scores for the whole group: 66–102; and for the subgroup: 85–102). We compared this SAD subgroup to a group of 27 healthy controls.

Experimental tasks

The three fMRI tasks have been described previously by Ziv et al. [10]. The tasks were composed of 'React' and 'Reappraise' conditions. Prior to scanning, participants were trained in how to react and to reappraise with stimuli not used in the MR scanner tasks. The instructions for the 'React' condition were to react normally without any attempt to control, modify, or regulate any reactions. During the 'Reappraise' condition, participants were instructed to try and down regulate negative emotion reactions by actively reinterpreting the meaning of the emotion inducing stimulus. We used reappraisal methods developed by Ochsner et al. [21].

After each trial, participants provided a negative emotion rating using a button response pad positioned in the participant's right hand inside the magnet by responding to 'How negative do you feel?' (1 = not at all to 5 = very much). All tasks were programmed in Eprime (Psychology Software Tools, Inc.).

Faces task

This task consisted of 24 trials during which the participants viewed color photos of faces displaying Ekman facial action coded anger and contempt facial expressions [22]. Each trial consisted of a cue (Look or Reframe) lasting 1.5 s, a single harsh facial stimulus presented in color and appearing to move closer to the participant to simulate looming (every 3 s over a total of 9 s), and a negative emotion rating after the face stimulus terminated (3 s) (Figure 1a). The length of the entire task was 516 TRs, which is 12 min and 54 s (774 s). Participants were trained prior to the baseline scan to either react to the faces by engaging in the picture ('Just let yourself feel') and thinking: 'This person is upset with me; angry with me', or to reappraise their emotion, for

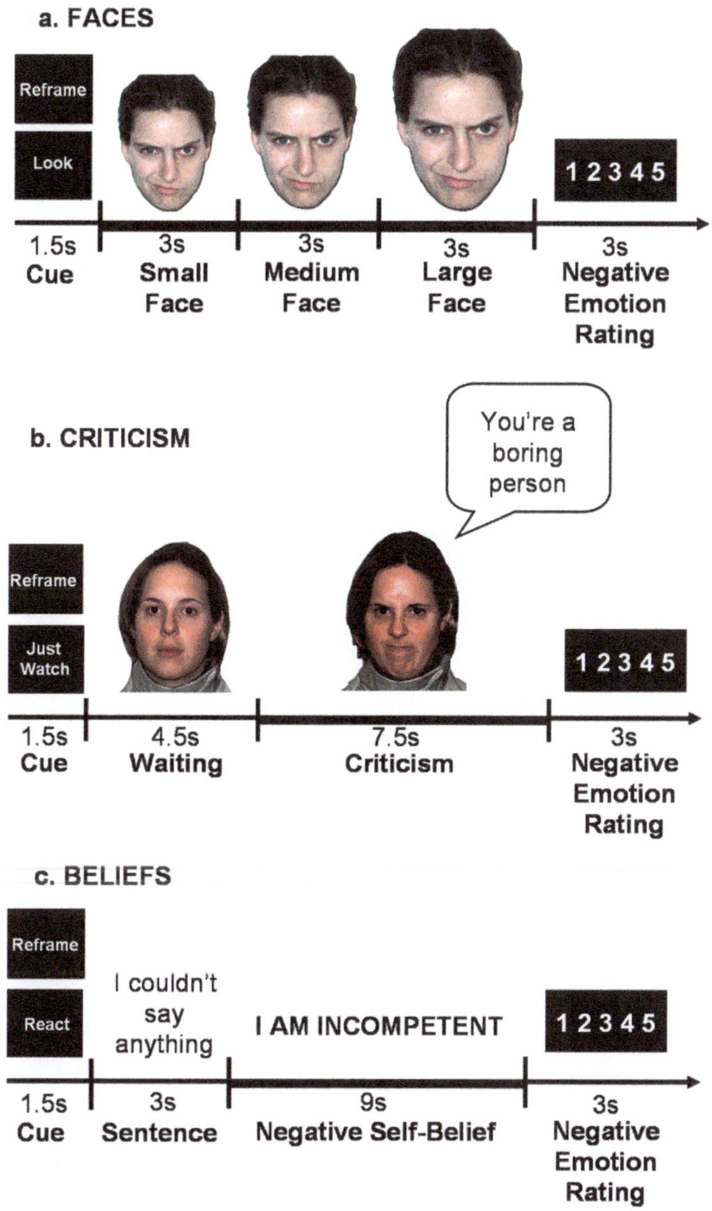

Figure 1 The three socio-emotional tasks. (a) Looming harsh faces (Faces); **(b)** Social criticism (Criticism); **(c)** Negative self-beliefs (Beliefs). Each task was composed of 'React' and 'Reappraise' trials, which consisted of: (1) a 1.5-s 'Cue'; (2) a socio-emotional stimulus (a looming harsh face/ a video-clip of an actor delivering social criticism/ an autobiographical sentence + negative self-beliefs); and (3) a negative emotion rating scale. Participants were instructed to either react normally to the stimuli without any attempt to control, modify, or regulate their reactions ('React'), or to try and down regulate negative emotion reactions by actively reinterpreting the meaning of the emotion inducing stimulus ('Reappraise').

example by thinking: 'Maybe this person just had a bad day'.

Criticism task

The task consisted of videotaped actors delivering social criticism and social praise and harsh or happy evaluation-congruent facial expressions (Figure 1b). The stimuli were delivered by five male and five female actors (seven Anglo-Americans and three Asian-Americans), with an age range of 23 to 50 years. In each trial the participants were asked to either 'Just Watch' or 'Reframe' their reaction (1.5 s) during the social evaluation video clip (12 s).

Each video clip had a 4.5-s waiting period during which the actor silently maintained a neutral facial expression followed by a 7.5-s evaluation period in which the actor delivered a social criticism or praise statement while displaying a harsh or positive facial expression. For the current study, only the 7.5-s evaluation period of the social criticism trials were included in the analysis. After each video clip, participants were cued to rate their current negative emotion (3 s). Each condition consisted of 16 trials delivered across two runs of 342 TRs, 8 min 35 s each (513 s). Participants were trained on the instructions prior to scanning. Participants were told to react to the social criticism by reflecting on how the statement represents something true about themselves, or to reappraise their emotion, for example by thinking: 'this is not always true', or 'this is only a thought, not a fact'.

Beliefs task

This task consisted of five situations. The first was an experimenter-composed neutral situation that was used to obtain baseline emotion ratings for reading neutral statements. The neutral situation was followed by four participant-generated autobiographical social anxiety situations that were characterized by social anxiety, humiliation, and/or embarrassment. Prior to scanning session, participants composed a single paragraph describing the events, thoughts, and feelings for each situation, and provided situation-specific negative self-beliefs (NSBs). At the scanner, the participants were asked to either React to the negative self-beliefs, or to Reframe their reaction.

Three situations were presented in a first run lasting 374 TRs, 9 min 21 s (561 s), followed by two situations in a second run of 256 TRs, 6 min 24 s (534 s). Each situation consisted of an instruction to react/reframe (1.5 s), 16 sentences (3 s each,) in white font against a black background describing the situation, 10 NSBs (9 s each) embedded in the unfolding story in uppercase letters that flashed nine times (850 ms on + 150 ms off), and a negative emotion rating after each NSB (3 s) (Figure 1c). Participants were trained prior to scanning to react to the NSBs by reflecting on how the NSB represents something that is true about themselves, or to reappraise their reaction by thinking of a positive coping statement that directly challenges the thoughts ('try to re-interpret the statement so it is less negative and toxic for you').

Image acquisition

Information about the fMRI image acquisition and data preprocessing have been described previously by Ziv et al. [8]. We used a General Electric 3-T Signa magnet with a T2*-weighted gradient echo spiral-in/out pulse sequence [23] and a custom-built quadrature 'dome' elliptical bird cage head-coil (GE Healthcare, Milwaukee, WI, USA). Head movements were minimized using a bite-bar and foam padding. Functional volumes (516 for faces, 684 for criticism, 630 for belief tasks) were obtained from 22 sequential axial slices (repetition time = 1500 ms, echo time = 30 ms, flip angle = 60°, field of view = 22 cm, matrix = 64 × 64, single-shot, resolution = 3.438 $mm^2 \times$ 4.5 mm). Three-dimensional high-resolution anatomical scans were acquired using a fast spin-echo spoiled gradient recall (resolution = 0.8594 $mm^2 \times 1.5$ mm; field of view = 22 cm, frequency encoding = 256).

FMRI data preprocessing

We used Analysis of Functional Neuroimages (AFNI) software [24] for preprocessing and statistical analysis. Preprocessing included an analysis of potential outliers, volume registration to a base image, motion correction, 4 mm^3 isotropic Gaussian spatial smoothing, high-pass filtering (0.011 Hz), linear detrending, and conversion into BOLD signal percentage change in each voxel. In addition, the first four images of each functional run were excluded, to allow for T2* equilibration effects. For the Criticism and Belief tasks, the two functional runs were concatenated prior to statistical analysis. No volumes demonstrated motion in the x, y, or z directions in excess of ±1 mm. There was no evidence of stimulus-correlated motion, as assessed by correlations between condition-specific reference functions and x, y, z motion correction parameters.

fMRI statistical analysis

Multiple-regression implemented with AFNI 3dDeconvolve included baseline parameters to remove mean, linear, and quadratic trends, and motion-related variance in the BOLD signal. Regressors for the React and Reappraise conditions were convolved with the Cohen's gamma variate model of the hemodynamic response function [25]. Functional MRI BOLD signal intensity was computed as percentage of signal change, an effect size measure [(MR signal per voxel per time point/mean MR signal in that voxel for the entire functional run) × 100].

Individual brain maps were converted to Talairach atlas space [26] and second-level group statistical parametric maps were produced according to a random-effects model. To correct for multiple comparisons, AlphaSim, a Monte Carlo simulation bootstrapping program in the AFNI library, was used to protect against false positives [27]. This method uses a voxel-wise and cluster volume joint-probability threshold to establish a cluster-wise false-positive cluster detection level. The cluster statistical threshold for the between-group analyses consisted of a voxel-wise $P < 0.005$ and cluster volume >244 mm^3 (6 voxels × 3.438 mm^3) to protect against false-positive cluster detection at $P < 0.01$.

To examine differential responses in BOLD signal magnitude, we conducted a whole-brain 2 Group (SAD, HC) between-group t-test of Reappraise *versus* React in SAD *versus* HC. To identify common responses, we ran a one-sample t-test of Reappraise *versus* React in SAD, and separately in HC.

To further examine the between-group differences in the BOLD responses during reappraisal, we ran between-group t-tests for early (first three time points, 0 to 4.5 s) and late (last two/three time points, 4.5 to 7.5 s or 4.5 to 9 s) BOLD responses for the contrast of Reappraise *versus* React. This analysis was conducted in each of the brain regions showing a between-group difference, and had several sub-steps: (1) creating masks from each of the clusters surviving the threshold of the between-group t-test, separately for each task; (2) extracting the percent signal change from each of these regions, at the individual subject level, for the Reappraise condition and for the React condition; (3) calculating the percent signal change for Reappraise minus React; (4) averaging (for each subject) the percent signal change for the first three time points, and for the last three time points; and (5) running between-group t-tests (SAD *versus* HC) separately for the early and late averaged responses, for each task.

In a secondary analysis, we examined brain regions showing BOLD responses common to SAD and HC across the three tasks, and ran between-group t-tests on the contrast of Reappraise *versus* React, for early and late responses, separately, for each task.

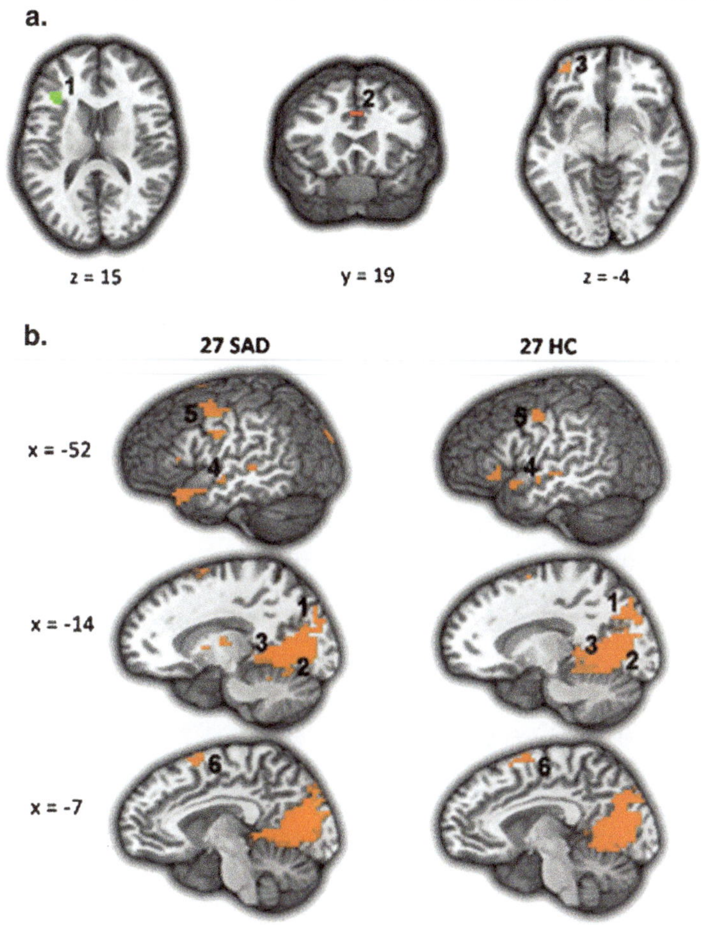

Figure 2 Faces task: brain responses during Reappraise *versus* React in SAD and HC. (a) Differential BOLD responses in patients with SAD *versus* healthy controls (HC > SAD). 1 = left inferior frontal gyrus, 2 = dorsal ACC, 3 = left lateral orbitofrontal cortex. **(b)** Common BOLD responses in patients with SAD and healthy controls. 1 = left cuneus, 2 = left lingual gyrus, 3 = left parahippocampus, 4 = left middle temporal gyrus, 5 = left precentral gyrus, 6 = dorsomedial PFC. Statistical threshold for BOLD responses: t-value threshold ≥2.93, voxel *P* <0.005, minimum cluster volume threshold ≥244 mm^3 (6 voxels × 3.438 mm^3), cluster-wise *P* <0.01.

Results

Faces task

Behavioral responses: negative emotion ratings

A between-group t-test revealed no significant differences ($P > 0.23$) in percent reduction in negative emotion between HC (30 %) and SAD (23 %) when reappraising faces (Additional file 1: Figure S1a).

Brain responses: BOLD signal magnitude

Differential responses Compared to HC, patients had lesser reappraisal-related BOLD responses in the left inferior frontal gyrus (IFG), dorsal anterior cingulate cortex (dACC), and left lateral orbitofrontal cortex (LOFC) (Figure 2a).

Common responses Separate one-sample t-tests of Reappraise *versus* React demonstrated increased BOLD responses in both groups in bilateral cuneus, precuneus, lingual gyrus, and hippocampus, and in left middle temporal gyrus, left precentral gyrus, and dorsomedial PFC (Figure 2b). See Table 2 for both differential and common responses.

Brain responses: BOLD signal temporal dynamics

To examine between-group differences in the BOLD responses during reappraisal, we conducted between-group t-tests for early (first three time points; 0–4.5 s) and late (last three time points; 4.5-9 s) BOLD responses for the Reappraise *versus* React contrast in the left IFG, dACC, and left LOFC. Between-group t-tests revealed a significantly greater late responses in HC, compared to SAD, in the left IFG (mean HC = 0.09 *vs.* mean SAD = −0.03, $t_{52} = -3.70$, $P < 0.0005$) and the dACC (mean HC = 0.07 *vs.* mean SAD = −0.11, $t_{52} = -3.26$, $P < 0.002$), with no between-group differences in early responses (Figures 3a, b). For the left LOFC, a between-group t-test showed that, compared to SAD, HC had greater early (mean HC = 0.09 *vs.* mean SAD = −0.05, $t_{50} = -2.34$, $P < 0.02$) and late (mean HC = 0.13 *vs.* mean SAD = −0.09, $t_{50} = -5.10$, $P < 0.0001$) responses for the Reappraisal *versus* React contrasts (Figure 3c).

Criticism task

Behavioral responses: negative emotion ratings

A between-group t-test revealed a trend towards greater percent reduction in negative emotion ratings for HC (23 %, SD = 18) than SAD (14 %, SD = 17; $t_{53} = -1.93$, $P < 0.059$) when reappraising criticism (Additional file 1: Figure S1b).

Brain responses: BOLD signal magnitude

Differential responses Compared to HC, patients had lesser reappraisal-related BOLD responses in bilateral fusiform gyrus, left lingual gyrus, left putamen, and right cerebellum (Figure 4a).

Table 2 Faces task: differential and common BOLD responses for Reappraise *versus* React

	x y z	Vol (mm³)	*t*-value
Between-group differential responses			
SAD > HC: Reappraise > React-none			
HC > SAD: Reappraise > React			
Left inferior frontal gyrus	-34, 25, 15	426	3.56
Dorsal anterior cingulate gyrus	0, 18, 33	372	3.46
Left lateral orbitofrontal cortex	-31, 52, -6	372	3.63
Within-group responses[1]			
SAD only: Reappraise > React			
Right cuneus	3, -82, 39	57,444	3.39
(Left cuneus, bilateral precuneus, bilateral lingual gyrus, bilateral parahippocampal gyrus)			
Left superior temporal gyrus BA38	-48, 28, -19	3,191	3.30
Left Superior Temporal Gyrus BA21	-65, -20, -2	1,330	3.76
Left dorsomedial PFC	-3, 11, 63	1,330	3.38
Left precentral gyrus BA6	-52, -3, 29	1,170	3.61
Right middle temporal gyrus BA21	55, -3, -9	1,117	3.64
Left putamen	-21, 4, 5	1,117	4.26
Right superior temporal gyrus BA38	45, 21, -16	1,011	3.56
Left inferior frontal gyrus BA45	-55, 31, 8	532	3.09
Left superior temporal gyrus	-65, -13, -2	479	3.72
Left thalamus	-14, -13, -8	426	4.05
Right thalamus	14, -13, 12	426	4.15
Right superior temporal gyrus	38, 7, -12	372	3.12
Left middle temporal gyrus	-55, -10, -9	372	3.75
HC only: Reappraise > React			
Left lingual gyrus	-3, -58, 5	67,125	7.08
(Right lingual gyrus, bilateral cuneus, bilateral precuneus, bilateral parahippocampus)			
Left dorsomedial PFC	-3, 4, 63	3,191	3.73
Left precentral gyrus BA4/6	-55, -3, 50	1,808	3.21
Left supramarginal gyrus BA40	-65, -48, 19	1,011	3.83
Left superior temporal gyrus	-55, -17, -2	798	5.05
Left inferior frontal gyrus	-52, 25, -6	745	3.62
Left superior temporal gyrus BA22	-62, -34, 12	745	3.10
Right superior temporal gyrus BA38	41, -24, 1	691	3.53
Left superior temporal gyrus BA38	-52, 14, -9	585	3.40
Right precentral gyrus BA6	62, 4, 19	426	3.69
Left middle temporal gyrus	-55, -6, -6	426	4.69

[1]Regions showing increased BOLD response during Reappraise *versus* React in both SAD and HC (common responses) are marked in italics.
Note. *t*-value threshold ≥2.932, voxel $P < 0.005$, minimum cluster volume threshold ≥244 mm^3 (6 voxels × 3.438 mm^3), cluster $P < 0.01$.
BA = Brodmann area, xyz = Talairach and Tournoux coordinates of maximum BOLD signal intensity voxel.

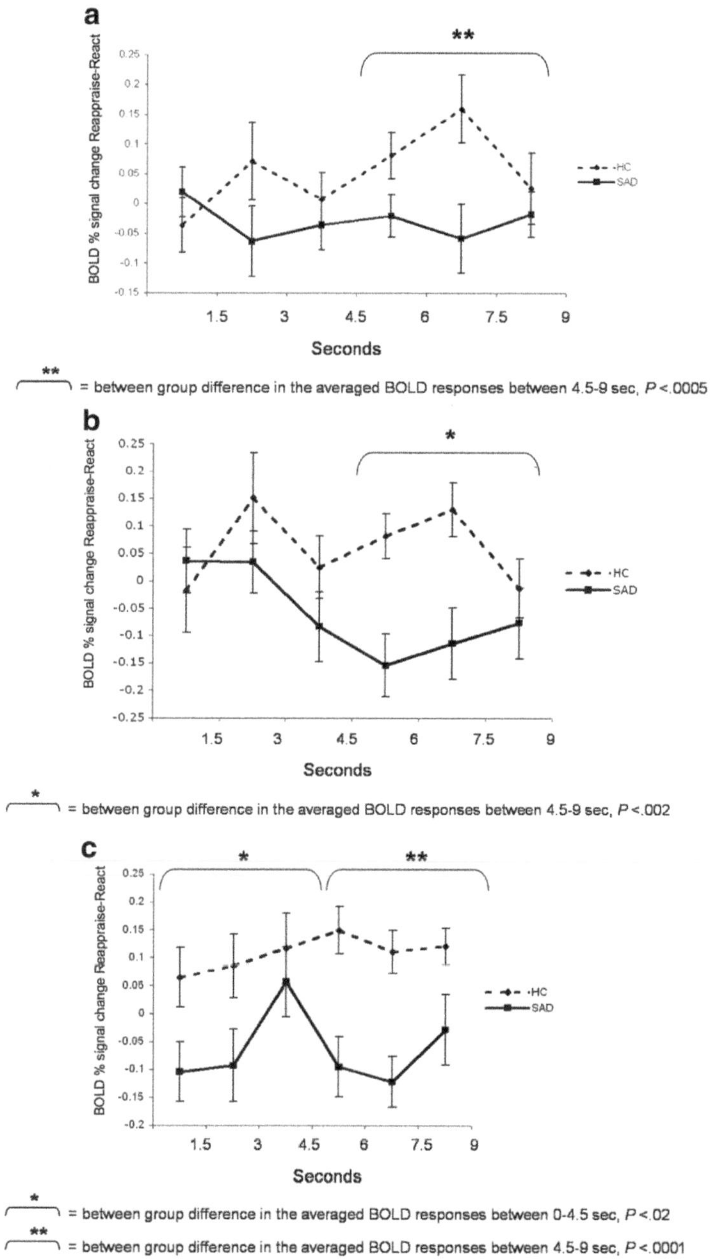

Figure 3 Faces task: temporal dynamics of the BOLD response during Reappraise *versus* React in SAD and HC. Asterisks represent a significant between-group difference in the average of the first three time points (early) or last three time points (late) BOLD responses. **(a)** Left inferior frontal gyrus; **(b)** Dorsal ACC; **(c)** Left lateral orbitofrontal cortex.

Common responses Separate one-sample t-tests of Reappraise *versus* React demonstrated increased BOLD responses in both groups in the right precuneus, dorsomedial PFC, and left dorsolateral PFC (Figure 4b). See Table 3 for both differential and common responses.

Brain responses: temporal dynamics

To examine the between-group differences in the BOLD signal timing during reappraisal, we conducted between-group t-tests for early (first three time points; 0–4.5 s) and late (last two time points; 4.5-7.5 s) BOLD responses

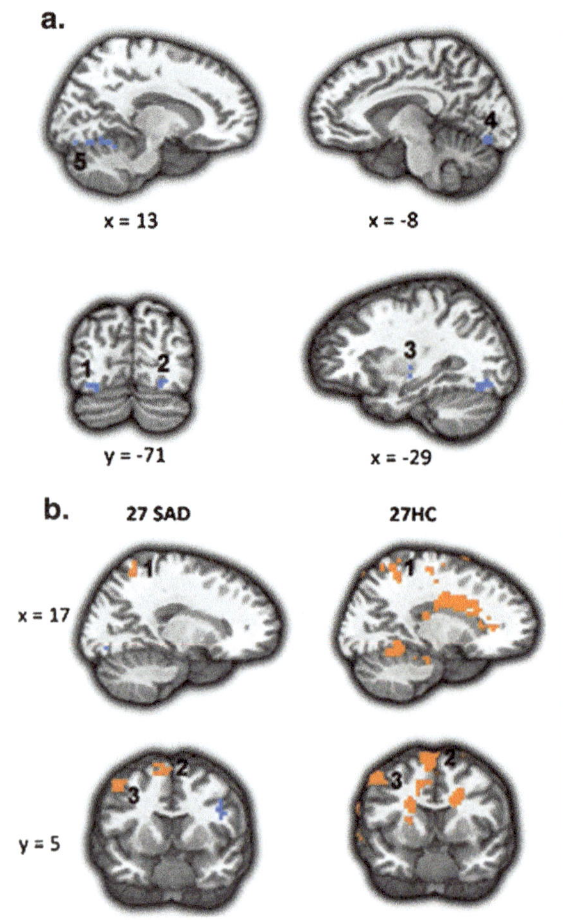

Figure 4 Criticism task: brain responses during Reappraise *versus* React in SAD and HC. (a) Differential BOLD responses in patients with SAD *versus* healthy controls (HC > SAD). 1 = left fusiform gyrus, 2 = right fusiform gyrus, 3 = left putamen, 4 = left lingual gyrus, 5 = right cerebellum. **(b)** Common BOLD responses in patients with SAD and healthy controls. 1 = right precuneus, 2 = dorsomedial PFC, 3 = left dorsolateral PFC. Statistical threshold for BOLD responses: t-value threshold ≥2.93, voxel P <0.005, minimum cluster volume threshold ≥244 mm^3 (6 voxels × 3.438 mm^3), cluster-wise P <0.01.

Table 3 Criticism task: differential and common BOLD responses for Reappraise *versus* React

	x y z	Vol (mm^3)	t-value
Between-group differential responses			
SAD > HC: Reappraise > React - none			
HC > SAD: Reappraise > React			
Left fusiform gyrus	-24, -68, -12	904	3.16
Right cerebellum	3, -68, -9	745	3.01
Right fusiform gyrus	24, -75, -12	585	4.13
Left putamen	-28, -13, -6	479	2.96
Left lingual gyrus	-7, -75, -12	426	3.28
Right cerebellum	24, -51, -16	372	2.94
Right cerebellum	17, -58, -12	372	3.04
Within-group responses[1]			
SAD only: Reappraise > React			
Left dorsomedial PFC	-3, 11, 60	2,500	4.27
Left dorsolateral PFC	-48, 7, 50	1,170	3.59
Right precuneus	17, -55, 63	745	3.36
Right parahippocampal gyrus	24, -44, -6	372	3.25
HC only: Reappraise > React			
Left lingual gyrus	-3, -58, 5	13,936	3.21
(Right lingual gyrus, bilateral fusiform gyrus, bilateral cerebellum)			
Right precentral gyrus BA6/BA4	28, -17, 63	9,308	3.14
Left dorsomedial PFC	-3, 11, 67	6,915	3.34
Left dorsolateral PFC	-52, 4, 50	3,776	3.83
Left supramarginal gyrus	-62, -58, 15	3,351	4.09
Left middle frontal gyrus	-45, 21, 29	2,234	3.42
Right superior parietal cortex/ precuneus	24, -55, 60	2,128	3.31
Left superior parietal cortex/ precuneus	-24, -75, 53	1,808	4.18
Left inferior frontal gyrus BA45	-55, 25, -2	1,755	3.25
Left medial frontal gyrus	-3, 7, 43	1,170	3.15
Right precuneus	28, -72, 22	1,064	3.45
Left superior temporal gyrus	-65, -174, -2	1,064	3.79
Left middle frontal gyrus	-31, 49, 12	851	3.14
Left precuneus	-31, -89, 19	745	3.34
Left anterior insula	-48, 11, 5	745	3.53
Left precentral gyrus BA4	-24, -24, 56	691	3.56
Left thalamus	-3, -3, 12	638	3.34
Left angular gyrus	-48, -61, 36	585	3.12
Left superior temporal gyrus	-38, -55, 29	319	3.38
Left putamen	-31, -10, -2	319	3.28
Left middle temporal gyrus	-52, -34, 5	319	3.33

[1]Regions showing increased BOLD response during Reappraise *versus* React in both SAD and HC (common responses) are marked in italics.
Note. *t*-value threshold ≥2.93, voxel P <0.005, minimum cluster volume threshold ≥244 mm^3 (6 voxels × 3.438 mm^3), cluster P <0.01.
BA = Brodmann area, xyz = Talairach and Tournoux coordinates of maximum BOLD signal intensity voxel.

for the Reappraise *versus* React conditions in left and right fusiform gyrus, left lingual gyrus, left putamen, and right cerebellum.

Between-group t-tests revealed a significant greater early response in HC, compared to SAD, in the left (mean HC = 0.03 *vs.* mean SAD = −0.09; $t_{48} = -2.20$, P <0.03) and right (mean HC = 0.05 *vs.* mean SAD = −0.19, $t_{48} = -2.78$, P <0.008) fusiform gyrus. For the left lingual gyrus, there were no early or late significant between-group differences (All Ps > 0.26). Significant increased late response in HC, compared to SAD, was found in the left putamen (mean HC = 0.05, mean SAD = −0.05, $t_{50} = -2.88$, P <0.006). Time course analyses for the right cerebellum

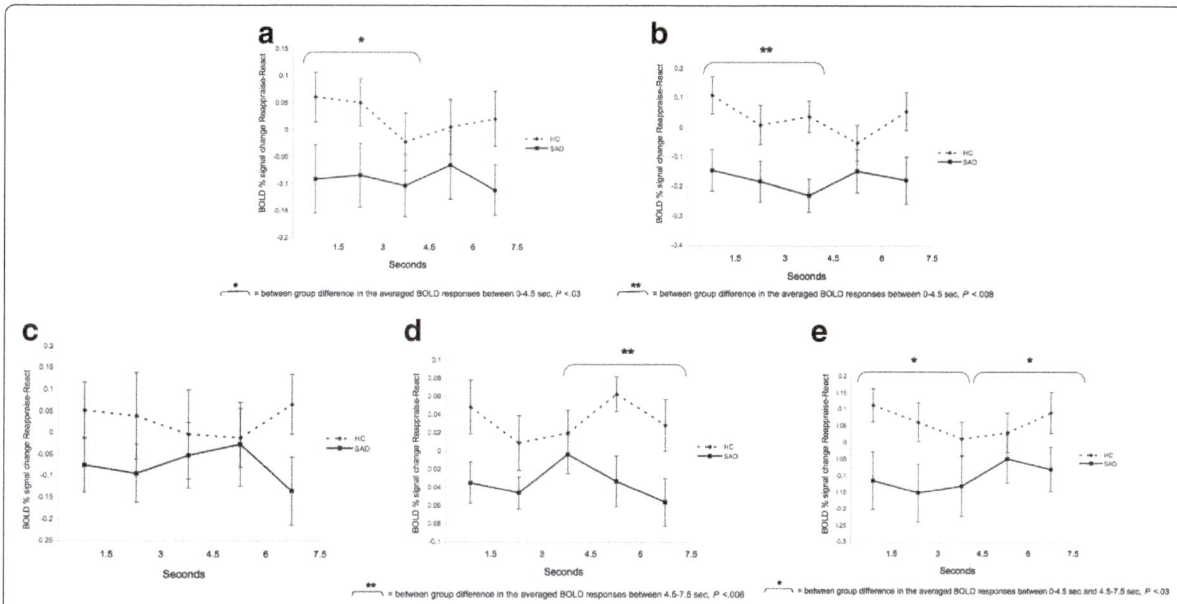

Figure 5 Criticism task: temporal dynamics of the BOLD response during Reappraise *versus* React in SAD and HC. Asterisks represent a significant between-group difference in the average of the first three time points (early) or last two time points (late) BOLD responses. **(a)** Left fusiform gyrus; **(b)** Right fusiform gyrus; **(c)** Left lingual gyrus; **(d)** Left putamen; **(e)** Right cerebellum.

showed both early (mean HC = 0.05 *vs.* mean SAD = −0.15, $t_{49} = -2.32$, $P < 0.03$) and late (mean HC = 0.05 *vs.* mean SAD = −0.15, $t_{49} = -2.22$, $P < 0.03$) increased responses in HC, compared to SAD, during reappraisal (Figure 5a-e)[a].

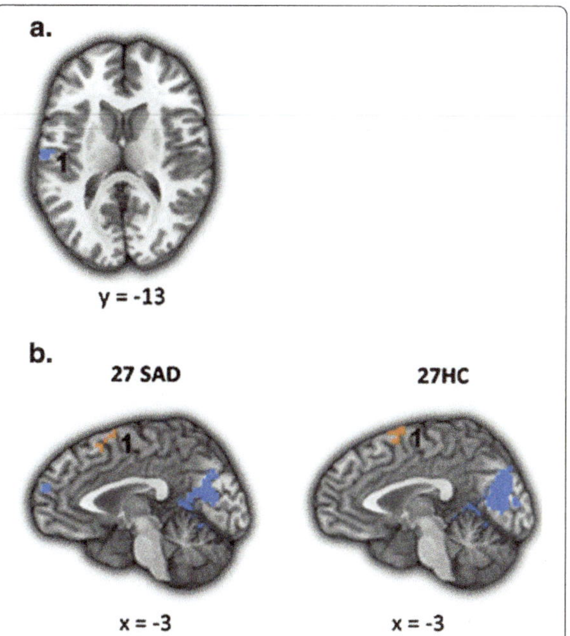

Figure 6 Beliefs task: brain responses during Reappraise *versus* React in SAD and HC. (a) Differential responses in patients with SAD *versus* healthy controls (HC > SAD). 1 = left superior temporal gyrus. **(b)** Common BOLD responses in patients with SAD and healthy controls. 1 = dorsomedial PFC. Statistical threshold for BOLD responses: t-value threshold ≥2.93, voxel $P < 0.005$, minimum cluster volume threshold ≥244 mm^3 (6 voxels × 3.438 mm^3), cluster-wise $P < 0.01$.

Beliefs task

Behavioral responses: negative emotion ratings

A between-group t-test revealed greater percent reduction in negative emotion ratings for HC (31%, SD = 16.2) than SAD (19%, SD = 19; $t49 = -2.52$, $P < 0.02$) when reappraising beliefs (Additional file 1: Figure S1c).

Brain responses: BOLD signal magnitude

Differential responses Compared to HC, patients had lesser BOLD responses in the left superior temporal gyrus (STG) (Figure 6a).

Common responses Separate one-sample t-tests of Reappraise *versus* React demonstrated increased response in both groups in the dorsomedial PFC (Figure 6b). See Table 4 for both differential and common responses.

Brain responses: temporal dynamics

To examine between-group differences in the BOLD responses during reappraisal of beliefs, we conducted between-group t-tests for early (first three time points; 0–4.5 s) and late (last three time points; 4.5-9 s) BOLD responses for the Reappraise *versus* React conditions in the left STG. This analysis revealed a significant

Table 4 Beliefs task: differential and common BOLD responses for Reappraise *versus* React

	x y z	Vol (mm^3)	*t*-value
Between-group differential responses			
SAD > HC: Reappraise > React - none			
HC > SAD: Reappraise > React			
Left superior temporal gyrus BA41	-58, -13, 12	585	2.96
Within-group responses[1]			
SAD only: Reappraise > React			
Left dorsomedial PFC	-3, 7, 60	1,596	3.16
Left inferior frontal gyrus BA45	-55, 25, 8	638	3.81
Left dorsolateral PFC	-41, 7, 50	638	3.57
HC only: Reappraise > React			
Left dorsomedial PFC	-3, 11, 63	1,170	3.09

[1]Regions showing increased BOLD response during Reappraise versus React in both SAD and HC (common responses) are marked in italics.
Note. *t*-value threshold ≥2.93, voxel *P* <0.005, minimum cluster volume threshold ≥244 mm^3 (6 voxels × 3.438 mm^3), cluster *P* <0.01.
BA = Brodmann area, xyz = Talairach and Tournoux coordinates of maximum BOLD signal intensity voxel.

increased late response in HC, compared to SAD (mean HC = 0.02 *vs.* mean SAD = −0.09, $t_{51} = -3.52$, *P* <0.0009) (Figure 7).

Secondary analyses

Examination of the reappraisal-related brain responses common for SAD and HC revealed only one region, the dorsomedial PFC (DMPFC), which showed reappraisal-related increased activity in both groups, in all three tasks (Figure 8). To examine the temporal dynamics of the BOLD response, and its potential association with between-group differences, we conducted two between-group t-tests: one for early and one for late BOLD responses during the Reappraise *versus* React conditions in this region, separately for each task.

There were no significant between-group differences in early or late responses for the contrast of Reappraise *versus* React Faces (*P*s >0.08) and Criticism (*P*s >0.26) (Figure 9a,b). However, for Beliefs, compared to HC, patients had lesser late BOLD responses (mean HC = 0.17, mean SAD = 0.07, $t_{50} = -2.12$, *P* <0.04) (Figure 9c).

Greater late DMPFC responses were associated with greater reduction in negative emotion ratings in SAD patients (r = 0.42, *P* <0.04), but not HC (r = −0.32, *P* = 0.13; Zdiff = 2.52, *P* <0.05) (Figure 10).

Discussion

We tested the hypothesis that dysfunctional emotion regulation processes in SAD patients are associated with altered reappraisal-related activity in prefrontal brain regions. We focused on both BOLD signal magnitude and temporal dynamics during reappraisal of three different socio-emotional stimuli in patients with SAD *versus* healthy controls. Results suggest distinct behavioral and neural effects related to each of the socio-emotional tasks.

Behavioral correlates of reappraisal in SAD

Behaviorally, the results of this study indicated a smaller percent reduction of negative emotion in patients with SAD compared to HC, but only during the reappraisal of idiographic social anxiety-related negative self-beliefs. Though it has long been thought that patients with SAD have problems with down regulating negative emotions [2,3,5,28], the behavioral findings in our study suggest a more nuanced picture of deficits in reappraisal. Specifically, the emotion regulation deficits were most pronounced when facing the negative self-beliefs. These idiographic stimuli, each linked to autobiographical social anxiety-related situations, are highly potent - in our previous report [10], using the same stimuli and the same

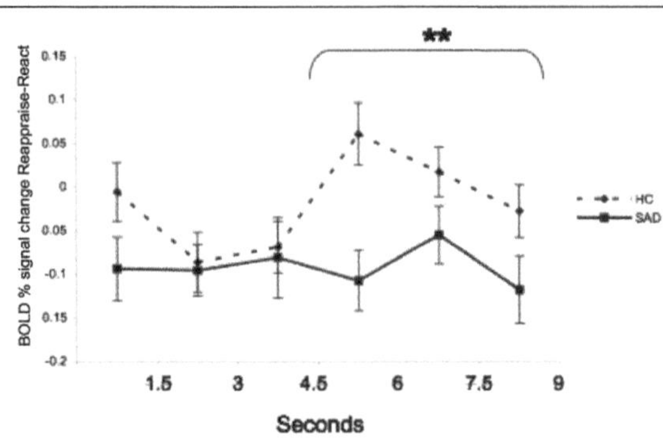

Figure 7 Beliefs task: temporal dynamics of the left STG BOLD responses during Reappraise *versus* React in SAD and HC. Asterisks represent a significant between-group difference in the average of the last three time points (late) BOLD responses.

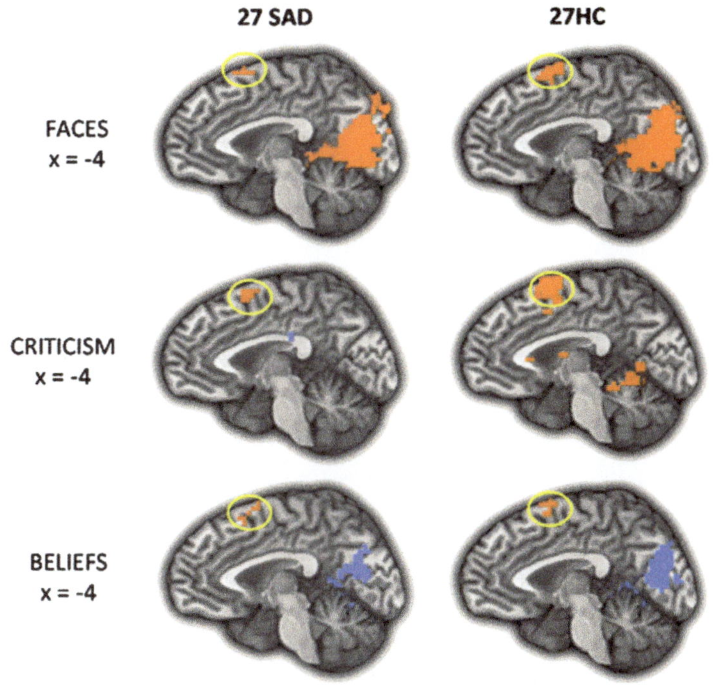

Figure 8 Dorsomedial PFC BOLD responses during the three socio-emotional tasks. The dorsomedial PFC (DMPFC) showed increased activity in both patients with SAD and HC, during reappraisal of faces, criticism, and beliefs.

sample, negative self-beliefs were associated with the greatest increase in negative emotion, compared to faces and criticism, in both SAD and HC. This suggests greater emotional effect for these stimuli, which might be related with the difficulty in down regulating its associated negative emotions.

Our finding is partially in line with the results of the one other study examining cognitive regulation of negative self-beliefs in SAD [3]. In that study, although no difference was found between patients and controls in the amount of reappraisal-related reduction of negative emotion, greater social anxiety symptom severity was associated with lesser down regulation of negative emotion in patients, suggesting that severity of social anxiety contributes to deficits in cognitive reappraisal of negative beliefs.

Neural correlates of reappraisal in SAD

Neurally, based on the prior findings in patients with SAD [3,5] and non-clinical populations [21], we hypothesized that, relative to HC, patients would have reduced recruitment of PFC regions during reappraisal. The between-group analyses partially confirmed our hypothesis. While there was PFC activation during reappraisal in both patients and controls during all three tasks, between-group differential PFC activation was found only during the reappraisal of faces, with no differential PFC responses when reappraising beliefs and criticism.

Reappraisal of looming harsh faces

When reappraising faces, compared to HC, patients had reduced activity in a PFC network that included left IFG, dACC, and lateral OFC. In these regions, time course analyses revealed greater BOLD response during the second half of the trial in HC compared to patients. This increased late responses in HC when reappraising looming harsh faces might be related to integrated cognitive processes that rely on linguistic (left IFG), cognitive control/attention (dACC), and evaluation/response selection (lateral OFC) processes [29]. In patients, the reduced late recruitment of prefrontal regulatory brain regions suggests deficits in reappraisal processes, especially of faces displaying contempt, anger, or disapproval. The use of harsh faces as an emotional probe in patients with SAD has ecological validity given that SAD is characterized by fear of interpersonal situations and a tendency to avoid eye contact [30]. Cognitive behavioral models of social anxiety suggest that patients with SAD manifest increased attentional focus on others' facial expressions and negative evaluation during social situations [31]. Supporting the models, behavioral studies have reported that patients with SAD tend to remember critical faces better than accepting ones [32], and scan faces with a

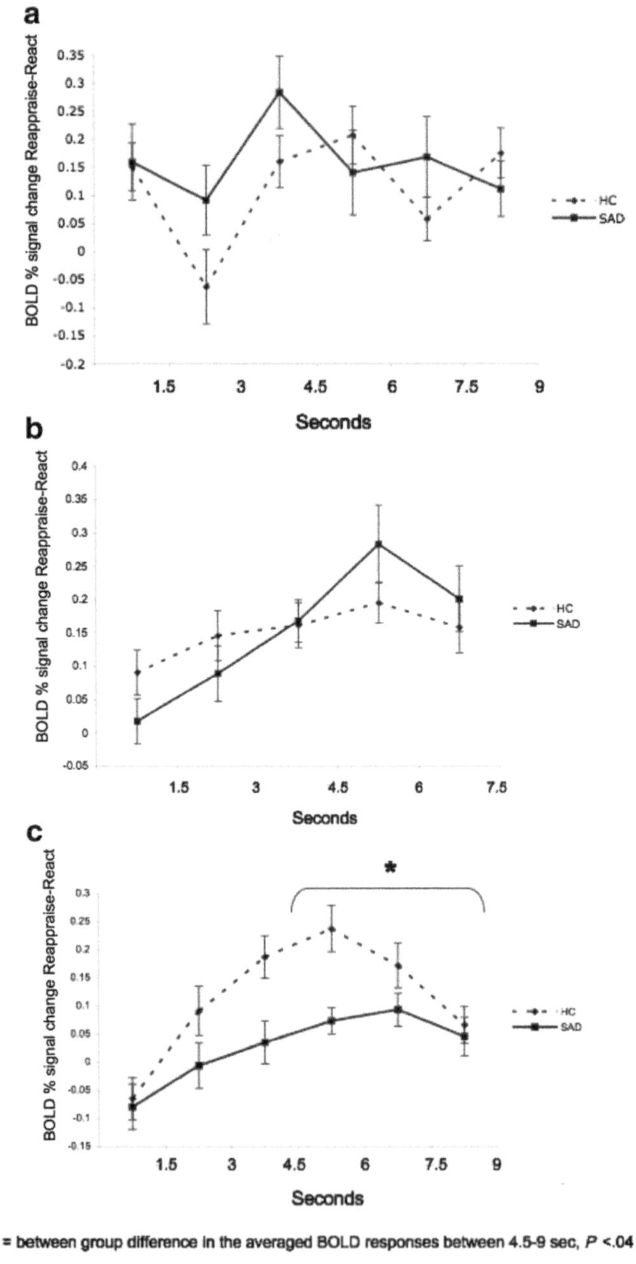

Figure 9 Temporal dynamics of the dorsomedial PFC BOLD responses during Reappraise *versus* React Faces (a), Criticism (b), and Beliefs (c) in SAD and HC. No significant between-group differences were found in early or late DMPFC activity when reappraising faces and criticism. A significant between-group difference was found in late DMPFC activity when reappraising beliefs (P <0.04).

different pattern of eye movements than is used by healthy controls [33]. The results of the current study accord with these models of social anxiety and extend the current theory by suggesting a delayed regulatory deficit in SAD.

Reappraisal of social criticism

During reappraisal of criticism, the left putamen exhibited increased reappraisal-related activity in HC, compared to SAD, during the second half of the trials. Previous studies implicated the putamen as involved in

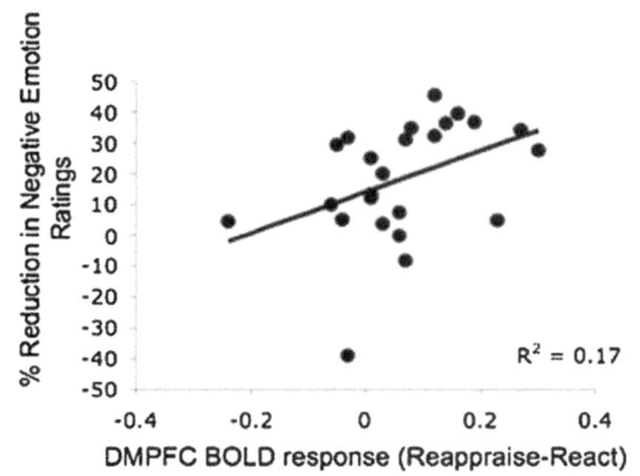

Figure 10 Beliefs task: association between dorsomedial PFC BOLD responses during Reappraise *versus* React and percent reduction in negative emotion ratings. When reappraising beliefs, DMPFC BOLD responses were positively correlated with % reduction in negative emotion ratings in SAD patients ($r = 0.42$, $P < 0.04$).

implicit learning, and specifically in prediction of future reward [34]. Recently, the left putamen was shown to be active when participants had to explicitly mirror observed emotional facial expressions [35]. The authors of this study suggested that the putamen is involved in the establishment of a successful social connection with another person. In the current study, it might be that HC, but not patients, were able to form a relatively more positive (or less negative) interpretation of the social feedback delivered by the actor following the reappraisal instruction. For patients with SAD, difficulties implementing cognitive reappraisal might make it harder for them to relate to the person in the video clip in a positive way, and prevent them from seeing the social situation as a potential rewarding event.

Interestingly, time course analyses of the fusiform gyrus, lingual gyrus, and cerebellum responses revealed that the between-group differences derived less from increased reappraisal-related responses in HC, and more from increased reactivity-related responses in patients with SAD. These results are in line with electrophysiological studies demonstrating early hyper-vigilance followed by attentional avoidance in adults with SAD when facing social threat stimuli [36]. Overall, this result confirms previous findings of increased activity in visual attention-related regions in SAD when reacting to social relevant stimuli [3].

Reappraisal of autobiographical negative self-beliefs

During reappraisal of beliefs, the between-group results indicated increased reappraisal-related activity in the left STG in healthy controls. The STG also manifested a late activity peak for HC, compared to SAD. The STG is related to social cognition, namely, the ability to attribute mental states to the self and others. During cognitive reappraisal, attending to one's own emotional state or to those of others is crucial to be able to monitor the process of changing the affective state [37]. Thus, greater activity in this region in HC, compared to patients, might be associated with the patients' reduced ability to regulate their cognitions when facing their self-created negative self-beliefs.

Temporal dynamics of reappraisal

Across the three tasks, the results of the temporal dynamics analyses converged, showing greater reappraisal-related neural responses in HC, compared to SAD, during the late reappraisal period. In the one previous paper that examined the temporal dynamics of neural responses during reappraisal, findings indicated greater reappraisal-related neural responses in HC, compared to HC, during the early reappraisal period [3]. That study utilized one of the three tasks reported in the current paper (negative self-beliefs) and tested reappraisal processes using similar reappraisal training methods. However, while the current study focused on between-group effects of the contrast of reappraise *versus* react, separately in the early and late responses, the goal of the previous study was to examine linear decreases in emotional reactivity and increases in regulatory responses during the whole 9-s trial. Thus, the previous study used linear regression to examine linear changes in BOLD responses over time, and compared early *versus* late BOLD responses on each trial, separately for reappraise and for react, in SAD compared to HC. In the present study, we ran between-group t-tests for early and late responses separately, but contrasted the reappraise and react conditions. In addition to these differences in data analytic approaches, the previous study examined one task, while three different contexts were tested in the current paper. Despite these dissimilarities, the results of both studies clearly suggest different timing of the brain responses in SAD and HC during reappraisal. The idea that differences in the temporal dynamics of the brain response are a key factor in regulation processes is consistent with recent findings by Goldin and colleagues, who showed changes in the timing of the BOLD responses in patients with SAD following an 8-week mindfulness-based stress reduction program, and following 16 sessions of individual CBT for SAD [14].

Task independent reappraisal responses

For each task separately, examination of reappraisal-related BOLD responses common to patients and HC revealed a task-specific network of regions. These regions are implicated in visual attention (cuneus, precuneus, lingual gyrus), working memory (dorsolateral PFC), cognitive regulation (dorsomedial PFC), memory (hippocampus), and language (left MTG, left precentral gyrus) processes, which all take part during reappraisal. Of these regions, the dorsomedial PFC was the only region showing increased activity for both HC and patients during all three tasks.

The DMPFC has been implicated in multiple cognitive functions, including strategic evaluation, introspection, and decision-making [38-40]. In the present study, though no group differences in DMPFC BOLD signal magnitude were found, time course analyses revealed increased late DMPFC activity in healthy controls, compared to SAD patients, when reappraising negative self-beliefs. This finding accords well with the study by Bruhl and colleagues [11], which found comparable MPFC activity in SAD patients who applied reality-checking to negative stimuli and in SAD patients who just perceived the stimuli with no regulation attempts. The researchers suggested that the lack of increased recruitment of MPFC activity due to cognitive control might point to deficits in emotion regulation processes in SAD.

This idea that the lack of additional recruitment of MPFC could be an important neural correlate of emotion regulation deficits in SAD is supported by the results of the current study, and more specifically by the convergence between the neural and behavioral findings: compared to SAD, HC manifested both greater late DMPFC activity, and greater percent reduction in negative emotion ratings, when reappraising negative self-beliefs. In addition, in patients with SAD, greater late DMPFC responses were associated with greater reduction in negative emotion ratings. Thus, decreased DMPFC activity in SAD might be associated with reduced emotion regulation capability, and consequently to reduced ability to down regulate negative reactivity.

Conclusions

The present study found reduced late BOLD responses in PFC regions in SAD, compared to healthy controls, when reappraising harsh faces. In addition, reduced late responses in the DMPFC in patients with SAD, compared to controls, were related to less reduction in negative emotion ratings when reappraising negative self-beliefs. Together, these results suggest deficient cognitive reappraisal processes in SAD. Importantly, these results indicate that probes with different stimulus dimensions (visual/linguistic, static/dynamic, general/idiographic) are associated with different reappraisal-related behavioral and brain responses. While reappraisal of faces was associated with increased prefrontal activity in HC when compared to patients with SAD, but with no between-group behavioral effects, reappraisal of beliefs was associated with less ability to down regulate negative emotions in patients, compared to HC, with much less robust between-group neural differences. It is important for future research to specifically examine which of these stimulus dimensions could be the most informative in studying reappraisal processes in SAD.

The results of this study suggest that when cued, patients with SAD do try to implement cognitive reappraisal, but their efforts are less efficient, leading to less than optimal emotional relief. Though reappraisal training is a crucial part of CBT for SAD, our results emphasize the importance of teaching patients how to improve the effectiveness of their reappraisal efforts. Mastering more adaptive regulation processes will help patients with SAD reduce the negative emotions they experience.

An interesting question arising from this study is whether, when no external cue exists, patients use cognitive reappraisal less frequently than healthy controls. To answer this question, future studies may examine the extent to which patients with SAD activate un-cued implicit emotion regulation, compared to healthy controls, in addition to examining the associated brain regions that are activated during implicit, *versus* explicit, emotion regulation processes.

One possible limitation of the current study is the specificity of the stimuli that were chosen to evoke negative emotional response. Because of the social nature of these stimuli, these stimuli were probably more emotionally evocative for patients than for HC. Future studies could examine whether regulatory deficits in SAD, behaviorally and in the brain, are specific to socially-related stimuli, or whether this is a more general deficit.

Finally, the current findings stress the importance of performing analyses that elucidate neural temporal change. Here we focused on temporal dynamics of cognitive reappraisal. However, when a patient with SAD enters a social situation, many other regulatory processes such as rumination, attention deployment, and expression suppression are activated. Although the theory suggests that distinct forms of emotion regulation have their own neural circuitry and temporal features [41], in SAD, the temporal dynamics of the BOLD response in regulatory brain regions are still not well understood. Future studies could examine brain activity related to different regulatory processes, taking place at different points in the emotion-generative process.

Endnote

[a]The increased reappraisal-related activity during criticism was found in two clusters identified as the left fusiform gyrus (1. x,y,z = −24, -68, -12, voxel size = 16; 2. x,y, z = −45, -65, -16, voxel size = 6) and in three clusters identified as the right cerebellum (1. x,y,z = 3, -68, -9, voxel size = 12; 2. x,y,z = 24, -51, -16, voxel size = 7; 3. x, y,z = 17, -58, -12, voxel size = 7). All demonstrated similar pattern of temporal dynamics. For simplicity, we report here only the effects of the biggest cluster in each region (16 voxels for the left fusiform, 12 voxels for the right cerebellum).

Additional file

Additional file 1: Figure S1. Negative emotion ratings in patients with SAD and in HC when reacting to and reappraising Faces (a), Criticism (b), and Beliefs (c). Left - Negative emotion ratings during the react and reappraise conditions. Right - Percent reduction in negative emotion ratings following reappraisal.

Competing interests

The authors declare that they have no competing interests.

Authors' contributions

MZ participated in the study's design and coordination, contributed to data acquisition, conducted the fMRI sessions, conducted the data analyses, and took the lead on writing the manuscript. PRG helped conceive of the design of the study, participated in the study's design and coordination, contributed to data acquisition, conducted the fMRI sessions, consulted on data analyses, and contributed to writing the manuscript. HJ participated in the study's design and coordination, contributed to data acquisition, conducted the fMRI sessions, consulted on data analyses, and contributed to writing the manuscript. KSH consulted on data analyses, and contributed to writing the manuscript. JJG helped conceive of the design of the study, consulted on data analyses, and contributed to writing the manuscript. All authors have read and approved the final manuscript.

Acknowledgements

We wish to thank Gary Glover, Ph.D. for his technical assistance with magnetic resonance imaging. This research was supported by an NIMH Grant R01 MH076074, awarded to James Gross. Michal Ziv had full access to all of the data in the study and takes responsibility for the integrity of the data and the accuracy of the data analysis.

References

1. Stein MB, Stein DJ: **Social anxiety disorder.** *Lancet* 2008, **371:**1115–1125.
2. Hofmann SG: **Cognitive mediation of treatment change in social phobia.** *J Consult Clin Psychol* 2004, **72:**393–399.
3. Goldin PR, Manber-Ball T, Werner K, Heimberg R, Gross JJ: **Neural mechanisms of cognitive reappraisal of negative self-beliefs in social anxiety disorder.** *Biol Psychiatry* 2009, **66:**1091–1099.
4. Gross JJ: *Handbook of emotion regulation.* New York, NY: Guilford Press; 2007.
5. Goldin PR, Manber T, Hakimi S, Canli T, Gross JJ: **Neural bases of social anxiety disorder: emotional reactivity and cognitive regulation during social and physical threat.** *Arch Gen Psychiatry* 2009, **66:**170–180.
6. Lorberbaum JP, Kose S, Johnson MR, Arana GW, Sullivan LK, Hamner MB, Ballenger JC, Lydiard RB, Brodrick PS, Bohning DE, George MS: **Neural correlates of speech anticipatory anxiety in generalized social phobia.** *Neuroreport* 2004, **15:**2701–2705.
7. Blair K, Geraci M, Devido J, McCaffrey D, Chen G, Vythilingam M, Ng P, Hollon N, Jones M, Blair RJ, Pine DS: **Neural response to self- and other referential praise and criticism in generalized social phobia.** *Arch Gen Psychiatry* 2008, **65:**1176–1184.
8. Guyer AE, Lau JY, McClure-Tone EB, Parrish J, Shiffrin ND, Reynolds RC, Chen G, Blair RJ, Leibenluft E, Fox NA, *et al*: **Amygdala and ventrolateral prefrontal cortex function during anticipated peer evaluation in pediatric social anxiety.** *Arch Gen Psychiatry* 2008, **65:**1303–1312.
9. Sripada CS, Angstadt M, Banks S, Nathan PJ, Liberzon I, Phan KL: **Functional neuroimaging of mentalizing during the trust game in social anxiety disorder.** *Neuroreport* 2009, **20:**984–989.
10. Ziv M, Goldin PR, Jazaieri H, Hahn KS, Gross JJ: **Is there less to social anxiety than meets the eye? Behavioral and neural responses to three socio-emotional tasks.** *Biol Mood Anxiety Disord* 2013, **3:**5.
11. Bruhl AB, Herwig U, Delsignore A, Jancke L, Rufer M: **General emotion processing in social anxiety disorder: neural issues of cognitive control.** *Psychiatry Res* 2013, **212:**108–115.
12. Freitas-Ferrari MC, Hallak JE, Trzesniak C, Filho AS, Machado-de-Sousa JP, Chagas MH, Nardi AE, Crippa JA: **Neuroimaging in social anxiety disorder: a systematic review of the literature.** *Prog Neuropsychopharmacol Biol Psychiatry* 2010, **34:**565–580.
13. Goldin PR, Gross JJ: **Effects of mindfulness-based stress reduction (MBSR) on emotion regulation in social anxiety disorder.** *Emotion* 2010, **10:**83–91.
14. Goldin P, Ziv M, Jazaieri H, Gross JJ: **Randomized controlled trial of mindfulness-based stress reduction versus aerobic exercise: effects on the self-referential brain network in social anxiety disorder.** *Front Hum Neurosci* 2012, **6:**295.
15. Campbell DW, Sareen J, Paulus MP, Goldin PR, Stein MB, Reiss JP: **Time-varying amygdala response to emotional faces in generalized social phobia.** *Biol Psychiatry* 2007, **62:**455–463.
16. DSM-IV-TR: *Diagnostic and statistical manual of mental disorders.* 4th edition. Washington, DC: American Psychiatric Association; 1994:2000.
17. DiNardo PA, Brown TA, Barlow DH: *Anxiety disorders interview schedule for DSM-IV: lifetime version (ADIS-IV-L).* Albany, NY: Graywind Publications, Inc; 1994.
18. Oldfield RC: **The assessment and analysis of handedness: the Edinburgh inventory.** *Neuropsychologia* 1971, **9:**97–113.
19. Liebowitz MR: **Social phobia.** *Mod Probl Pharmacopsychiatry* 1987, **22:**141–173.
20. Fresco DM, Coles ME, Heimberg RG, Liebowitz MR, Hami S, Stein MB, Goetz D: **The Liebowitz social anxiety scale: a comparison of the psychometric properties of self-report and clinician-administered formats.** *Psychol Med* 2001, **31:**1025–1035.
21. Ochsner KN, Ray RD, Cooper JC, Robertson ER, Chopra S, Gabrieli JD, Gross JJ: **For better or for worse: neural systems supporting the cognitive down-and up-regulation of negative emotion.** *Neuroimage* 2004, **23:**483–499.
22. Ekman P, Friesen W: *Facial action coding system: a technique for the measurment of facial movement.* Palo Alto, CA: Consulting Psychologists Press; 1978.
23. Glover GH, Law CS: **Spiral-in/out BOLD fMRI for increased SNR and reduced susceptibility artifacts.** *Magn Reson Med* 2001, **46:**515–522.
24. Cox RW: **AFNI: software for analysis and visualization of functional magnetic resonance neuroimages.** *Comput Biomed Res* 1996, **29:**162–173.
25. Cohen MS: **Parametric analysis of fMRI data using linear systems methods.** *Neuroimage* 1997, **6:**93–103.
26. Talairach J, Tournoux P: *Co-planar stereotaxic atlas of the human brain.* New York, NY: Thieme; 1988.
27. Forman SD, Cohen JD, Fitzgerald M, Eddy WF, Mintun MA, Noll DC: **Improved assessment of significant activation in functional magnetic resonance imaging (fMRI): use of a cluster-size threshold.** *Magn Reson Med* 1995, **33:**636–647.
28. Mcclure EB, Pine DS: **Social anxiety and emotion regulation: A model for developmental psychopathology perspectives on anxiety disorders.** In *Developmental Psychopathology, Risk, Disorder, and Adaptation.* 2nd edition. Edited by Cicchetti D, Cohen DJ. Hoboken, New Jersey: John Wiley & Sons; 2006:470–50.
29. Ochsner KN, Silvers JA, Buhle JT: **Functional imaging studies of emotion regulation: a synthetic review and evolving model of the cognitive control of emotion.** *Ann N Y Acad Sci* 2012, **1251:**E1–E24.
30. Stein MB, Goldin PR, Sareen J, Zorrilla LT, Brown GG: **Increased amygdala activation to angry and contemptuous faces in generalized social phobia.** *Arch Gen Psychiatry* 2002, **59:**1027–1034.
31. Schultz LT, Heimberg RG: **Attentional focus in social anxiety disorder: potential for interactive processes.** *Clin Psychol Rev* 2008, **28:**1206–1221.
32. Lundh LG, Ost LG: **Recognition bias for critical faces in social phobics.** *Behav Res Ther* 1996, **34:**787–794.
33. Horley K, Williams LM, Gonsalvez C, Gordon E: **Face to face: visual scanpath evidence for abnormal processing of facial expressions in social phobia.** *Psychiatry Res* 2004, **127:**43–53.
34. O'Doherty J, Dayan P, Schultz J, Deichmann R, Friston K, Dolan RJ: **Dissociable roles of ventral and dorsal striatum in instrumental conditioning.** *Science* 2004, **304:**452–454.
35. Vrticka P, Simioni S, Fornari E, Schluep M, Vuilleumier P, Sander D: **Neural substrates of social emotion regulation: a FMRI study on imitation and expressive suppression to dynamic facial signals.** *Front Psychol* 2013, **4:**95.
36. Mueller EM, Hofmann SG, Santesso DL, Meuret AE, Bitran S, Pizzagalli DA: **Electrophysiological evidence of attentional biases in social anxiety disorder.** *Psychol Med* 2009, **39:**1141–1152.
37. McRae K, Gross JJ, Weber J, Robertson ER, Sokol-Hessner P, Ray RD, Gabrieli JD, Ochsner KN: **The development of emotion regulation: an fMRI study**

of cognitive reappraisal in children, adolescents and young adults. *Soc Cogn Affect Neurosci* 2012, **7**:11–22.
38. Van der Meer L, Costafreda S, Aleman A, David AS: **Self-reflection and the brain: a theoretical review and meta-analysis of neuroimaging studies with implications for schizophrenia.** *Neurosci Biobehav Rev* 2010, **34**:935–946.
39. Northoff G, Bermpohl F: **Cortical midline structures and the self.** *Trends Cogn Sci* 2004, **8**:102–107.
40. Lemogne C, Delaveau P, Freton M, Guionnet S, Fossati P: **Medial prefrontal cortex and the self in major depression.** *J Affect Disord* 2012, **136**:e1–e11.
41. Goldin PR, McRae K, Ramel W, Gross JJ: **The neural bases of emotion regulation: reappraisal and suppression of negative emotion.** *Biol Psychiatry* 2008, **63**:577–586.

8

Genetic moderation of the association between regulatory focus and reward responsiveness: a proof-of-concept study

Elena L Goetz[1*], Ahmad R Hariri[1,2], Diego A Pizzagalli[3] and Timothy J Strauman[1]

Abstract

Background: Recent studies implicate individual differences in regulatory focus as contributing to self-regulatory dysfunction, particularly not responding to positive outcomes. How such individual differences emerge, however, is unclear. We conducted a proof-of-concept study to examine the moderating effects of genetically driven variation in dopamine signaling, a key modulator of neural reward circuits, on the association between regulatory focus and reward cue responsiveness.

Method: Healthy Caucasians (N=59) completed a measure of chronic regulatory focus and a probabilistic reward task. A common functional genetic polymorphism impacting prefrontal dopamine signaling (*COMT* rs4680) was evaluated.

Results: Response bias, the participants' propensity to modulate behavior as a function of reward, was predicted by an interaction of regulatory focus and *COMT* genotype. Specifically, self-perceived success at achieving promotion goals predicted total response bias, but only for individuals with the *COMT* genotype (Val/Val) associated with relatively increased phasic dopamine signaling and cognitive flexibility.

Conclusions: The combination of success in promotion goal pursuit and Val/Val genotype appears to facilitate responding to reward opportunities in the environment. This study is among the first to integrate an assessment of self-regulatory style with an examination of genetic variability that underlies responsiveness to positive outcomes in goal pursuit.

Keywords: Regulatory focus, Self-regulation, Reward responsiveness, Dopamine, *COMT*

Background

The concept of *self-regulation* describes a broad set of cognitive and behavioral processes by which individuals pursue their goals and respond dynamically to their perceived progress toward them [1]. There is increasing evidence that self-regulatory dysfunction constitutes a vulnerability factor for mood disorders and related forms of psychopathology [2,3]. Variability in goal pursuit strategies and the effectiveness of those strategies reflect differences in both top-down and bottom-up mechanisms as well as the characteristics of the interpersonal context in which goals are being pursued [4]. Although self-regulation has been studied at multiple levels of analysis, little research has examined how those mechanisms interact to influence people's responsiveness to opportunities for goal attainment. Behavioral scientists are beginning to turn their attention to interactions between psychological mechanisms of self-regulation and neurobiological factors that underlie goal pursuit [5]. In this proof-of-concept study, we sought to examine the independent and interactive contributions of a psychological construct relevant to self-regulation of personal goal pursuit and a genetically-based neurobiological individual difference that affects reward-related cognitive processing. Specifically, we investigated whether individual differences in regulatory focus – a preference for pursuing desired end-states via strategic approach vs. avoidance, and/or variation in prefrontal dopamine signaling associated with *COMT* rs4680 genotype, predic-

* Correspondence: elena.goetz@duke.edu
[1]Department of Psychology & Neuroscience, Duke University, Durham, NC, USA
Full list of author information is available at the end of the article

ted performance on a well-validated measure of reward responsiveness.

Regulatory focus and goal pursuit

Regulatory focus theory (RFT) [6,7] proposes two cognitive/motivational systems for personal goal pursuit, the *promotion* and *prevention* systems. Both systems serve the purpose of pursuing positive end-states, but they differ in sensitivity to environmental cues as well as in goal pursuit means and strategies. The promotion system operates by approaching a match with the desired positive outcome and "making good things happen," using eagerness as a means of pursuit. The prevention system operates by avoiding a mismatch with the positive outcome and "keeping bad things from happening," using vigilance as a means of pursuit. RFT proposes that a history of success with one class of goal-pursuit strategies would be expected to induce a bias toward using those strategies, leading an individual to seek out contexts where preferred goals and strategies would be available [8]. RFT thus postulates stable individual differences in goal responsiveness based on the individual's history of promotion and/or prevention socialization and goal pursuit experiences [9,10].

Individual differences in promotion and prevention orientation have dissociable neural correlates. For example, Eddington et al. [11] found that priming of individuals' promotion (but not prevention) goals was associated with activation of the left orbitofrontal cortex (OFC), and magnitude of activation correlated with strength of orientation to promotion goal pursuit. Thus, relative preference for promotion goals is manifested in intensity of neural responses to personalized cues for such goals, suggesting that neurobiological differences could moderate the association between regulatory focus and sensitivity to cues for positive outcomes. Furthermore, chronic perceived failure to attain promotion goals is associated with dysphoric symptoms (e.g., [12]), and Eddington et al. [13] observed that individuals meeting DSM-IV criteria for major depressive disorder manifested attenuated left OFC activation in response to promotion goals. Thus, delineating the neurobiological mechanisms associated with self-regulatory dysfunction may provide new insights into the onset and maintenance of mood disorders [14].

COMT genotype, dopaminergic signaling, and goal pursuit

Several lines of research have established the role of dopamine (DA) signaling in a mesocorticostriatal circuit to update reinforcement information, encode new reward contingencies, and facilitate incentive motivation [15,16]. DA signaling in the prefrontal cortex (PFC) is also important for working memory and attentional processes [17], underlying its role in goal pursuit. A common functional missense polymorphism (rs4680) in the gene for catechol-O-methyltransferase (COMT) – an enzyme responsible for the degradation of catecholamines including DA – is known to affect PFC synaptic DA availability [18-20] as well as relative DA signaling in the mesocorticostriatal circuit [21]. Specifically, the low-activity Methionine (Met) allele of rs4680 results in relatively higher tonic dopamine levels in the PFC, facilitating sustained DA firing and improved maintenance of activity states, as well as a higher threshold to switch activity states. In contrast, the Valine (Val) allele is associated with relatively decreased tonic PFC DA, and higher phasic activity in mesocorticostriatal circuits [21].

Several studies have probed moderating effects of rs4680 on mechanisms of self-regulation, including executive control, learning and adaptability, and affective processing. Both the Met and Val alleles are associated with improved performance and processing efficiency in different contexts, representing a *trade-off* in functionality [22,23]. Research on task switching and reversal learning has found that the Met/Met genotype is associated with increased cognitive stability while the Val/Val genotype is associated with increased cognitive flexibility [24,25]. Thus, the Met allele is associated with improved executive cognition, more efficient PFC function [26], increased attentional control (e.g., [27]), as well as reward-related activation in the PFC [28,29]. In contrast, the Val allele is associated with better adaptability to new contingencies and efficient shifting between informational states, allowing for better reversal learning and serving a protective function against stress and negative affect in the face of failure (e.g., [30,31]). However, the association between rs4680 genotype and reward responding is not straightforward: Val allele carriers have been found to better differentiate win and loss experiences, which can facilitate learning (e.g., [32]), while Met allele carriers have been shown to have potentiated responsiveness to rewards due to higher DA availability (e.g., [29,33]).

Given the importance of task parameters and motivational context in determining which allele is advantageous for regulating goal pursuit, a main effect of rs4680 genotype is unlikely. There is no particular rs4680 genotype that is uniformly advantageous across circumstances and no categorical "risk" genotype; instead, the particular mechanisms, tendencies, and vulnerabilities associated with each genotype are best considered as a trade-off where the outcome depends on the contingencies in the environment. Both proximal and long-term environmental conditions interact with genetic variability to produce particular context-specific advantages and disadvantages in task performance, behavior, and affect.

A similar cost/benefit framework can be found in psychological theories of self-regulation, such as RFT. For example, individuals differ in their capacity to self-regulate and have different styles and strategies of pursuing their goals. They also differ in their responsiveness to feedback about their strategies and their resilience in the face of set-backs. These individual differences may prove to be adaptive or maladaptive depending on the circumstances in which goal pursuit occurs.

Given the commonality that psychological mechanisms of self-regulation and underlying behavioral genetics both frequently involve trade-offs, it is essential to integrate behavioral theories of individual differences in goal pursuit with knowledge about underlying genetic variability. In particular, these factors are likely to interact to produce responses to reward not predictable from either mechanism alone, and potentially constitute pathways to disordered behavior and psychopathology. The present study examined whether the interaction between rs4680 genotype and individual differences in regulatory focus predicted responses to cues for reward.

Modeling the interactive effects of regulatory focus and *COMT* genotype

To measure reward responsiveness, we selected a well-validated laboratory probabilistic reward task designed to provide an experimentally-derived operationalization of reward responsiveness and learning. This task has been used to assess reward responsiveness in healthy populations [34], individuals under stress [35,36], and individuals with depression [37]. In this task, reward responsiveness is operationalized as the tendency to preferentially select a more frequently rewarded stimulus and thus to develop a response bias.

The task offers several advantages as an index of responsiveness to cues for goal attainment. First, it has been characterized as a signal detection task (e.g., [34]), and the signal detection framework has been previously applied to describe the promotion and prevention systems [38,39]. Individuals in a promotion focus seek to achieve "hits" and ensure against errors of omission, resulting in a bias of saying "yes" to a cue that might signify an opportunity for reward. Conversely, individuals in a prevention focus are concerned with making correct rejections and ensuring against errors of commission, resulting in a bias of saying "no" to a potential reward and avoiding incorrect responses. This task in particular is promotion-consistent because the goal is to earn money (rather than to "avoid losing" money) and the payoff structure is framed as gain versus non-gain. Since promotion focus entails a preference for opportunities to make good things happen and a relative attention to cues for reward as well as increased use of approach strategies, the task is a "fit" [7] for a chronic orientation toward promotion goals. Second, the task has been shown to measure reward-related cognitive processes directly relevant to self-regulation of goal pursuit, such as responding to positive feedback and capitalizing on opportunities for gain [34]. Finally, the task provides an efficient way to quantify goal-directed behavior, namely, an accumulation of trial-by-trial responding in pursuit of monetary rewards.

We hypothesized that individual differences in promotion system strength would predict reward-related behavior in our experimental task. However, we also hypothesized that DA signaling in the PFC as modeled by rs4680 genotype would moderate the association between promotion goal pursuit orientation and reward learning. Specifically, we predicted that the rs4680 Val allele would be associated with greater behavioral modulation and flexibility in reward-responsive behavior for individuals with different experiences of promotion goal pursuit. On the other hand, we predicted that the rs4680 Met allele would be associated with a more stable profile of reward responsiveness, regardless of previous goal pursuit experiences or promotion system strength.

Method

Participants

To minimize possible population stratification due to different rs4680 allele frequencies across ethnic groups, our study sample was restricted to Caucasian participants. Study participants (N=67) were recruited via on-campus flyers. All participants were healthy volunteers between 18 and 30 years of age and were self-reported non-smokers, due to previous reports that nicotine has significant effects on reward responsiveness as assessed by the current probabilistic reward task [40]. Participants provided written informed consent, were compensated $10 per hour, and earned a pre-determined amount between $5.80 and $6.20 in the computer task.

Four participants were excluded for non-compliance (N=3) or computer malfunction (N=1). One subject was excluded due to high levels of depressive symptoms, and three subjects were excluded from analyses due to outlier scores (see Data Analysis section for details). Thus, complete and valid data were available for N=59 subjects (35 female). The participants had a mean age = 21.3 ± 2.7 and 92% were right-handed as per self-report. The participants were generally free of psychological distress (mean Beck Depression Inventory-II (BDI-II) score = 5.93, SD = 4.86, range = 1 to 18), although information about medication use and psychiatric history was not collected.

Procedures

Participants completed the 20-min probabilistic reward task and a set of self-report questionnaires, including the Regulatory Focus Questionnaire (RFQ) [8], the BDI-II [41], and the trait version of the Positive and Negative Affect Schedule (PANAS) [42]. In addition, participants gave a saliva sample for genetic analysis. All procedures were approved by the Duke University Institutional Review Board for Non-Medical Research.

Probabilistic reward task

This computerized task is a probabilistic reward-based learning paradigm where participants are asked to identify which of two stimulus images is being presented on each trial. This task has been described in detail elsewhere (e.g., [34]) and has been adopted from Tripp and Alsop [43]. Briefly, participants are instructed press a button on the keyboard to indicate whether a long (13 mm) or short (11.5 mm) mouth is presented (100 ms) within a schematic face. They are told that for *some* of their correct responses, they will receive a monetary reward of 5 cents. One of the images is rewarded more frequently, with a 3:1 reward ratio between the "rich" stimulus and the "lean" stimulus. The task consists of three blocks of 100 trials each, with up to 40 trials per block receiving a reward. The two mouth types are presented with equal frequency, but, unknown to the participants, the reward feedback is asymmetrical in favor of the "rich" stimulus (30 rich versus 10 lean rewards). This paradigm has been found to reliably produce a response bias such that as the task proceeds, the "rich" or more frequently rewarded stimulus is preferentially selected [34,36].

Response bias and discriminability scores were calculated according to the following formulae [34]:

$$\log b = \frac{1}{2}\log\left(\frac{Rich_{correct} * Lean_{incorrect}}{Rich_{incorrect} * Lean_{correct}}\right)$$

$$\log d = \frac{1}{2}\log\left(\frac{Long_{correct} * Short_{correct}}{Long_{incorrect} * Short_{incorrect}}\right)$$

Both formulae were adjusted by adding 0.5 to each value of correct or incorrect responses to eliminate zero values in the denominator (see [37]). Discriminability scores were used to ensure that any findings observed for response bias were not artifacts of task difficulty or individual variability in skill. Response bias towards the more frequently rewarded stimulus can be interpreted as the degree to which an individual engages in the task based on her/his reinforcement history, and as an index of the capacity to respond to reward information and maintain the bias even when reinforcement is intermittent [34,43]. A high response bias results if a participant has a high hit rate for the rich stimulus and a high miss rate for the lean stimulus, reflecting a strategy where participants try to ensure "hits" where they are rewarded for their response (gains), and to ensure against errors of omission (non-gains).

To capture participants' propensity to modulate behavior as a function of prior reward, total response bias across the three blocks of the task was used as the outcome variable. Bias and discriminability were calculated across all valid trials, defined as one where the response reaction time (RT) was between 150 and 2500 msec, and the natural log transformation of RT was within 3 standard deviations of the mean for each participant, as in previous studies using this task (e.g., [34]). A total of 1.43% of the trials were excluded.

Individual differences in regulatory focus

The Regulatory Focus Questionnaire (RFQ) [8] is a 22-item, self-report Likert-style measure designed to assess individual differences in orientation toward promotion and prevention. The questionnaire has four subscales, two that measure individuals' recollection of their early experiences in being oriented toward a promotion or prevention focus by their parents ("history" subscales), and two that measure individuals' subjective assessment of their experiences achieving goals of either a promotion or prevention nature ("success" subscales). Sample items include "My parents encouraged me to try new things" (promotion history), "My parents kept order in our house by having a lot of rules and regulations for me" (prevention history), "I feel like I have made progress towards being successful in life" (promotion success), and "Not being careful enough has gotten me into trouble at times" (prevention success, reverse-scored). Responses are made on a 5-point scale ranging from "never or seldom" or "certainly false" to "very often" or "certainly true," and the item responses within each subscale are averaged to produce four scores: promotion history, prevention history, promotion success, and prevention success. Higgins et al. [8] reported good internal reliability for the promotion success scale (α = 0.73) and prevention success scale (α = 0.80), and the scales showed a two month test-retest reliability of 0.79 correlation or higher. There are no published psychometric data for the history scales, although in the current sample, the reliability scores for the history subscales were α = 0.70 for promotion history, and α = 0.80 for prevention history.

Genotyping

Saliva samples were collected via Oragene kits (Oragene, DNA Genotek; Ottawa, Ontario, Canada). The samples were purified and DNA was extracted and rehydrated according to standard protocols (www.dnagenotek.com). Genotyping of rs4680 was performed using TaqMan allele-specific polymerase chain reaction (PCR) as per Caspi et al. [44]. All genotype calls were ascertained by two independent raters using sequence verified standards with 100% agreement.

Data analysis

Extreme response bias scores (>3 standard deviations from the mean) of two participants were removed to improve the normality of the data. One participant had two

RFQ subscale scores that were >3 standard deviations from the mean and these exerted moderate to high influence on the association of those subscale scores and response bias scores. To prevent statistical distortion due to these outlier scores, this participant was also removed from the final analyses. Genotypes were coded as the number of Met alleles for rs4680.

Results

Distribution of genotypes in the sample

The sample was split into three groups on the basis of genotype: Met/Met (N=14, 24% of sample), Val/Met (N=28, 47%), and Val/Val (N=17, 29%). The three groups were in Hardy-Weinberg equilibrium ($\chi^2(2)=.14$, $p=.93$). The Pearson correlations among the RFQ scores, PANAS trait scores, and response bias are displayed in Table 1.

Discriminability and accuracy

A set of regression analyses examined whether any of the RFQ variables or genotypes predicted total discriminability or accuracy scores as main effects or interactions, and all models and interaction effects were non-significant (all $p > .1$).

Regulatory focus and genotype predicting response bias

We conducted a series of analyses to determine whether individual differences in regulatory focus and/or *COMT* rs4680 genotype predicted total response bias on the reward task. First, a one-way ANOVA was performed to examine whether response bias differed by genotype group; this test was not significant ($F(2, 56) = 0.52$, $p > .5$). In addition, ANOVAs were performed to examine whether any of the regulatory focus variables differed by genotype group, using a Bonferroni correction to control for Type 1 error (4 tests, α threshold =.0125). Only prevention history was found to differ by rs4680 group, $F(2,56) = 4.73$, $p < .05$. A post-hoc Tukey pairwise comparison test revealed that the rs4680 Val/Val group had significantly higher prevention history scores than the Val/Met group (group means = 4.17 versus 3.56 respectively, $p < .05$) but not the Met/Met group (group mean = 4.11, $p > .9$). See Table 2 for descriptive statistics of key study variables by *COMT* rs4680 genotype group.

Next, hierarchical regression analysis was used to test the prediction that regulatory focus and rs4680 genotype interacted to predict response bias. In the first step, the four RFQ variables were entered. This step was non-significant, $F(4, 54) = .56$, $p = .69$, and all βs were non-significant (all $p > .4$). In the second step, rs4680 genotype was added to the model but did not significantly improve fit, $\Delta F(1, 53) = 1.04$, $p = .31$. For the third step, the RFQ variables were mean-centered and regulatory focus X rs4680 interaction terms were created. Each interaction term was entered into the model to evaluate its unique contribution above the main effects of all RFQ variables and the main effect of rs4680. The interaction terms for prevention history, promotion history, and prevention success did not provide significant incremental improvement in model fit: all ΔF $p > .60$. However, the promotion success X rs4680 interaction was a significant predictor of response bias: $\Delta F(1, 52) = 4.13$, $p < .05$, $\Delta R^2 = 0.07$ (see Additional file 1: Table S1). In a reduced model where only promotion success, rs4680 genotype, and the interaction were entered, the overall model fit was marginally significant: $F(3, 55) = 2.39$, $p < .08$, $R^2 = 0.12$.

Next, the promotion success X rs4680 interaction was decomposed by dividing the sample into genotype

Table 1 Correlation matrix for study variables

	Promotion history	Prevention success	Promotion success	PANAS PA	PANAS NA	Total RB
Prevention History	0.05	-.27*	-.34**	-.11	-.33*	-.13
	p>.1	p=.036	p=.008	p>.1	p=.012	p>.1
Promotion History		.38**	.15	.27*	-.26*	-.07
		p=.003	p>.1	p=.038	p=.048	p>.1
Prevention Success			.74**	.11	-.04	.13
			p<.001	p>.1	p>.1	p>.1
Promotion Success				.15	-.06	.14
				p>.1	p>.1	p>.1
PANAS PA					.04	-.14
					p>.1	p>.1
PANAS NA						.19
						p>.1
Total RB						1

* $p<.05$, ** $p<.01$; PANAS = Positive and Negative Affect Schedule, PA = Positive Affect, NA = Negative Affect, RB = Response Bias.

Table 2 Descriptive statistics (means and standard deviations) for study variables by *COMT* genotype group

COMT group	Prevention history	Promotion history	Prevention success	Promotion success	BDI-II	PANAS PA	PANAS NA	Total RB
Val/Val	4.17 (0.58)	3.81 (0.93)	2.92 (0.99)	3.29 (0.86)	5.00 (3.94)	32.06 (6.16)	13.41 (4.17)	0.11 (0.15)
Val/Met	3.56 (0.78)	3.99 (0.68)	2.93(1.04)	3.39 (0.81)	6.93 (5.13)	34.46 (5.47)	14.29 (3.79)	0.11 (0.14)
Met/Met	4.11 (0.78)	4.13 (0.59)	2.87(1.15)	3.25 (1.14)	5.07 (5.24)	32.50 (6.43)	13.57 (3.80)	0.16 (0.18)

PANAS = Positive and Negative Affect Schedule, PA = Positive Affect, NA = Negative Affect, RB = Response Bias.

groups and examining the linear association between promotion success and response bias within each group. These regression analyses revealed that a significant association between promotion success and response bias was present only in the Val/Val genotype group: $F(1, 15) = 9.85$, $p < .01$, adjusted $R^2 = .36$. The Val/Met and Met/Met groups did not manifest any association between promotion success and response bias (both $F < .15$; see Figure 1).

Finally, a tertiary split was performed on promotion success scores in order to compare mean response bias across the range of promotion success. The *COMT* rs4680 genotype groups Val/Met and Met/Met were combined. Total response bias was significantly lower for the Val/Val group compared to Met allele carriers in the lowest third of promotion scores, $t(18) = -2.30$, $p = .034$ (Additional file 2: Figure S1). There were no significant differences in response bias across genotype groups between those participants in the middle ($p > .82$) or highest third ($p > .50$) of promotion success.

Discussion

The goal of this proof-of-concept study was to examine how regulatory focus and a common functional polymorphism affecting DA signaling predicted behavior in a probabilistic reward task. The results confirmed our hypothesis that rs4680 genotype, which biases COMT function and associated DA signaling in the PFC, moderates the degree to which a particular pattern of self-regulatory success experiences affects reward responsiveness. Specifically, our results showed that the combination of success in promotion goal pursuit and Val/Val genotype appears to facilitate responding to reward opportunities in the environment. On the other hand, Met allele carriers did not show an association between regulatory success in pursuing promotion goals and developing a reward-related response bias in our task.

Research examining the nature and consequences of self-regulation may provide a context for interpreting the present findings, both from the perspective of basic science and in regard to potential pathways of vulnerability for mood disorders. For example, we suggest that it is important to recognize that the observed associations among regulatory focus, rs4680 genotype, and reward responsiveness are not readily apparent at the phenotypic level. There was no broad association found between rs4680 genotype and self-regulatory style. This finding is consistent with previous research indicating that regulatory orientation is primarily shaped by accumulated experience with success or failure in goal pursuit and is independent from

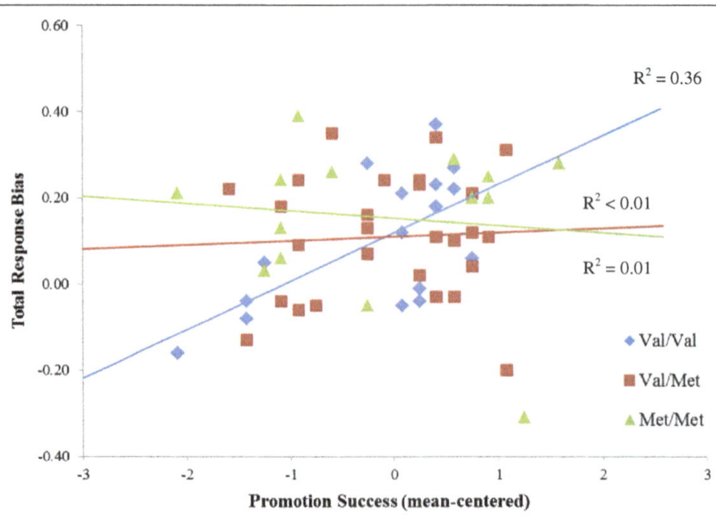

Figure 1 Total response bias as a function of promotion success score, across *COMT* rs4680 genotype groups. Promotion success predicted response bias only for the Val/Val participants, $p < .01$, adjusted $R^2 = .36$.

biological factors such as temperament [9], and also with the fact that variability in both mechanisms involves trade-offs that manifest in context-specific ways.

In this study, we hypothesized that an interaction of rs4680 genotype and self-regulatory style would result in predictable effects on responses to probabilistic reward feedback. The reward task yielded a reliably quantifiable measure of reward responsiveness, that is, participants' propensity to modulate behavior as a function of prior reward. Individuals who are more responsive to reward feedback will preferentially select the more frequently rewarded stimulus and thus manifest a stronger response bias across the task. As noted previously, the task is promotion-consistent because outcomes are presented to participants as gain/non-gain – to earn money (instead of to "avoid losing" money). Therefore, individuals who believe that they are successful at achieving promotion goals should manifest a response bias that favors the more rewarded or "rich" stimulus. Interestingly, we did not observe a main effect of rs4680 genotype or promotion orientation on reward responsiveness. Rather, the effect of a history of promotion success on reward responsiveness was found to be moderated by rs4680 genotype (specific to the Val/Val genotype group).

The pattern of findings revealed a terminative interaction, where among individuals reporting relatively low levels of success pursuing promotion goals, the Val/Val genotype was associated with significantly lower response bias than in Met allele carriers. However, among individuals reporting frequent success experiences in the promotion domain, the Val/Val genotype was associated with mean response bias that did not significantly differ than that observed for Val/Met or Met/Met genotypes. Self-reported promotion success did not predict response bias among Val/Met or Met/Met genotypes, which also did not differ from each either. Thus, no Met allele dose effect was observed either as a main effect or as an interaction.

This pattern of results corresponds with the trade-off framework for interpreting *COMT*-related variability in reward sensitivity that was described above. The Val/Val individuals who reported low levels of promotion success demonstrated significantly lower total response bias scores than Met allele carriers. There is the possibility that Val/Val individuals are more susceptible to fluctuations in DA when rewards are omitted and therefore have greater difficulty integrating reward-related information over time. This would be an example of flexibility and behavioral adaptability being disadvantageous within a particular context, and such a neurobiological profile would be especially maladaptive given a personal history of low promotion success. Thus, Val/Val individuals with low promotion success might constitute a group of individuals who would be particularly vulnerable to anhedonia or reward insensitivity in the face of chronic promotion failure experiences. There is evidence that Val/Val individuals show decreased responsiveness to reinforcers [28,29], and reduced motivational drive to pursue reinforcers would interfere with successful promotion goal pursuit.

The fact that Met allele carriers did not show modulation of their response bias based on their degree of success in pursuing their promotion goals fits with a "resilience" model. Even in the context of low promotion success, individuals with higher tonic PFC dopamine (Met allele carriers) did not manifest low levels of reward-responsive behavior. However, there is a competing interpretation: that Met allele carriers are not able to increase reward-related responding based on their previous goal-pursuit experiences, which might adversely affect the pursuit of promotion goals. Such an alternative hypothesis is consistent with previous findings of cognitive [24,25] and affective [30] inflexibility associated with the Met allele. There may be some relative deficits in reward-related responding for Met allele carriers who have had successful self-regulatory experiences, because those individuals with high promotion success scores exhibited only average response bias scores. The Met allele carriers might have an inability to update or adapt behavior via reward feedback that could create some vulnerability in the face of future self-regulatory challenges or failure experiences.

The results from this study illustrate that an integrative approach to *COMT* variability and self-regulation has the potential to reveal novel pathways of psychological vulnerability. Self-regulation involves a complex set of processes including goal selection and pursuit, cognitive and emotional control, and ongoing decision-making [45]. Factors such as reward responsiveness, impulsivity/distractibility, and affective resilience can impact how goals are pursued and how feedback about progress is managed, and individual variability in *COMT* has been shown to affect all of these processes. A research strategy that applies individual differences information from genetic sources to studies of ongoing, situationally-embedded self-regulation might yield context-sensitive examples of when these processes break down and produce regulatory dysfunction and, possibly, clinical disorders.

Regions in the PFC, particularly the OFC, are involved in responsiveness to motivationally salient feedback and shifts in goal pursuit originating from bottom-up processes (e.g., [28]) as well as top-down processes (e.g., [11]). Thus, the OFC is likely to be a site that mediates the interaction between individual differences in regulatory focus and rs4680 genotype to produce reward-related behavior, and at least one study [13] has observed that clinically depressed individuals manifest attenuated left OFC activation in response to their own promotion goals.

The significant interaction between promotion success and rs4680 genotype was detected even in the hierarchical multiple regression models that included other regulatory focus variables as covariates. These analyses were particularly important to differentiate promotion success from prevention success, which were substantially correlated ($r=.74$, $p<.001$). Despite the intercorrelation, it was success in attaining promotion goals, and not successful prevention goal attainment, that predicted reward responsiveness for the Val/Val genotype. RFT postulates fundamental differences between the promotion and prevention systems with regard to the targets of goal pursuit (e.g., "ideals" vs. "oughts"), the strategies used to pursue them ("making good things happen" vs. "keeping bad things from happening"), and the motivational impetus that underlies goal pursuit (eagerness vs. vigilance). These behavioral and cognitive distinctions appear to be accompanied by differences in cortical activation when promotion vs. prevention goals are primed [11,13], although additional research is needed to characterize the shared and unique neural circuitry associated with these two hypothetical cognitive/motivational systems. Such research, in combination with a genetic/neurobiological level of analysis, could help to elucidate pathways by which self-regulatory dysfunction could lead to the onset and maintenance of mood disorders.

There are several limitations of this study that should be acknowledged. First, the relatively small sample size leaves us vulnerable to statistical noise including false positives. However, this is more problematic in the absence of significant effects (i.e., false negatives), which could simply reflect inadequate power, and thus one should use caution when interpreting non-significant results such as the lack of main effects. The fact that we found significant effects robust to the influence of covariates suggests the observed interaction between self-regulatory style and rs4680 genotype is valid. Nevertheless, replication of the effects described herein is necessary to further the possible utility of our interaction model for understanding clinically relevant outcomes (e.g., risk for mood disorders). Second, because the genetic analyses were restricted to a Caucasian-only sample, generalizability may be limited. It will be of interest to examine this effect in non-Caucasian samples. Third, although the task provided a well-validated operationalization of the experience of responding to reward feedback, its external validity as a proxy of goal pursuit behavior is understandably limited. Previous studies of the neurobiological substrates underlying regulatory focus relied on idiographic stimuli that captured individuals' personal goals [11,13], and the degree to which earning money was a goal of the participants in this study was implied by their participation but not explicitly verified. A future study could extend these findings by obtaining genetic information on participants who undergo neuroimaging when exposed to their goals, or using another kind of goal-pursuit task such as anagram solving that is related to perseverance and conscious decision-making about effort and motivation. In addition, a future exploration of these effects should include measures of potential important contributory variables such as stressful life events (particularly during development) and state-level anxiety, as these both could impact the development and manifestation of one's regulatory focus.

Conclusions

This study used a research strategy that integrated neurobiological variability (as indexed by a common functional genetic polymorphism) and trait-like differences in cognitive/motivational systems to predict reward-related behavior in a novel way. Our findings showed that – consistent with a trade-off model – rs4680 genotype interacts with self-regulatory success experiences to predict reward responsive behavior only in individuals with a Val/Val genotype, and this pattern could be adaptive at high levels of success or maladaptive at low levels of success. By contrast, the response profiles of Met allele carriers indicated that previous goal pursuit success does not impact their development of a reward-related response bias. Our approach extends our understanding of how top-down self-regulatory mechanisms affect behavior by examining the moderating influence of bottom-up biological mechanisms. This interaction of mechanisms and methodologies is likely to be a fruitful avenue of future inquiry to elaborate the individual differences affecting complex behaviors and psychiatric phenotypes, such as reward dysfunction in depression or addiction [46].

Additional files

Additional file 1: Table S1. Regression results: Regulatory focus variables, *COMT* rs4680 genotype, and interactions predicting total response bias.

Additional file 2: Figure S1. *COMT* rs4680 Val/Val verses Met-carrier response bias scores by promotion success groups. The * indicates that mean response bias values were significantly different, $p<.05$.

Abbreviations

(RFT): Regulatory focus theory; (COMT): Catechol-o-methyltransferase; (DA): Dopamine; (RFQ): Regulatory Focus Questionnaire.

Competing interests

DAP has received consulting fees from ANT North America Inc. (Advanced Neuro Technology), AstraZeneca, Shire, and Ono PharmaUSA, and honoraria from AstraZeneca for studies unrelated to this project. The authors declare that they have no other competing interests.

Authors' contributions

ELG helped conceive of the design of the study, collected data and conducted genotyping, performed data analysis, and took the lead on writing the manuscript. ARH helped conceive of the design of the study, oversaw genetic analysis, and contributed to writing the manuscript. DAP contributed to the design of the study and data interpretation, as well as consulted on the implementation of the experimental task and provided feedback on the manuscript. TJS helped conceive of the design of the study, contributed to data analysis, and contributed to writing the manuscript. All authors read and approved the final manuscript.

Acknowledgements

The authors would like to thank Yuliya Nikolova, Karen Sugden, and Ben Williams for their assistance with genotyping, and Matthew Hoyle for his assistance with data collection. This work was supported by the National Institute on Drug Abuse [R01 DA031579 to Timothy J. Strauman, which is supported by the NIH Common Fund and managed by the OD/Office of Strategic Coordination, and P30 DA023026 to Kenneth Dodge and Philip Costanzo]; by Duke University funding to Ahmad R. Hariri; and an NSF Graduate Research Fellowship to Elena L. Goetz.

Author details

[1]Department of Psychology & Neuroscience, Duke University, Durham, NC, USA. [2]Institute for Genome Sciences and Policy, Duke University, Durham, NC, USA. [3]Department of Psychiatry, Harvard University Medical School, Boston, MA, USA.

References

1. Carver CS, Scheier MF: **Origins and functions of positive and negative affect: a control- process view.** *Psychol Rev* 1990, **97:**19–35.
2. Karoly P: **Mechanisms of self-regulation: a systems view.** *Annu Rev Psychol* 1993, **44:**23–52.
3. Strauman TJ: **Self-regulation and depression.** *Self and Identity* 2002, **1:**151–157.
4. Strauman TJ, Wilson WA: **Individual differences in approach and avoidance: Behavioral activation/inhibition and regulatory focus as distinct systems.** In *Handbook of Self- Regulation and Personality.* Edited by Hoyle R. New York: Guilford Press; 2010:447–473.
5. Carver CS, Johnson SL, Joormann J: **Two-mode models of self-regulation as a tool for conceptualizing effects of the serotonin system in normal behavior and diverse disorders.** *Curr Dir Psychol Sci* 2009, **18:**195–199.
6. Higgins ET: **Beyond pleasure and pain.** *Am Psychol* 1997, **52:**1280–1300.
7. Higgins ET: **Promotion and prevention: Regulatory focus as a motivational principle.** In *Advances in Experimental Social Psychology, Volume 30.* Edited by Zanna MP. New York: Academic; 1998,1–46.
8. Higgins ET, Friedman RS, Harlow RE, Idson LC, Ayduk ON, Taylor A: **Achievement orientations from subjective histories of success: promotion pride versus prevention pride.** *Eur J Soc Psych* 2001, **31:**3–23.
9. Manian N, Papadakis AA, Strauman TJ, Essex MJ: **The development of children's ideal and ought self-guides: parenting, temperament, and individual differences in guide strength.** *J Pers* 2006, **74:**1619–1645.
10. Strauman TJ: **Stability within the self: a longitudinal study of the implications of self discrepancy theory.** *J Pers Soc Psychol* 1996, **71:**1142 1153.
11. Eddington KM, Dolcos F, Cabeza R, Krishnan KRR, Strauman TJ: **Neural correlates of promotion and prevention goal activation: an fMRI study using an idiographic approach.** *J Cogn Neurosci* 2007, **19:**1152–1162.
12. Miller AK, Markman KD: **Depression, regulatory focus, and motivation.** *Pers Individ Dif* 2007, **43:**427–436.
13. Eddington KM, Dolcos F, McLean AN, Cabeza R, Krishnan KRR, Strauman TJ: **Neural correlates of idiographic goal priming in depression: goal-specific dysfunctions in the orbitofrontal cortex.** *Soc Cogn Affect Neurosci* 2009, **4:**238–246.
14. Hasler G, Drevets WC, Manji HK, Charney DS: **Discovering endophenotypes for major depression.** *Neuropsychopharmacology* 2004, **29:**1765–1781.
15. Depue RA, Collins PF: **Neurobiology of the structure of personality: dopamine, facilitation of incentive motivation, and extraversion.** *Behav Brain Sci* 1999, **22:**491–517.
16. Schultz W: **Getting formal with dopamine and reward.** *Neuron* 2002, **36:**241–263.
17. Goldman-Rakic PS, Muly EC III, Williams GV: **D(1) receptors in prefrontal cells and circuits.** *Brain Res Rev* 2000, **31:**295–301.
18. Chen J, Lipska BK, Halim N, Ma QD, Matsumoto M, Melhem S, Kolachana BS, Hyde TM, Herman MM, Apud J, Egan MF, Kleinman JE, Weinberger DR: **Functional analysis of genetic variation in catechol-O-methyltransferase (COMT): effects on mRNA, protein, and enzyme activity in postmortem human brain.** *Am J Hum Genet* 2004, **75:**807–821.
19. Matsumoto M, Weickert CS, Akil M, Lipska BK, Hyde TM, Herman MM, Kleinman JE, Weinberger DR: **Catechol O-methyltransferase mRNA expression in human and rat brain: evidence for a role in cortical neuronal function.** *Neuroscience* 2003, **116:**127–137.
20. Tunbridge EM, Harrison PJ, Weinberger DR: **Catechol-*o*-methyltransferase, cognition, and psychosis: Val^{158}Met and beyond.** *Biol Psychiatry* 2006, **60:**141–151.
21. Bilder RM, Volavka J, Lachman HM, Grace AA: **The catechol-*O*-methyltransferase polymorphism: relations to the tonic-phasic dopamine hypothesis and neuropsychiatric phenotypes.** *Neuropsychopharmacology* 2004, **29:**1943–1961.
22. Barnett JH, Scoriels L, Munafò MR: **Meta-analysis of the cognitive effects of the catechol-*O*-methyltransferase gene val158/108met polymorphism.** *Biol Psychiatry* 2008, **64:**137–144.
23. Mier D, Kirsch P, Meyer-Lindenberg A: **Neural substrates of pleiotropic action of genetic variation in COMT: a meta-analysis.** *Mol Psychiatry* 2010, **15:**918–927.
24. Colzato LS, Waszak F, Nieuwenhuis S, Posthuma D, Hommel B: **The flexible mind is associated with the catechol-O-methyltransferase (*COMT*) Val^{158}Met polymorphism: evidence for a role of dopamine in the control of task-switching.** *Neuropsychologia* 2010, **48:**2764–2768.
25. Krugel LK, Biele G, Mohr PN, Li SC, Heekeren HR: **Genetic variation in dopaminergic neuromodulation influences the ability to rapidly and flexibly adapt decisions.** *Proc Natl Acad Sci USA* 2009, **106:**17951–17956.
26. Egan MF, Goldberg TE, Kolachana BS, Callicott JH, Mazzanti CM, Straub RE, Goldman D, Weinberger DR: **Effect of COMT Val108/158 Met genotype on frontal lobe function and risk for schizophrenia.** *Proc Natl Acad Sci USA* 2001, **98:**6917–6922.
27. Blasi G, Mattay VS, Bertolino A, Elvevåg B, Callicott JH, Das S, Kolachana BS, Egan MF, Goldberg TE, Weinberger DR: **Effect of catechol-O-methyltransferase val158met genotype on attentional control.** *J Neurosci* 2005, **25:**5038–5045.
28. Dreher JC, Kohn P, Kolachana B, Weinberger DR, Berman KF: **Variation in dopamine genes influences responsivity of the human reward system.** *Proc Natl Acad Sci USA* 2009, **106:**617–622.
29. Yacubian J, Sommer T, Schroeder K, Gläscher J, Kalisch R, Leuenberger B, Braus DF, Büchel C: **Gene-gene interaction associated with neural reward sensitivity.** *Proc Natl Acad Sci* 2007, **104:**8125–8130.
30. Drabant EM, Hariri AR, Meyer-Lindenberg A, Munoz KE, Mattay VS, Kolachana BS, Egan MF, Weinberger DR: **Catechol O-methyltransferase val158met genotype and neural mechanisms related to affective arousal and regulation.** *Arch Gen Psychiatry* 2006, **63:**1396–1406.
31. Smolka MN, Schumann G, Wrase J, Grüsser SM, Flor H, Mann K, Braus DF, Goldman D, Büchel C, Heinz A: **Catechol-*O*-methyltransferase*val^{158}met* genotype affects processing of emotional stimuli in the amygdala and prefrontal cortex.** *J Neurosci* 2005, **25:**836–842.
32. Camara E, Krämer UM, Cunillera T, Marco-Pallarés J, Cucurell D, Nager W, Mestres-Missé A, Bauer P, Schüle R, Schöls L, Tempelmann C, Rodriguez-Fornells A, Münte TF: **The effects of COMT (Val108/158Met) and DRD4 (SNP −521) dopamine genotypes on brain activations related to valence and magnitude of rewards.** *Cereb Cortex* 2010, **20:**1985–1996. doi:10.1093/cercor/bhp263.
33. Schmack K, Schlagenhauf F, Sterzer P, Wrase J, Beck A, Dembler T, Kalus P, Puls I, Sander T, Heinz A, Gallinat J: **Catechol-O-methyltransferase val158met genotype influences neural processing of reward anticipation.** *Neuroimage* 2008, **42:**1631–1638. doi:10.1016/j.neuroimage.2008.06.019.
34. Pizzagalli DA, Jahn AL, O'Shea JP: **Toward an objective characterization of an anhedonic phenotype: a signal-detection approach.** *Biol Psychiatry* 2005, **57:**319–327.
35. Bogdan R, Pizzagalli DA: **Acute stress reduces reward responsiveness: implications for depression.** *Biol Psychiatry* 2006, **60:**1147–1154.
36. Pizzagalli DA, Bogdan R, Ratner KG, Jahn AL: **Increased perceived stress is associated with blunted hedonic capacity: potential implications for depression research.** *Behav Res Ther* 2007, **45:**2742–2753.
37. Pizzagalli DA, Iosifescu D, Hallett LA, Ratner KG, Fava M: **Reduced hedonic capacity in major depressive disorder: evidence from a probabilistic reward task.** *J Psychiatr Res* 2008, **43:**76–87.
38. Crowe E, Higgins ET: **Regulatory focus and strategic inclinations: promotion and prevention in decision-making.** *Organ Behav Hum Decis Process* 1997, **69:**117–132.
39. Cunningham WA, Raye CL, Johnson MK: **Neural correlates of evaluation associated with promotion and prevention regulatory focus.** *Cogn Affect Behav Neurosci* 2005, **5:**202–211.

40. Barr RS, Pizzagalli DA, Culhane MA, Goff DC, Evins AE: **A single dose of nicotine enhances reward responsiveness in non-smokers: implications for development of dependence.** *Biol Psychiatry* 2008, **63:**1061–1065.
41. Beck AT, Steer RA, Brown GK: *Beck Depression Inventory Manual.* 2nd edition. San Antonio: The Psychological Corporation; 1996.
42. Watson D, Clark LA, Tellegen A: **Development and validation of brief measures of positive and negative affect: the PANAS scales.** *J Pers Soc Psychol* 1988, **54:**1063–1070.
43. Tripp G, Alsop B: **Sensitivity to reward frequency in boys with attention deficit hyperactivity disorder.** *J Clin Child Psychol* 1999, **28:**366–375.
44. Caspi A, Langley K, Milne B, Moffitt TE, O'Donovan M, Owen MJ, Polo Tomas M, Poulton R, Rutter M, Taylor A, Williams B, Thapar A: **A replicated molecular genetic basis for subtyping antisocial behavior in children with attention-deficit/hyperactivity disorder.** *Arch Gen Psychiatry* 2008, **65:**203–210.
45. Carver CS, Scheier MF: **Self-regulatory perspectives on personality.** In *Handbook of psychology: Personality and social psychology, Volume 5.* Edited by Millon T, Lerner MJ. New York: Wiley; 2003,185–208.
46. Hariri AR: **The neurobiology of individual differences in complex behavioral traits.** *Annu Rev Neurosci* 2009, **32:**225–247.

9

Imaging the pathophysiology of major depressive disorder - from localist models to circuit-based analysis

Michael T Treadway* and Diego A Pizzagalli*

Abstract

The neuroimaging literature of Major Depressive Disorder (MDD) has grown substantially over the last several decades, facilitating great advances in the identification of specific brain regions, neurotransmitter systems and networks associated with depressive illness. Despite this progress, fundamental questions remain about the pathophysiology and etiology of MDD. More importantly, this body of work has yet to directly influence clinical practice. It has long been a goal for the fields of clinical psychology and psychiatry to have a means of making objective diagnoses of mental disorders. Frustratingly little movement has been achieved on this front, however, and the 'gold-standard' of diagnostic validity and reliability remains expert consensus. In light of this challenge, the focus of the current review is to provide a critical summary of key findings from different neuroimaging approaches in MDD research, including structural, functional and neurochemical imaging studies. Following this summary, we discuss some of the current conceptual obstacles to better understanding the pathophysiology of depression, and conclude with recommendations for future neuroimaging research.

Keywords: Major Depression, Neuroimaging, PET, MRI, Serotonin, Dopamine, MRS, Glutamate, GABA, Inflammation

Introduction

The neuroimaging literature of Major Depressive Disorder (MDD) has exploded in recent years, with the current pace of research including over 250 new articles listed each year in PubMed alone. A substantial majority of these studies have been focused on identifying putative biological and neural variables that differentiate individuals with MDD from psychiatrically healthy controls. This program of research has been successful in demonstrating a large number of abnormalities in MDD samples, including alterations across measures of brain structure and function; endocrine, immune and neurotransmitter systems; and large-scale network organization. Despite this progress, however, fundamental questions remain about the pathophysiology and etiology of MDD as well as the strengths and pitfalls of neuroimaging methodologies in attempting to answer them.

Even more importantly, this body of work has yet to influence clinical practice in any substantive way. A longstanding goal of clinical psychology and biological psychiatry research has been the development of objective tests for diagnosing mental disorders. Frustratingly little progress has been made on this front, however, and the 'gold-standard' of diagnostic validity and reliability remains expert consensus, a practice that is essentially unchanged from Meehl's day [1]. Despite our capacity to measure an astonishing array of biological signals in MDD patients, we have yet to find a single measure - or a combination of variables - that tracks symptom expression with the requisite specificity and sensitivity to be reliably meaningful in the clinic.

It is against this backdrop that we present the current review. First, we provide a (non-exhaustive) summary of the major findings that have emerged from different neuroimaging approaches. This includes a review of structural, functional, neurochemical, neuroendocrine and neuroimmune imaging studies in MDD. Following this summary, we discuss some of the current conceptual obstacles to better understanding the pathophysiology of

* Correspondence: mtreadway@mclean.harvard.edu; dap@mclean.harvard.edu
Center for Depression Anxiety and Stress Research, McLean Hospital/Harvard Medical School, 115 Mill Street, Belmont, MA 02478, USA

depression, and present the use of circuit-based analysis as a methodological path forward.

Review

Neuroimaging and the pathophysiology of MDD

Morphometric neuroimaging studies

A large number of studies in MDD patients to date have identified structural alterations across multiple tissue classes. These findings have been summarized using me ta-analytic approaches reporting on structural alterations observed using regions-of-interest (ROI) tracing-based methods [2,3], voxel-based methods (VBM) [4], post-mortem tissue analysis [5], and diffusion tensor imaging of white-matter integrity [6]. Tracer-based methods have provided especially strong evidence for reduced hippocampal volume and enlarged ventricles in MDD [3]. These results have been recapitulated by voxel-based methods, which additionally implicate a more distributed network of structural alterations associated with MDD, including the anterior cingulate cortex (ACC), medial prefrontal cortex (mPFC), orbitofrontal cortex (OFC), dorsolateral prefrontal cortex (dlPFC), the striatum, and the amygdala. A limitation of these findings is that they are mostly drawn from cross-sectional designs. Therefore, it is difficult to know whether such structural differences represent a biological diathesis, a compensatory adaptation, or a consequence of the illness.

A handful of longitudinal studies have addressed this significant limitation by investigating structural changes as a function of depressive state and treatment outcome. \For some regions, including the hippocampus and medial prefrontal areas, several studies have suggested that grey-matter volume may decline monotonically over multiple depressive episodes [7,8]. In contrast, the amygdala may become enlarged prior to a first depressive episode [9]. Structural integrity of these regions has also been found to partially predict symptom remission. Specifically, hippocampal volumes have been found to prospectively correlate with treatment outcome at both one- and three-year follow-ups [10,11], and longitudinal studies have found that decreased hippocampal volumes were partially restored following successful treatment or spontaneous remission [11-13]. Importantly, similar morphometric changes in these regions have also been associated with high levels of trait negative affect in non-depressed individuals who have an elevated polygenic risk profile for developing MDD. This has been observed using both genome-wide analysis [14] and examinations of non-depressed individuals with a family history of MDD [15,16], consistent with the hypothesis that these structural decreases likely reflect an endophenotype marker [17].

Taken together, structural imaging studies have found robust evidence for group-level differences in grey-matter volume across cortical and sub-cortical areas. Longitudinal studies provide the strongest evidence linking these changes to the onset and remission of a depressive state, suggesting that they are either causally involved in MDD or that they at least meaningfully fluctuate with illness progression. Future longitudinal work, especially with prospective-cohort designs, will help further elucidate the role of these morphometric alterations in the etiopathophysiology of MDD.

Functional neuroimaging studies

Functional imaging studies of MDD have also grown substantially over the last two decades, with a wide variety of functional domains probed using a large number of tasks. We will therefore limit our focus to two general domains that have been most frequently examined in depression studies: (1) emotion processing and regulation, and (2) reward processing (Figure 1). For a more comprehensive discussion of other aspects of the functional neuroimaging literature in major depression, we refer readers to several excellent recent reviews and meta-analyses: [18-20].

Functional neuroimaging of emotion processing Arguably the most common domain assessed by functional imaging studies of depression is responses to emotional stimuli. Examples include studies of responses to both explicit and implicit presentations of affect-laden stimuli [21-23], recruitment of cognitive control mechanisms required to gate out affective 'distractors' during simple working memory and attention tasks [24,25], and deliberate top-down control of affective responses to positive and negative stimuli [26-29]. The most replicated result observed during passive presentation of emotional stimuli is a heightened responsivity in limbic regions - especially the amygdala - to negatively valenced stimuli in depressed individuals. For tasks that require subjects to efficiently 'gate-out' affective content in order to better attend to non-emotional aspects of a task or stimulus, elevated limbic activity is often accompanied by hypo-activation in prefrontal areas, including aspects of ventromedial PFC, ventrolateral prefrontal cortex (vlPFC), ACC, and dlPFC. It is noteworthy that these same regions frequently exhibit volumetric abnormalities.

While prefrontal hypo-activations are commonly interpreted as evidence of a top-down control 'deficit', it is unclear whether they reflect a local deficit in network recruitment or simply a failure to engage in the task as effectively as controls. Interestingly, when task performance is matched across depressed and non-depressed individuals, there is evidence for hyper-response in prefrontal areas [30,31], possibly indicating cortical inefficiency. In addition, the specificity of alterations in amygdalar and prefrontal networks to depression is unclear, as similar patterns are frequently observed in studies of anxiety, and

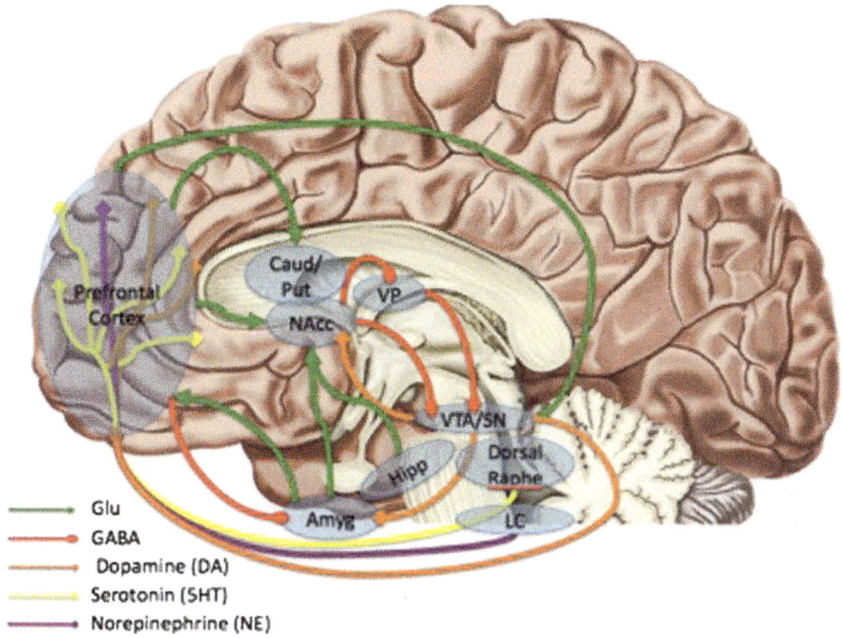

Figure 1 Regions, transmitters and circuits implicated in the pathology of major depressive disorder (MDD) by human neuroimaging studies. Past studies have identified alterations in monoamine levels and receptor availability as well as alterations in glutamate and GABA. These neurotransmitter systems participate in larger circuits involved in the experience and regulation of emotion, responses to stress, and processing of rewards. Note: placement of structure labels is approximate. Amyg = amygdala; Caud = Caudate; GABA = GABAergic projections; Glu = glutamatergic projections; Hipp = hippocampus; NAcc = nucleus accumbens; Put = Putamen; SN = substantia nigra; VP = ventral pallidum; VTA = ventral tegmental area. Republished with permission from Treadway and Zald [49].

only a few direct comparison studies have been conducted to date [32,33]. Future research is needed to further isolate the specific alterations in cortico-limbic responses to emotion in MDD, and to determine the extent to which these effects are specific to a depressed mood or rather represent a common mechanism associated with other forms of internalizing psychopathology.

In contrast to experimental paradigms that require either passive emotional processing or implicit emotion regulation in the form of attentional control, findings of studies of directed emotion regulation in MDD are highly variable. In healthy controls, down-regulation of negative emotion has been consistently associated with increased activation in medial and dlPFC areas and reduced activity in the amygdala [34]. These observations, combined with observations of impaired functional coupling between mPFC and amygdala during passive viewing of affective stimuli [35], led investigators to hypothesize that depressed patients would be less successful in reducing amygdala reactivity - and associated negative emotions - when explicitly regulating emotional responses to negative stimuli. Empirical support for this hypothesis, however, has been mixed. Only one study has reported that depressed patients experience more difficulty in decreasing sadness than controls [26], while others have found no differences [27-29]. These studies have also generally failed to observe impaired cortico-amygdala interactions during explicit emotion regulation in MDD. Consequently, these data suggest that emotion regulation deficits in MDD do not reflect a true inability to regulate emotion when explicitly directed to do so, at least not in the context of typical laboratory-based affective stimuli.

Functional neuroimaging of reward processing Another primary area of functional neuroimaging research in MDD involves responses to rewarding stimuli. While early functional magnetic resonance imaging (fMRI) (and non-imaging) studies frequently operationalized reward in terms of the passive viewing or consumption of positively valenced stimuli (for example [36-38]), more recent work has increasingly emphasized constructs of reward anticipation [39-42], reinforcement learning [43,44] and motivation [45-47], which are psychologically and neurobiologically distinct. This shift has been motivated largely by the enhanced understanding of functional segregation of dopaminergic cortico-striatal systems in reward processing, which have been found to underlie anticipation, learning, and salience of rewards, rather than affective responses to them [48]. Indeed, reward-related symptoms are especially amenable to a translational neuroscience approach, given how well characterized reward-related pathways are by both preclinical and human neuroeconomic studies (see [49] for a longer discussion). The most common observation from this body of work is hypo-recruitment in MDD patients of striatal regions associated with reward salience, anticipation and learning, possibly reflecting alterations in the availability of pre-synaptic pools in dopaminergic afferents to striatal sub-regions [50-52] (see also discussion of dopamine imaging studies below). In addition, altered crosstalk between cortical and ventral striatal regions has been associated with rapid habituation to rewarding stimuli, which is also consistent with anhedonic presentation [53].

In sum, these studies highlight cortico-striatal pathways as critically involved in specific symptom domains of MDD. Of note, there is arguably greater consistency in studies of reward processing in MDD than of other cognitive processes. This may reflect the fact that reward processing studies have focused on a more homogeneous symptom domain and that the neurobiology of normative reward functioning is better understood.

Neurochemical imaging studies in MDD

The hypothesis that specific neurotransmitter systems represent a core pathology of mood disorders is among the oldest in biological psychiatry (see, for example, Schildkraut [54]). For most of modern psychiatric history, this line of work has emphasized alterations in monoamines, given early observations that administration of various monoamine-reducing drugs or pharmacological manipulations could induce depressive symptoms. It was only decades later, however, when the *in vivo* visualization of these signaling pathways could be achieved.

Currently, the two most widely used approaches to neurochemical imaging in psychiatric populations are Positron Emission Tomography (PET) and Magnetic Resonance Spectroscopy (MRS). A less commonly used technique is Single Photon Emission Computed Tomography (SPECT). Both PET and SPECT rely on the measurement of radioactive decay from an injected isotope as the basis of targeting the spatial distribution of a particular receptor or protein. In contrast, MRS takes advantage of the different magnetic resonance signatures associated with distinct molecular compounds, and can be useful for quantifying the availability of relatively abundant neurotransmitters such as glutamate (Glu) and γ-aminobutyric acid (GABA). Both of these methods have contributed to the study of pathophysiology in MDD, and are notable for both their positive and null findings. In this section, we review some of the primary neurotransmitter systems that have been investigated in MDD using these techniques.

Neurochemical imaging of serotonin systems in MDD

Interest in serotonin (5-HT) has been central to depression research over the last three decades, owing primarily to reported success of antidepressant pharmacotherapies that selectively target the serotonergic system in both humans and animal models. Evidence from preclinical studies further supports a role for serotonin in MDD symptoms, particularly those related to the processing of stress. Under normal conditions of wakefulness, serotonin neurons are tonically active [55] and the distribution of serotonergic tone is relatively even across most brain regions [56] - a pattern that has been found to support normal network functioning for a variety of cognitive and goal-directed behaviors. In contrast, exposure to stress can produce a surge in 5-HT signaling, which has been found to disrupt the emotion-regulatory functions of cortico-amygdalar networks [57]. Further, evidence suggests that medial prefrontal projections to serotonin-releasing neurons in the dorsal raphe play a crucial role in determining adaptive versus non-adaptive responses to stress [58,59]. Consequently, impaired serotonin signaling may be a substrate involved in stress vulnerability and a key risk factor in the development of MDD [60-62].

For these reasons, serotonin is among the most widely imaged neurochemical systems in MDD, with over 35 studies exploring group differences in the expression of serotonin receptor sub-types as well as the serotonin transporter (for recent reviews, see [63,64]). To date, however, results have been mixed, with investigators frequently reporting higher or lower serotonin receptor or transporter expression in MDD participants than in controls [63]. For example, of the 15 studies investigating expression of 5-HT_{1A} receptor in depressed patients relative to healthy controls, nine reported decreased expression in MDD, four reported increased expression, and two observed no change. Similar discrepancies have been observed for other proteins involved in 5-HT signaling pathways, including the 5-HT_{2A} receptor, 5-HT_{1B} receptor, and the serotonin transporter (SERT).

It is important to note that most of these studies are relatively small in size (between 9 and 22 MDD patients) and are, therefore, underpowered to explore within-sample relations between serotonin function and specific symptom dimensions. This is a potentially critical limitation, as the substantial heterogeneity of MDD is likely to be associated with divergent effects on neurotransmitter systems. In addition, most of these studies have not investigated the function of serotonin signaling systems, compared to baseline expression. Moreover, no longitudinal studies have been performed. Therefore, as with cross-sectional studies of structure or function, it is difficult to know whether 5HT abnormalities should be interpreted as a primary deficit, a downstream consequence, a risk factor, or a compensatory mechanism.

What is clear, however, is that to the extent that the 5-HT system is involved in the etiopathophysiology, its effect size is modest, and likely dependent on interactions with numerous other systems.

Neurochemical imaging of catecholamine systems in MDD Other monoamines that have long been associated with MDD are the catecholamines dopamine (DA) and norepinephrine (NE) [65,66]. DA is well established as being necessary for motivation, reward-based learning, and goal-directed behavior [48,67,68] and, therefore, is believed to be a substrate of reward-related symptoms such as anhedonia, fatigue, and anergia in psychiatric disorders [69,70]. Unlike 5-HT, which is relatively uniform in its distribution across the brain, DA expression is densest in the striatum, a key structure involved in valuation, decision-making and action.

Neuroimaging evidence for altered DA systems in MDD comes primarily from PET, SPECT and pharmacological challenge studies. This research has found that MDD is associated with changes in DA synthesis capacity as indexed by L-3,4-dihydroxyphenylalanine (L-DOPA) uptake [71], as well as changes in the regional distribution and availability of DA receptors, and the DA transporter (DAT). As with the 5-HT studies summarized above, however, imaging studies of DA systems have produced conflicting results. In PET and SPECT studies of DAT, MDD has been associated with both lower [72] and higher [73-75] binding potential in the striatum. Interestingly, all studies reporting DAT increases have used SPECT, which has much lower sensitivity than PET [76] and often employed tracers that have equal affinity for the SERT and DAT (for example, β-CIT) and thus do not allow conclusive interpretations. Moreover, post-mortem studies support the observation of reduced DAT expression [77].

Studies of DA receptor availability in MDD have also yielded mixed results. In some cases, increased striatal D2/D3 receptor binding has been shown to occur in heterogeneous depressed samples [78,79]. This increase in D2/D3 receptor availability appears to contradict animal data in which antidepressant responses are associated with increased D2-like binding in the striatum [80]. Other studies using medication-naïve or medication-free patients have failed to find group differences in striatal receptor binding [81,82], while one additional small study reported variable changes in D2-like binding following treatment with selective serotonin reuptake inhibitors (SSRIs) with patients who showed increased binding exhibiting more clinical improvement than those who did not [83]. With respect to the D1 receptor, fewer studies have examined this system given the lack of available ligands that reliably distinguish between the D1 and serotonin 5-HT_{2A} receptor, especially in extrastriatal areas where the receptor density of D1 and $5HT_{2A}$ is roughly equivalent. One study reported reduced D1 availability in left middle caudate [84], but this finding has not yet been replicated. Taken together, these studies suggest a possible role of D2-like receptors in downstream effects of antidepressant treatment, although the precise nature of the effect and how alterations in D2-like receptor availability may be related to DA function are unclear.

As with other conflicting reports in neuroimaging studies of MDD, part of the discrepancy across studies likely reflects the heterogeneity of the disorder. Supporting this assertion is the observation of slightly more consistent effects when MDD samples are selected on the basis of a particular symptom profile. For example, one study that restricted its MDD patient sample to individuals with anhedonic symptoms reported decreased DAT binding [85]. In addition, L-DOPA alterations in the striatum are present in depressed individuals with flat affect or psychomotor slowing, but not in depressed individuals without these symptoms [86,87]. Decreases in DA synthesis have also been observed in patients who develop depressive symptoms after undergoing IFN-α therapy [50]. This therapy stimulates inflammation signaling cascades, which have been found to disrupt DA synthesis, and may provide a link between elevated inflammation in MDD and specific symptoms related to perturbances of DA signaling, such as motivation and anhedonia [50,88]. Overall, these studies provide mixed evidence for general DA alterations in MDD, with additional evidence highlighting the importance of examining links between DA systems and specific symptoms in MDD, rather than in the disorder as a whole.

In contrast to DA, molecular imaging methods of NE signaling pathways have been much slower to develop. Currently, only studies of the NE transporter (NET) have been performed in MDD [89], with no studies examining NE receptors in MDD due to a lack of available ligands. Pharmacological functional imaging studies have also been used to indirectly explore effects of NE-increasing agents, though many of these studies have used drugs such as duloxetine, which simultaneously target both 5-HT and NE transporters. Duloxetine reduced connectivity within resting-state and task-positive networks, [90], and boosted ventral striatal responses during a reward task [91], while the NET-selective agent reboxetine increased thalamic dorsolateral prefrontal responsivity to emotional pictures [92,93]. While these studies provide promising leads, insufficient functional or molecular imaging work of NE function in the context of MDD is available, despite significant evidence for its role in the disorder [94].

Neurochemical imaging of glutamatergic and GABAergic systems in MDD In recent years there has been substantial interest in the contribution of non-monoamine neurotransmitters to the pathophysiology of MDD, particularly the excitatory and inhibitory amino acid transmitters of glutamate (Glu) and GABA, respectively. At an intuitive level, the hypothesis that these systems would be implicated in depression holds significant appeal; the innervation of Glu- and GABA-releasing neurons vastly outnumbers all other neurotransmitter systems in the brain, making these two neurochemicals responsible for the bulk of information processing related to learning, cognition, memory, and decision-making [95]. When considering the scope of this diverse functional anatomy, it is difficult to imagine that Glu and GABA would not be directly, or at least indirectly, involved.

Evidence for alterations of Glu transmission in MDD have long been reported, but findings have been mixed, with increased Glu levels observed in plasma samples and post-mortem tissue as compared to decreased levels found in neuroimaging studies [96-98]. These discrepancies may be due in part to the multiple roles that Glu plays in the brain (for a more extended discussion, see [99]). A recent meta-analysis or MRS imaging studies found that MDD was associated with a substantial decrease in Glu levels within the mPFC/ACC [100], though it should be noted that not all studies were able to distinguish between Glu and glutamine, a common metabolite of astrocyte reuptake processes. Studies published after this meta-analysis provided additional evidence of reduced Glu concentration in the mPFC of MDD subjects [101-103], and similar alterations have also been detected in children with depressive symptoms [104] as well as remitted MDD subjects [102], raising the possibility that they constitute a trait-like vulnerability factor for MDD. Highlighting the clinical significance of these findings, among MDD subjects, increased pre-treatment Glu levels predicted better electroconvulsive therapy (ECT) response [103].

PET imaging studies of metabotropic Glu receptors have also revealed changes in Glu signaling pathways in MDD [105] and in relation to MDD symptoms [106]. The rapid antidepressant effects of ketamine, an N-methyl-D-aspartate (NMDA) partial agonist [107,108] further implicate the Glu pathway. Finally, aberrations in Glu signaling and Glu neurotoxicity have been associated with mPFC volumetric reductions discussed above [95]. In sum, while investigation of Glu dysfunction in MDD is relatively new, given the near ubiquitous distribution of Glu signaling throughout the brain, it is likely that many of the alterations in neural circuit function observed using fMRI studies partially reflect Glu-related pathology.

In contrast to Glu, studies of GABA are less frequent in MDD. GABA alterations have been documented in MDD [17,109], including reports of reduced GABA levels in plasma and cerebrospinal fluid [110-112], as well as specific GABA reductions in the mPFC as assessed with MRS [113,114]. Moreover, GABA function in this region has been suggested to play a critical role in mediating negative feedback of hypothalamic-pituitary-adrenal (HPA)-axis activity [115,116]. Thus, decreased GABAergic tone may foment excess glucocorticoid exposure in mPFC, as reviewed above. The combination of increased glucocorticoid exposure and elevated GABA has been hypothesized to be a combination that may lead to increased excitotoxicity in these regions, thereby partially explaining the structural alterations in these areas summarized in the preceding section. To date, however, the number of studies focused on GABA is relatively small, making it difficult to draw firm conclusions.

Imaging neuroendocrine and neuroimmune systems in MDD Lastly, there has been growing interest in using neuroimaging to study the functional and structural consequence of other neurochemicals, such as hormones, factors and other endogenous signaling molecules. While technical limitations generally prevent the imaging of such molecules directly, their effects on structure and metabolism can nevertheless be observed using MRI. In the case of MDD, this work has focused most heavily on pro-inflammatory factors, including families of cytokines such as interleukins and interferons, hormones such as glucocorticoids (cortisol), thyroid stimulating hormone (TSH), and ghrelin [117,118].

Dysregulation of stress hormones has been widely reported in MDD (albeit with significant variance), and is believed to partially mediate some of the observed structural alterations associated with the disorder, especially within the hippocampus and mPFC [119,120]. These regions are well known for playing a critical role in the regulation of stress hormones via direct and indirect projections to the hypothalamus, and have been shown to be structurally vulnerable to glucocorticoid-mediated excitotoxicity. Animal studies using either chronic stress protocols or local corticosteroid injections have repeatedly demonstrated tissue damage following excessive glucocorticoid exposure, including loss of dendritic spines and de-arborization [121-124]. In human studies, comparable relationships have been observed between daily cortisol levels and grey-matter volume in depressed patients [125]. Given that elevated stress is a major precipitant of first-time depressive episodes [60], the association between stress and regional microdamage is highly relevant.

In addition to stress hormones, depressive states have been strongly associated with an elevated inflammatory load [126,127], and there has been growing interest in signaling pathways related to the metabolic syndrome and excess adipose tissue as potential mediators of chronic low-grade inflammation [128,129]. Neuroimaging has therefore been employed as an aid to understanding the possible consequences of altered inflammatory and metabolic factors on neural systems [130,131]. Animal models suggest that elevations of peripheral cytokines and subsequent CNS microglia activation can disrupt the synthesis of both 5-HT and DA [132,133], and induce symptoms of fatigue and motivational anhedonia [134,135]. While direct evidence of increased microglia activity in MDD has not been detected using available PET ligands [136], functional neuroimaging studies have sought to better understand the downstream consequences of increased cytokine activity by examining correlations between peripheral cytokine levels and resting or task-induced fluctuations in Blood-Oxygen-Level Dependent (BOLD) signals. Of note, healthy controls receiving an endotoxin challenge exhibited blunted neural responses to reward anticipation in the ventral striatum during a Monetary Incentive Delay (MID) task [137], similar to what is observed in MDD [42]. Further evidence comes from imaging studies of patients receiving IFN-α therapy. Following IFN-α treatment - which robustly increases inflammation - subjects exhibited decreased DA turnover within the striatum, as measured using a pre/post PET imaging of DA uptake with [^{18}F] Dopa (F-DOPA) [50]. By beginning to localize the functional architecture of brain regions that are affected by stress hormones and inflammation and by linking such abnormalities to specific cardinal symptoms of MDD (for example, anhedonia), these studies are playing a critical role in advancing a more precise understanding of depression symptomatology.

Summary of neuroimaging studies In review of the findings above, several themes emerge. The most promising result is that regardless of imaging modality, neuroimaging studies repeatedly isolate a similar network of regions in which MDD patients differ from controls. Indeed, the greatest success of neuroimaging studies in MDD has been to identify core nodes involved in the expression of depressive symptoms. Neural responses in cortico-striato-limbic circuits have been shown to discriminate between responders to different treatment modalities [20,138] and have been the empirical foundation for new treatment techniques, such as deep brain stimulation (DBS) [139,140] and transcranial magnetic stimulation (TMS) [141].

But this is perhaps where the good news ends; for while the same regions are often implicated, the direction of the effects is often contradictory (for example, greater or lesser BOLD signal, depending on the task). Moreover, some of this consistency is undoubtedly due to confirmatory bias in ROI selection; that is, reports of group differences in a given region increase the probability that future studies will focus on the region, either with targeted measurement (for example, volumetric tracing) or with more liberal statistical thresholds in voxel-based studies (for example, small-volume correction). Even when group differences emerge, they are often present only at the level of group average, with comparable ranges for both groups (for example, [142]). As a result, the field has been unable to identify any neural signature that may serve as useful biomarker in the diagnosis of MDD, and guide treatment selection.

The lack of stable pathophysiological markers of MDD after so many neuroimaging studies raises the possibility that the biological origins of depressive symptoms are simply too dynamic to produce consistent patterns using case–control designs. For example, many receptor subtypes, including those of monoamine, Glu and GABA pathways show rapid, activity-dependent changes in expression and ligand affinity [143]. This plasticity may be affected by the time of day, the amount of sleep someone received two nights before, and how much they have been taxing their working memory in recent weeks just as much as it is affected by MDD ([105,143]). Against all these additional sources of variance, it is perhaps unsurprising that cross-sectional designs have been unable to identify reliable biomarkers.

As a result, an increasing number of researchers have called for a better understanding of specific circuits that may mediate transdiagnostic symptom expression [144,145]. While much of this discussion has rightly emphasized the importance of animal models [146,147], the final section presents several conceptual and methodological approaches to clinical imaging studies that we feel may aid in the identification of circuits rather than regions.

Future directions and circuit-based analysis

A clear limitation of current neuroimaging studies in MDD has been the tendency to assess particular measures of brain function independently, despite clear evidence that these measures are highly inter-related. In contrast to measures of specific brain regions, chemicals, or tissue classes, circuit-based analysis provides a conceptual framework that is organized around a specific behavioral process. Circuits are defined by the combined structural and functional properties that enable a specific set of computations to be performed on a discrete set of inputs. As such, circuit-analysis integrates across many different levels and measures of brain function, but eschew the complexity of simultaneous whole-brain analysis. By focusing on discrete computations with a circumscribed array of possible inputs and outputs, circuit analysis meets the basic scientific requirement of simplification, but does so without neglecting biological complexity.

One of the most powerful and readily available methods for circuit-analysis in patient populations is functional connectivity. Whereas much of the first two decades of neuroimaging research emphasized localization of function to a particular brain region while individuals were either at rest or performing a particular task, growing appreciation for the role of functional networks has emerged in recent years. This shift reflects a broader recognition in the field of neuroimaging that the brain is comprised of discrete networks, which show local properties (for example, 'small-worldness') and can rapidly re-configure themselves to adapt to current environmental demands [148,149]. Consequently, focusing on task-driven changes within a single brain area provides only limited insight into the specific computations being performed. Indeed, significant progress has been made in the characterization of several stable networks that support domain-general functions, including attentional control, novelty and threat detection, default-mode and social cognition, and reinforcement learning and decision-making, all of which have been implicated in MDD [150] (Figure 2).

Complementing functional connectivity as a path towards understanding MDD from a systems-level approach is the growing use of multi-modal imaging. The most common example is the combined use of structural and function neuroimaging data. Such data are often collected together, as standard preprocessing pipelines for functional neuroimaging data typically require high-resolution structural scans [151]. More recently, the scope of multi-modal imaging studies has been expanded to include neurotransmitters such as monoamines, Glu and GABA. In an important study by Northoff and colleagues, researchers identified shifts in neurotransmitter availability of Glu and GABA as major drivers of altered functional responses to emotional stimuli in MDD [152]. Similarly, decreases in pre-synaptic striatal DA as measured using F-DOPA were associated with blunted ventral striatal BOLD signal during reward anticipation in depressed subjects, demonstrating a clear link between DA bioavailability and striatal responses to reward [50].

Another essential benefit of circuit-based analysis is the bridge it creates to behavioral and molecular neuroscience. Animal models play a pivotal role in testing causal hypotheses about brain function [146]. Such models are not only useful in aiding the interpretation of correlative neuroimaging data, they can also help refine the mapping of psychiatric symptom definitions to discrete and dissociable circuits. For example, the symptom of anhedonia - which was once perceived as a unitary construct tapping into the experience of pleasure - has gradually come to be recognized as involving multiple sub-components, including motivation and hedonic response, each of which involves distinct neural substrates [69,70,153]. However, because these sub-components in humans are often heavily correlated with each other at the level of symptom expression,

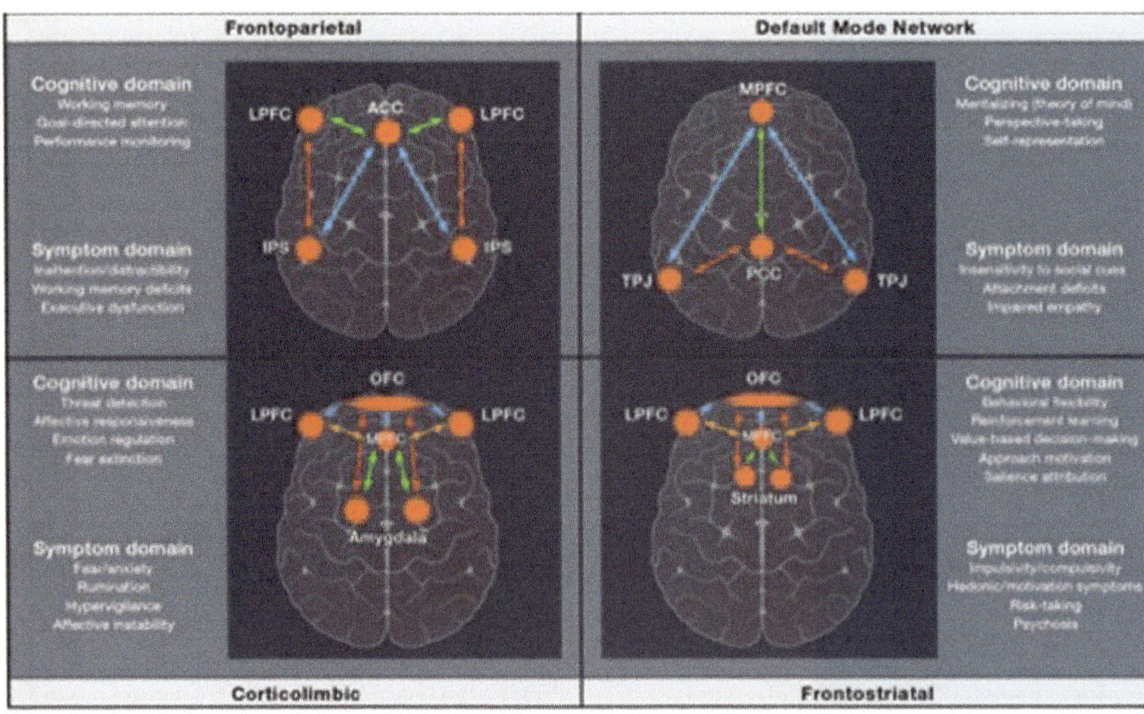

Figure 2 Schematic depiction of commonly identified functional networks and their associated cognitive and symptom domains. Republished with permission from Buckholtz and Meyer-Lindenberg [150].

animal models were required to demonstrate that motivational and hedonic aspects of reinforcement were indeed neurobiologically dissociable [48,67].

Pharmacological manipulations and other interventional techniques also provide tremendous advantages over imaging measures alone; these studies can identify plasticity dynamics that can help unpack some of the cross-sectional observations. For example, behavioral pharmacology studies of DA in MDD suggest that patients experience a much stronger euphoria response to amphetamine than controls [154,155], possibly indicating an up-regulation of post-synaptic DA receptors sites and/or DAT. The cross-sectional imaging studies discussed above, however, suggest down-regulation of both D1 and D2 as well as DAT proteins. Since the expression of these proteins is dynamic, imaging studies done in conjunction with pharmacological challenges (within-subject) hold the promise for stronger mechanistic inferences regarding how neurotransmitter systems are able to adapt to changing conditions in MDD. Such pharmacological challenges can therefore greatly aid in the understanding of plasticity within circuits, and help shift away from a focus on the identification of a stable, persistent pathological marker, which appears unlikely to exist.

Finally, circuit-based analysis may help facilitate a shift in the conceptualization and measurement of psychiatric symptom inventories that are often used to define groups and regress against imaging data. Psychiatric measurement largely relies on subjective self-reporting of distress as they *sine qua non* of symptom diagnosis. When it comes to reporting how one feels, however, studies in healthy populations have increasingly observed dissociation between the 'believing self' and the 'experiencing self' [156-158]. Accordingly, while the former describes how an individual summarizes their experience over a period of time, the latter refers to experiential reports made 'in the moment'. Whereas these constructs would theoretically be expected to correlate highly, growing evidence suggests that they are only moderately correlated at best [157,159]. This is in part due to the presence of well-known retrospective biases that reflect a heightened sensitivity to recency or maximum intensity of emotional experiences (so-called 'peak and end' effects) [160]. In disorders like schizophrenia, such retrospective biases can result in almost completely uncorrelated findings of emotional response across retrospective and in-the-moment reports [161].

This renders significantly liable the common practice of regressing symptom severity measures (for example, the BDI-II) against imaging data [162], as both the independent and dependent measures likely reflect a complex mix of 'believing self' and 'experiencing self'. For example, if someone has reported severe depression over the past week, but happens to have a brief lifting during the two- to three-hour window in which the lab experiment occurs, it may be more important to consider the 'in the moment' affect rather than feelings aggregated over the past weeks when trying to interpret associated imaging data; this stands in contrast with the traditional assumption that individuals with shared symptom severity over a one-week period will have more variance in common than individuals with shared experience of a particular experimental task. One approach to addressing this challenge is the development of measures that seek to tease apart 'believing self' and 'experiencing self', with the aim of identifying separate biological correlates. It is likely that both are implicated in the maintenance of depressive symptoms [163], but current symptom assessment inventories are poorly suited to distinguish between these distinct modes of types of subjective report.

In sum, clinical imaging studies can contribute to circuit-based analysis through a focus on network-based analytical techniques, such as functional connectivity, multi-modal imaging methods, the use of within-subject pharmacological challenge designs, and greater sensitivity to potential discrepancies between 'believing self' and 'experiencing self' that may mask important distinctions in the relationships between subjective report and neuroimaging data.

Conclusion

The neuroimaging literature of depression has grown tremendously over the last several decades. The primary fruit of these efforts has been the identification of brain regions and structures that are most critical to the expression of depressive symptomatology, while also increasing our knowledge of how these regions interact with particular neurotransmitter systems, neurochemicals, hormones, and other signaling proteins. Despite a wealth of positive findings, translations to treatment remain elusive. Moving forward, the integration of these various methods through the use of circuit-based analysis will be critical for the development of a biologically-based nosology and personalized medicine in psychiatry.

Abbreviations

5-HT: Serotonin; ACC: anterior cingulate cortex; BOLD: blood-oxygen level-dependent; CNS: central nervous system; DA: dopamine; DAT: dopamine transporter; DBS: deep-brain stimulation; dlPFC: dorsolateral prefrontal cortex; Glu: glutamate; GABA: gamma-aminobutyric acid; HPA axis: hypothalamic-pituitary-adrenal axis; IFN: interferon; MDD: major depressive disorder; MID: monetary incentive delay; mPFC: medial prefrontal cortex; MRI: magnetic resonance imaging; MRS: magnetic resonance spectroscopy; NE: norepinephrine; NET: norepinephrine transporter; OFC: orbitofrontal cortex; PET: positron emission tomography; PFC: prefrontal cortex; ROI: region of interest; SPECT: single photon emission computed tomography; SERT: serotonin transporter; TMS: transcranial magnetic stimulation; TSH: thyroid stimulating hormone; VBM: voxel-based morphometry; vlPFC: ventrolateral prefrontal cortex.

Competing interests
The authors declare no competing interests. Over the past three years, Dr. Pizzagalli received consulting/honoraria from AstraZeneca, Ono Pharma USA, Pfizer, Servier, and Shire for activities unrelated to the current review.

Authors' contributions
MTT and DAP developed the outline, MTT reviewed the relevant literature, and MTT and DAP wrote the manuscript. Both authors read and approved the final manuscript.

Acknowledgements
This work was funded by R01MH068376, R01MH06376S1, and R01MH095809 to DAP, and a McLean Corneel Fellowship to MTT. The authors also wish to thank two anonymous reviewers for their helpful comments.

References

1. Kapur S, Phillips AG, Insel TR: **Why has it taken so long for biological psychiatry to develop clinical tests and what to do about it?** *Mol Psychiatry* 2012, **17**:1174–1179.
2. Koolschijn PC, van Haren NE, Lensvelt-Mulders GJ, Hulshoff Pol HE, Kahn RS: **Brain volume abnormalities in major depressive disorder: a meta-analysis of magnetic resonance imaging studies.** *Hum Brain Mapp* 2009.
3. Kempton MJ, Salvador Z, Munafo MR, Geddes JR, Simmons A, Frangou S, Williams SC: **Structural neuroimaging studies in major depressive disorder. Meta-analysis and comparison with bipolar disorder.** *Arch Gen Psychiatry* 2011, **68**:675–690.
4. Bora E, Fornito A, Pantelis C, Yucel M: **Gray matter abnormalities in Major Depressive Disorder: a meta-analysis of voxel based morphometry studies.** *J Affect Disord* 2011, **138**:9–18.
5. Cotter D, Mackay D, Landau S, Kerwin R, Everall I: **Reduced glial cell density and neuronal size in the anterior cingulate cortex in major depressive disorder.** *Arch Gen Psychiatry* 2001, **58**:545–553.
6. Liao Y, Huang X, Wu Q, Yang C, Kuang W, Du M, Lui S, Yue Q, Chan RC, Kemp GJ, Gong Q: **Is depression a disconnection syndrome? Meta-analysis of diffusion tensor imaging studies in patients with MDD.** *J Psychiatry Neurosci* 2013, **38**:49–56.
7. Yucel K, McKinnon MC, Chahal R, Taylor VH, Macdonald K, Joffe R, MacQueen GM: **Anterior cingulate volumes in never-treated patients with major depressive disorder.** *Neuropsychopharmacology* 2008, **33**:3157–3163.
8. McKinnon MC, Yucel K, Nazarov A, MacQueen GM: **A meta-analysis examining clinical predictors of hippocampal volume in patients with major depressive disorder.** *J Psychiatry Neurosci* 2009, **34**:41–54.
9. van Eijndhoven P, van Wingen G, van Oijen K, Rijpkema M, Goraj B, Jan Verkes R, Oude Voshaar R, Fernandez G, Buitelaar J, Tendolkar I: **Amygdala volume marks the acute state in the early course of depression.** *Biol Psychiatry* 2009, **65**:812–818.
10. Frodl T, Meisenzahl EM, Zetzsche T, Hohne T, Banac S, Schorr C, Jager M, Leinsinger G, Bottlender R, Reiser M, Moller HJ: **Hippocampal and amygdala changes in patients with major depressive disorder and healthy controls during a 1-year follow-up.** *J Clin Psychiatry* 2004, **65**:492–499.
11. Frodl T, Jager M, Smajstrlova I, Born C, Bottlender R, Palladino T, Reiser M, Moller HJ, Meisenzahl EM: **Effect of hippocampal and amygdala volumes on clinical outcomes in major depression: a 3-year prospective magnetic resonance imaging study.** *J Psychiatry Neurosci* 2008, **33**:423–430.
12. Arnone D, McKie S, Elliott R, Juhasz G, Thomas EJ, Downey D, Williams S, Deakin JF, Anderson IM: **State-dependent changes in hippocampal grey matter in depression.** *Mol Psychiatry* 2012.
13. Schermuly I, Wolf D, Lieb K, Stoeter P, Fellgiebel A: **State dependent posterior hippocampal volume increases in patients with major depressive disorder.** *J Affect Disord* 2011, **135**:405–409.
14. Holmes AJ, Lee PH, Hollinshead MO, Bakst L, Roffman JL, Smoller JW, Buckner RL: **Individual differences in amygdala-medial prefrontal anatomy link negative affect, impaired social functioning, and polygenic depression risk.** *J Neurosci* 2012, **32**:18087–18100.
15. Saleh K, Carballedo A, Lisiecka D, Fagan AJ, Connolly G, Boyle G, Frodl T: **Impact of family history and depression on amygdala volume.** *Psychiatry Res* 2012, **203**:24–30.
16. Amico F, Meisenzahl E, Koutsouleris N, Reiser M, Moller HJ, Frodl T: **Structural MRI correlates for vulnerability and resilience to major depressive disorder.** *J Psychiatry Neurosci* 2011, **36**:15–22.
17. Hasler G, Northoff G: **Discovering imaging endophenotypes for major depression.** *Mol Psychiatry* 2011, **16**:604–619.
18. Diener C, Kuehner C, Brusniak W, Ubl B, Wessa M, Flor H: **A meta-analysis of neurofunctional imaging studies of emotion and cognition in major depression.** *Neuroimage* 2012, **61**:677–685.
19. Hamilton JP, Etkin A, Furman DJ, Lemus MG, Johnson RF, Gotlib IH: **Functional neuroimaging of major depressive disorder: a meta-analysis and new integration of base line activation and neural response data.** *Am J Psychiatry* 2012, **169**:693–703.
20. Pizzagalli DA: **Frontocingulate dysfunction in depression: toward biomarkers of treatment response.** *Neuropsychopharmacology* 2011, **36**:183–206.
21. Victor TA, Furey ML, Fromm SJ, Ohman A, Drevets WC: **Relationship between amygdala responses to masked faces and mood state and treatment in major depressive disorder.** *Arch Gen Psychiatry* 2010, **67**:1128–1138.
22. Fu CH, Williams SC, Cleare AJ, Brammer MJ, Walsh ND, Kim J, Andrew CM, Pich EM, Williams PM, Reed LJ, Mitterschiffthaler MT, Suckling J, Bullmore ET: **Attenuation of the neural response to sad faces in major depression by antidepressant treatment: a prospective, event-related functional magnetic resonance imaging study.** *Arch Gen Psychiatry* 2004, **61**:877–889.
23. Siegle GJ, Steinhauer SR, Thase ME, Stenger VA, Carter CS: **Can't shake that feeling: event-related fMRI assessment of sustained amygdala activity in response to emotional information in depressed individuals.** *Biol Psychiatry* 2002, **51**:693–707.
24. Mitterschiffthaler MT, Williams SC, Walsh ND, Cleare AJ, Donaldson C, Scott J, Fu CH: **Neural basis of the emotional Stroop interference effect in major depression.** *Psychol Med* 2008, **38**:247–256.
25. Siegle GJ, Thompson W, Carter CS, Steinhauer SR, Thase ME: **Increased amygdala and decreased dorsolateral prefrontal BOLD responses in unipolar depression: related and independent features.** *Biol Psychiatry* 2007, **61**:198–209.
26. Beauregard M, Paquette V, Levesque J: **Dysfunction in the neural circuitry of emotional self-regulation in major depressive disorder.** *Neuroreport* 2006, **17**:843–846.
27. Dillon DG, Pizzagalli DA: **Evidence of successful modulation of brain activation and subjective experience during reappraisal of negative emotion in unmedicated depression.** *Psychiatry Res* 2013, **212**:99–107.
28. Erk S, Mikschl A, Stier S, Ciaramidaro A, Gapp V, Weber B, Walter H: **Acute and sustained effects of cognitive emotion regulation in major depression.** *J Neurosci* 2010, **30**:15726–15734.
29. Johnstone T, van Reekum CM, Urry HL, Kalin NH, Davidson RJ: **Failure to regulate: counterproductive recruitment of top-down prefrontal-subcortical circuitry in major depression.** *J Neurosci* 2007, **27**:8877–8884.
30. Matsuo K, Glahn DC, Peluso MA, Hatch JP, Monkul ES, Najt P, Sanches M, Zamarripa F, Li J, Lancaster JL, Fox PT, Gao JH, Soares JC: **Prefrontal hyperactivation during working memory task in untreated individuals with major depressive disorder.** *Mol Psychiatry* 2007, **12**:158–166.
31. Wagner G, Sinsel E, Sobanski T, Kohler S, Marinou V, Mentzel HJ, Sauer H, Schlosser RG: **Cortical inefficiency in patients with unipolar depression: an event-related FMRI study with the Stroop task.** *Biol Psychiatry* 2006, **59**:958–965.
32. Etkin A, Schatzberg AF: **Common abnormalities and disorder-specific compensation during implicit regulation of emotional processing in generalized anxiety and major depressive disorders.** *Am J Psychiatry* 2011, **168**:968–978.
33. Beesdo K, Lau JY, Guyer AE, McClure-Tone EB, Monk CS, Nelson EE, Fromm SJ, Goldwin MA, Wittchen HU, Leibenluft E, Ernst M, Pine DS: **Common and distinct amygdala-function perturbations in depressed versus anxious adolescents.** *Arch Gen Psychiatry* 2009, **66**:275–285.
34. Ochsner KN, Ray RD, Cooper JC, Robertson ER, Chopra S, Gabrieli JD, Gross JJ: **For better or for worse: neural systems supporting the cognitive down- and up-regulation of negative emotion.** *Neuroimage* 2004, **23**:483–499.
35. Matthews SC, Strigo IA, Simmons AN, Yang TT, Paulus MP: **Decreased functional coupling of the amygdala and supragenual cingulate is related to increased depression in unmedicated individuals with current major depressive disorder.** *J Affect Disord* 2008, **111**:13–20.

36. Mitterschiffthaler MT, Kumari V, Malhi GS, Brown RG, Giampietro VP, Brammer MJ, Suckling J, Poon L, Simmons A, Andrew C, Sharma T: **Neural response to pleasant stimuli in anhedonia: an fMRI study.** *Neuroreport* 2003, **14**:177–182.
37. Surguladze S, Brammer MJ, Keedwell P, Giampietro V, Young AW, Travis MJ, Williams SC, Phillips ML: **A differential pattern of neural response toward sad versus happy facial expressions in major depressive disorder.** *Biol Psychiatry* 2005, **57**:201–209.
38. Keedwell PA, Andrew C, Williams SC, Brammer MJ, Phillips ML: **A double dissociation of ventromedial prefrontal cortical responses to sad and happy stimuli in depressed and healthy individuals.** *Biol Psychiatry* 2005, **58**:495–503.
39. Gotlib IH, Hamilton JP, Cooney RE, Singh MK, Henry ML, Joormann J: **Neural processing of reward and loss in girls at risk for major depression.** *Arch Gen Psychiatry* 2010, **67**:380–387.
40. Dichter GS, Felder JN, Petty C, Bizzell J, Ernst M, Smoski MJ: **The effects of psychotherapy on neural responses to rewards in major depression.** *Biol Psychiatry* 2009, **66**:886–897.
41. Forbes EE, Hariri AR, Martin SL, Silk JS, Moyles DL, Fisher PM, Brown SM, Ryan ND, Birmaher B, Axelson DA, Dahl RE: **Altered striatal activation predicting real-world positive affect in adolescent major depressive disorder.** *Am J Psychiatry* 2009, **166**:64–73.
42. Pizzagalli DA, Holmes AJ, Dillon DG, Goetz EL, Birk JL, Bogdan R, Dougherty DD, Iosifescu DV, Rauch SL, Fava M: **Reduced caudate and nucleus accumbens response to rewards in unmedicated individuals with major depressive disorder.** *Am J Psychiatry* 2009, **166**:702–710.
43. Kumar P, Waiter G, Ahearn T, Milders M, Reid I, Steele JD: **Abnormal temporal difference reward-learning signals in major depression.** *Brain* 2008, **131**:2084–2093.
44. Pizzagalli DA, Iosifescu D, Hallett LA, Ratner KG, Fava M: **Reduced hedonic capacity in major depressive disorder: evidence from a probabilistic reward task.** *J Psychiatr Res* 2008, **43**:76–87.
45. Clery-Melin ML, Schmidt L, Lafargue G, Baup N, Fossati P, Pessiglione M: **Why don't you try harder? An investigation of effort production in major depression.** *PLoS One* 2011, **6**:e23178.
46. Sherdell L, Waugh CE, Gotlib IH: **Anticipatory pleasure predicts motivation for reward in major depression.** *J Abnorm Psychol* 2011.
47. Treadway MT, Bossaller NA, Shelton RC, Zald DH: **Effort-based decision-making in major depressive disorder: a translational model of motivational anhedonia.** *J Abnorm Psychol* 2012.
48. Berridge KC: **The debate over dopamine's role in reward: the case for incentive salience.** *Psychopharmacology (Berl)* 2007, **191**:391–431.
49. Treadway MT, Zald DH: **Reconsidering anhedonia in depression: lessons from translational neuroscience.** *Neurosci Biobehav Rev* 2011, **35**:537–555.
50. Capuron L, Pagnoni G, Drake DF, Woolwine BJ, Spivey JR, Crowe RJ, Votaw JR, Goodman MM, Miller AH: **Dopaminergic mechanisms of reduced basal ganglia responses to hedonic reward during interferon alfa administration.** *Arch Gen Psychiatry* 2012, **69**:1044–1053.
51. Hasler G, Fromm S, Carlson PJ, Luckenbaugh DA, Waldeck T, Geraci M, Roiser JP, Neumeister A, Meyers N, Charney DS, Drevets WC: **Neural response to catecholamine depletion in unmedicated subjects with major depressive disorder in remission and healthy subjects.** *Arch Gen Psychiatry* 2008, **65**:521–531.
52. Hasler G, Luckenbaugh DA, Snow J, Meyers N, Waldeck T, Geraci M, Roiser J, Knutson B, Charney DS, Drevets WC: **Reward processing after catecholamine depletion in unmedicated, remitted subjects with major depressive disorder.** *Biol Psychiatry* 2009, **66**:201–205.
53. Heller AS, Johnstone T, Shackman AJ, Light SN, Peterson MJ, Kolden GG, Kalin NH, Davidson RJ: **Reduced capacity to sustain positive emotion in major depression reflects diminished maintenance of fronto-striatal brain activation.** *Proc Natl Acad Sci U S A* 2009, **106**:22445–22450.
54. Schildkraut JJ: **The catecholamine hypothesis of affective disorders: a review of supporting evidence.** *Am J Psychiatry* 1965, **122**:509–522.
55. Jacobs BL, Fornal CA: **Activity of serotonergic neurons in behaving animals.** *Neuropsychopharmacology* 1999, **21**:9S–15S.
56. Daubert EA, Condron BG: **Serotonin: a regulator of neuronal morphology and circuitry.** *Trends Neurosci* 2010, **33**:424–434.
57. Jasinska AJ, Lowry CA, Burmeister M: **Serotonin transporter gene, stress and raphe-raphe interactions: a molecular mechanism of depression.** *Trends Neurosci* 2012, **35**:395–402.
58. Amat J, Baratta MV, Paul E, Bland ST, Watkins LR, Maier SF: **Medial prefrontal cortex determines how stressor controllability affects behavior and dorsal raphe nucleus.** *Nat Neurosci* 2005, **8**:365–371.
59. Amat J, Paul E, Watkins LR, Maier SF: **Activation of the ventral medial prefrontal cortex during an uncontrollable stressor reproduces both the immediate and long-term protective effects of behavioral control.** *Neuroscience* 2008, **154**:1178–1186.
60. Hammen C: **Stress and depression.** *Annu Rev Clin Psychol* 2005, **1**:293–319.
61. Kessler RC: **The effects of stressful life events on depression.** *Annu Rev Psychol* 1997, **48**:191–214.
62. Kendler KS, Karkowski LM, Prescott CA: **Causal relationship between stressful life events and the onset of major depression.** *Am J Psychiatry* 1999, **156**:837–841.
63. Savitz JB, Drevets WC: **Neuroreceptor imaging in depression.** *Neurobiol Dis* 2013, **52**:49–65.
64. Smith DF, Jakobsen S: **Molecular neurobiology of depression: PET findings on the elusive correlation with symptom severity.** *Front Psychiatry* 2013, **4**:8.
65. Willner P: **Dopamine and depression: a review of recent evidence. I. Empirical studies.** *Brain Res* 1983, **287**:211–224.
66. van Praag HM, Korf J, Schut D: **Cerebral monoamines and depression. An investigation with the probenecid technique.** *Arch Gen Psychiatry* 1973, **28**:827–831.
67. Salamone JD, Correa M: **The mysterious motivational functions of mesolimbic dopamine.** *Neuron* 2012, **76**:470–485.
68. Schultz W: **Behavioral dopamine signals.** *Trends Neurosci* 2007, **30**:203–210.
69. Barch DM, Dowd EC: **Goal representations and motivational drive in schizophrenia: the role of prefrontal-striatal interactions.** *Schizophr Bull* 2010, **36**:919–934.
70. Treadway MT, Zald DH: **Parsing anhedonia translational models of reward-processing deficits in psychopathology.** *Curr Dir Psychol Sci* 2013, **22**:244–249.
71. Agren H, Reibring L: **PET studies of presynaptic monoamine metabolism in depressed patients and healthy volunteers.** *Pharmacopsychiatry* 1994, **27**:2–6.
72. Meyer JH, Kruger S, Wilson AA, Christensen BK, Goulding VS, Schaffer A, Minifie C, Houle S, Hussey D, Kennedy SH: **Lower dopamine transporter binding potential in striatum during depression.** *Neuroreport* 2001, **12**:4121–4125.
73. Yang YK, Yeh TL, Yao WJ, Lee IH, Chen PS, Chiu NT, Lu RB: **Greater availability of dopamine transporters in patients with major depression - a dual-isotope SPECT study.** *Psychiatry Res* 2008, **162**:230–235.
74. Amsterdam JD, Newberg AB: **A preliminary study of dopamine transporter binding in bipolar and unipolar depressed patients and healthy controls.** *Neuropsychobiology* 2007, **55**:167–170.
75. Laasonen-Balk T, Kuikka J, Viinamaki H, Husso-Saastamoinen M, Lehtonen J, Tiihonen J: **Striatal dopamine transporter density in major depression.** *Psychopharmacology (Berl)* 1999, **144**:282–285.
76. Rahmim A, Zaidi H: **PET versus SPECT: strengths, limitations and challenges.** *Nucl Med Commun* 2008, **29**:193–207.
77. Klimek V, Schenck JE, Han H, Stockmeier CA, Ordway GA: **Dopaminergic abnormalities in amygdaloid nuclei in major depression: a postmortem study.** *Biol Psychiatry* 2002, **52**:740–748.
78. Shah PJ, Ogilvie AD, Goodwin GM, Ebmeier KP: **Clinical and psychometric correlates of dopamine D2 binding in depression.** *Psychol Med* 1997, **27**:1247–1256.
79. D'Haenen HA, Bossuyt A: **Dopamine D2 receptors in depression measured with single photon emission computed tomography.** *Biol Psychiatry* 1994, **35**:128–132.
80. Gershon AA, Vishne T, Grunhaus L: **Dopamine D2-like receptors and the antidepressant response.** *Biol Psychiatry* 2007, **61**:145–153.
81. Parsey RV, Oquendo MA, Zea-Ponce Y, Rodenhiser J, Kegeles LS, Pratap M, Cooper TB, Van Heertum R, Mann JJ, Laruelle M: **Dopamine D(2) receptor availability and amphetamine-induced dopamine release in unipolar depression.** *Biol Psychiatry* 2001, **50**:313–322.
82. Hirvonen J, Karlsson H, Kajander J, Markkula J, Rasi-Hakala H, Nagren K, Salminen JK, Hietala J: **Striatal dopamine D2 receptors in medication-naive patients with major depressive disorder as assessed with [11C]raclopride PET.** *Psychopharmacology (Berl)* 2008, **197**:581–590.
83. Klimke A, Larisch R, Janz A, Vosberg H, Muller-Gartner HW, Gaebel W: **Dopamine D2 receptor binding before and after treatment of major depression measured by [123I]IBZM SPECT.** *Psychiatry Res* 1999, **90**:91–101.

84. Cannon DM, Klaver JM, Peck SA, Rallis-Voak D, Erickson K, Drevets WC: **Dopamine type-1 receptor binding in major depressive disorder assessed using positron emission tomography and [11C]NNC-112.** *Neuropsychopharmacology* 2009, **34:**1277–1287.
85. Sarchiapone M, Carli V, Camardese G, Cuomo C, Di Giuda D, Calcagni ML, Focacci C, De Risio S: **Dopamine transporter binding in depressed patients with anhedonia.** *Psychiatry Res* 2006, **147:**243–248.
86. Martinot M, Bragulat V, Artiges E, Dolle F, Hinnen F, Jouvent R, Martinot J: **Decreased presynaptic dopamine function in the left caudate of depressed patients with affective flattening and psychomotor retardation.** *Am J Psychiatry* 2001, **158:**314–316.
87. Bragulat V, Paillere-Martinot ML, Artiges E, Frouin V, Poline JB, Martinot JL: **Dopaminergic function in depressed patients with affective flattening or with impulsivity: [18 F]fluoro-L-dopa positron emission tomography study with voxel-based analysis.** *Psychiatry Res* 2007, **154:**115–124.
88. Haroon E, Raison CL, Miller AH: **Psychoneuroimmunology meets neuropsychopharmacology: translational implications of the impact of inflammation on behavior.** *Neuropsychopharmacology* 2011, **37:**137–162.
89. Takano H, Arakawa R, Nogami T, Suzuki M, Nagashima T, Fujiwara H, Kimura Y, Kodaka F, Takahata K, Shimada H: **Norepinephrine transporter occupancy by nortriptyline in patients with depression: a positron emission tomography study with (S, S)-[18F] FMeNER-D2.** *Int J Neuropsychopharmaco* 2013:1–8.
90. van Wingen GA, Tendolkar I, Urner M, van Marle H, Denys D, Verkes R-J, Fernandez G: **Short-term antidepressant administration reduces default mode and task-positive network connectivity in healthy individuals during rest.** *Neuroimage* 2013.
91. Ossewaarde L, Verkes RJ, Hermans EJ, Kooijman SC, Urner M, Tendolkar I, van Wingen GA, Fernandez G: **Two-week administration of the combined serotonin-noradrenaline reuptake inhibitor duloxetine augments functioning of mesolimbic incentive processing circuits.** *Biol Psychiatry* 2011, **70:**568–574.
92. Bruhl AB, Jancke L, Herwig U: **Differential modulation of emotion processing brain regions by noradrenergic and serotonergic antidepressants.** *Psychopharmacology (Berl)* 2011, **216:**389–399.
93. Bruhl AB, Kaffenberger T, Herwig U: **Serotonergic and noradrenergic modulation of emotion processing by single dose antidepressants.** *Neuropsychopharmacology* 2010, **35:**521.
94. Ressler KJ, Nemeroff CB: **Role of norepinephrine in the pathophysiology and treatment of mood disorders.** *Biol Psychiatry* 1999, **46:**1219–1233.
95. Sanacora G, Treccani G, Popoli M: **Towards a glutamate hypothesis of depression: an emerging frontier of neuropsychopharmacology for mood disorders.** *Neuropharmacology* 2012, **62:**63–77.
96. Altamura CA, Mauri MC, Ferrara A, Moro AR, D'Andrea G, Zamberlan F: **Plasma and platelet excitatory amino acids in psychiatric disorders.** *Am J Psychiatry* 1993, **150:**1731–1733.
97. Kim JS, Schmid-Burgk W, Claus D, Kornhuber HH: **Increased serum glutamate in depressed patients.** *Arch Psychiatr Nervenkr* 1982, **232:**299–304.
98. Hashimoto K, Sawa A, Iyo M: **Increased levels of glutamate in brains from patients with mood disorders.** *Biol Psychiatry* 2007, **62:**1310–1316.
99. Yuksel C, Ongur D: **Magnetic resonance spectroscopy studies of glutamate-related abnormalities in mood disorders.** *Biol Psychiatry* 2010, **68:**785–794.
100. Luykx JJ, Laban KG, van den Heuvel MP, Boks MP, Mandl RC, Kahn RS, Bakker SC: **Region and state specific glutamate downregulation in major depressive disorder: a meta-analysis of (1)H-MRS findings.** *Neurosci Biobehav Rev* 2011, **36:**198–205.
101. Jarnum H, Eskildsen SF, Steffensen EG, Lundbye-Christensen S, Simonsen CW, Thomsen IS, Frund ET, Theberge J, Larsson EM: **Longitudinal MRI study of cortical thickness, perfusion, and metabolite levels in major depressive disorder.** *Acta Psychiatr Scand* 2011, **124:**435–446.
102. Portella MJ, de Diego-Adelino J, Gomez-Anson B, Morgan-Ferrando R, Vives Y, Puigdemont D, Perez-Egea R, Ruscalleda J, Enric A, Perez V: **Ventromedial prefrontal spectroscopic abnormalities over the course of depression: a comparison among first episode, remitted recurrent and chronic patients.** *J Psychiatr Res* 2010, **45:**427–434.
103. Merkl A, Schubert F, Quante A, Luborzewski A, Brakemeier EL, Grimm S, Heuser I, Bajbouj M: **Abnormal cingulate and prefrontal cortical neurochemistry in major depression after electroconvulsive therapy.** *Biol Psychiatry* 2010, **69:**772–779.
104. Kondo DG, Hellem TL, Sung YH, Kim N, Jeong EK, Delmastro KK, Shi X, Renshaw PF: **Review: magnetic resonance spectroscopy studies of pediatric major depressive disorder.** *Depress Res Treat* 2011, **2011:**650450.
105. Deschwanden A, Karolewicz B, Feyissa AM, Treyer V, Ametamey SM, Johayem A, Burger C, Auberson YP, Sovago J, Stockmeier CA, Buck A, Hasler G: **Reduced metabotropic glutamate receptor 5 density in major depression determined by [11C]ABP688 PET and postmortem study.** *Am J Psychiatry* 2011, **168:**727–734.
106. Hefti K, Holst SC, Sovago J, Bachmann V, Buck A, Ametamey SM, Scheidegger M, Berthold T, Gomez-Mancilla B, Seifritz E: **Increased metabotropic glutamate receptor subtype 5 availability in human brain after one night without sleep.** *Biol Psychiatry* 2013.
107. Berman RM, Cappiello A, Anand A, Oren DA, Heninger GR, Charney DS, Krystal JH: **Antidepressant effects of ketamine in depressed patients.** *Biol Psychiatry* 2000, **47:**351–354.
108. Zarate CA Jr, Singh JB, Carlson PJ, Brutsche NE, Ameli R, Luckenbaugh DA, Charney DS, Manji HK: **A randomized trial of an N-methyl-D-aspartate antagonist in treatment-resistant major depression.** *Arch Gen Psychiatry* 2006, **63:**856–864.
109. Luscher B, Shen Q, Sahir N: **The GABAergic deficit hypothesis of major depressive disorder.** *Mol Psychiatry* 2010, **16:**383–406.
110. Petty F, Schlesser MA: **Plasma GABA in affective illness. A preliminary investigation.** *J Affect Disord* 1981, **3:**339–343.
111. Petty F, Sherman AD: **GABAergic modulation of learned helplessness.** *Pharmacol Biochem Behav* 1981, **15:**567–570.
112. Gerner RH, Hare TA: **CSF GABA in normal subjects and patients with depression, schizophrenia, mania, and anorexia nervosa.** *Am J Psychiatry* 1981, **138:**1098–1101.
113. Hasler G, van der Veen JW, Tumonis T, Meyers N, Shen J, Drevets WC: **Reduced prefrontal glutamate/glutamine and gamma-aminobutyric acid levels in major depression determined using proton magnetic resonance spectroscopy.** *Arch Gen Psychiatry* 2007, **64:**193–200.
114. Gabbay V, Mao X, Klein RG, Ely BA, Babb JS, Panzer AM, Alonso CM, Shungu DC: **Anterior cingulate cortex gamma-aminobutyric acid in depressed adolescents: relationship to anhedonia.** *Arch Gen Psychiatry* 2012, **69:**139–149.
115. Radley JJ, Sawchenko PE: **A common substrate for prefrontal and hippocampal inhibition of the neuroendocrine stress response.** *J Neurosci* 2011, **31:**9683–9695.
116. Radley JJ, Gosselink KL, Sawchenko PE: **A discrete GABAergic relay mediates medial prefrontal cortical inhibition of the neuroendocrine stress response.** *J Neurosci* 2009, **29:**7330–7340.
117. Homan P, Drevets WC, Hasler G: **Neural correlates of free T3 alteration after catecholamine depletion in subjects with remitted major depressive disorder and in controls.** *Psychopharmacology (Berl)* 2014, **231:**409–417.
118. Homan P, Grob S, Milos G, Schnyder U, Hasler G: **Reduction in total plasma ghrelin levels following catecholamine depletion: relation to bulimic and depressive symptoms.** *Psychoneuroendocrinology* 2013.
119. McEwen BS: **Physiology and neurobiology of stress and adaptation: central role of the brain.** *Physiol Rev* 2007, **87:**873–904.
120. Sapolsky RM: **Glucocorticoids and hippocampal atrophy in neuropsychiatric disorders.** *Arch Gen Psychiatry* 2000, **57:**925–935.
121. Radley JJ, Rocher AB, Miller M, Janssen WG, Liston C, Hof PR, McEwen BS, Morrison JH: **Repeated stress induces dendritic spine loss in the rat medial prefrontal cortex.** *Cereb Cortex* 2006, **16:**313–320.
122. Cook SC, Wellman CL: **Chronic stress alters dendritic morphology in rat medial prefrontal cortex.** *J Neurobiol* 2004, **60:**236–248.
123. Cerqueira JJ, Pego JM, Taipa R, Bessa JM, Almeida OF, Sousa N: **Morphological correlates of corticosteroid-induced changes in prefrontal cortex-dependent behaviors.** *J Neurosci* 2005, **25:**7792–7800.
124. McEwen BS: **Stress and hippocampal plasticity.** *Annu Rev Neurosci* 1999, **22:**105–122.
125. Treadway MT, Grant MM, Ding Z, Hollon SD, Gore JC, Shelton RC: **Early adverse events, HPA activity and rostral anterior cingulate volume in MDD.** *PLoS One* 2009, **4:**e4887.
126. Dowlati Y, Herrmann N, Swardfager W, Liu H, Sham L, Reim EK, Lanctot KL: **A meta-analysis of cytokines in major depression.** *Biol Psychiatry* 2010, **67:**446–457.
127. Zorrilla EP, Luborsky L, McKay JR, Rosenthal R, Houldin A, Tax A, McCorkle R, Seligman DA, Schmidt K: **The relationship of depression and stressors to**

immunological assays: a meta-analytic review. *Brain Behav Immun* 2001, **15**:199–226.
128. Shelton RC, Miller AH: **Eating ourselves to death (and despair): the contribution of adiposity and inflammation to depression.** *Prog Neurobiol* 2010, **91**:275–299.
129. Papakostas GI, Shelton RC, Kinrys G, Henry ME, Bakow BR, Lipkin SH, Pi B, Thurmond L, Bilello JA: **Assessment of a multi-assay, serum-based biological diagnostic test for major depressive disorder: a Pilot and Replication Study.** *Mol Psychiatry* 2011.
130. Miller AH, Maletic V, Raison CL: **Inflammation and its discontents: the role of cytokines in the pathophysiology of major depression.** *Biol Psychiatry* 2009, **65**:732–741.
131. Dantzer R, O'Connor JC, Freund GG, Johnson RW, Kelley KW: **From inflammation to sickness and depression: when the immune system subjugates the brain.** *Nat Rev Neurosci* 2008, **9**:46–56.
132. Dantzer R, Meagher MW, Cleeland CS: **Translational approaches to treatment-induced symptoms in cancer patients.** *Nat Rev Clin Oncol* 2012, **9**:414–426.
133. Felger JC, Mun J, Kimmel HL, Nye JA, Drake DF, Hernandez CR, Freeman AA, Rye DB, Goodman MM, Howell LL: **Chronic interferon-α decreases dopamine 2 receptor binding and striatal dopamine release in association with anhedonia-like behavior in nonhuman primates.** *Neuropsychopharmacology* 2013.
134. Felger JC, Alagbe O, Hu F, Mook D, Freeman AA, Sanchez MM, Kalin NH, Ratti E, Nemeroff CB, Miller AH: **Effects of interferon-alpha on rhesus monkeys: a nonhuman primate model of cytokine-induced depression.** *Biol Psychiatry* 2007, **62**:1324–1333.
135. Nunes EJ, Randall PA, Estrada A, Epling B, Hart EE, Lee CA, Baqi Y, Mueller CE, Correa M, Salamone JD: **Effort-related motivational effects of the pro-inflammatory cytokine interleukin 1-beta: studies with the concurrent fixed ratio 5/chow feeding choice task.** *Psychopharmacology (Berl)* 2014, **231**:727–736.
136. Hannestad J, DellaGioia N, Gallezot J-D, Lim K, Nabulsi N, Esterlis I, Pittman B, Lee J-YO, Pelletier D, ÄôConnor KC: **The neuroinflammation marker translocator protein is not elevated in individuals with mild-to-moderate depression: A [< sup > 11</sup > C] PBR28 PET study.** *Brain Behav Immun* 2013, **33**:131–138.
137. Eisenberger NI, Berkman ET, Inagaki TK, Rameson LT, Mashal NM, Irwin MR: **Inflammation-induced anhedonia: endotoxin reduces ventral striatum responses to reward.** *Biol Psychiatry* 2010, **68**:748–754.
138. McGrath CL, Kelley ME, Holtzheimer PE, Dunlop BW, Craighead WE, Franco AR, Craddock RC, Mayberg HS: **Toward a neuroimaging treatment selection biomarker for major depressive disorder.** *JAMA Psychiatry* 2013, **70**:821–829.
139. Malone DA Jr, Dougherty DD, Rezai AR, Carpenter LL, Friehs GM, Eskandar EN, Rauch SL, Rasmussen SA, Machado AG, Kubu CS, Tyrka AR, Price LH, Stypulkowski PH, Giftakis JE, Rise MT, Malloy PF, Salloway SP, Greenberg BD: **Deep brain stimulation of the ventral capsule/ventral striatum for treatment-resistant depression.** *Biol Psychiatry* 2009, **65**:267–275.
140. Mayberg HS, Lozano AM, Voon V, McNeely HE, Seminowicz D, Hamani C, Schwalb JM, Kennedy SH: **Deep brain stimulation for treatment-resistant depression.** *Neuron* 2005, **45**:651–660.
141. Carpenter LL, Janicak PG, Aaronson ST, Boyadjis T, Brock DG, Cook IA, Dunner DL, Lanocha K, Solvason HB, Demitrack MA: **Transcranial magnetic stimulation (TMS) for major depression: a multisite, naturalistic, observational study of acute treatment outcomes in clinical practice.** *Depress Anxiety* 2012, **29**:587–596.
142. Raison CL, Miller AH: **Is depression an inflammatory disorder?** *Curr Psychiatry Rep* 2011, **13**:467–475.
143. Cooper JC, Bloom FE, Roth RH: *The Biochemical Basis of Neuropharmacology.* 8th edition. New York: Oxford University Press; 2003.
144. Insel T, Cuthbert B, Garvey M, Heinssen R, Pine DS, Quinn K, Sanislow C, Wang P: **Research domain criteria (RDoC): toward a new classification framework for research on mental disorders.** *Am J Psychiatry* 2010, **167**:748–751.
145. Akil H, Brenner S, Kandel E, Kendler KS, King MC, Scolnick E, Watson JD, Zoghbi HY: **Medicine. The future of psychiatric research: genomes and neural circuits.** *Science* 2010, **327**:1580–1581.
146. Nestler EJ, Hyman SE: **Animal models of neuropsychiatric disorders.** *Nat Neurosci* 2010, **13**:1161–1169.
147. Deisseroth K: **Circuit dynamics of adaptive and maladaptive behaviour.** *Nature* 2014, **505**:309–317.
148. Bullmore ET, Bassett DS: **Brain graphs: graphical models of the human brain connectome.** *Annu Rev Clin Psychol* 2011, **7**:113–14.
149. Bullmore E, Sporns O: **Complex brain networks: graph theoretical analysis of structural and functional systems.** *Nat Rev Neurosci* 2009, **10**:186–198.
150. Buckholtz JW, Meyer-Lindenberg A: **Psychopathology and the human connectome: toward a transdiagnostic model of risk for mental illness.** *Neuron* 2012, **74**:990–1004.
151. Friston KJ, Ashburner JT, Kiebel SJ, Nichols TE, Penny WD: *Statistical Parametric Mapping: the Analysis of Functional Brain Images.* Academic; 2011.
152. Walter M, Henning A, Grimm S, Schulte RF, Beck J, Dydak U, Schnepf B, Boeker H, Boesiger P, Northoff G: **The relationship between aberrant neuronal activation in the pregenual anterior cingulate, altered glutamatergic metabolism, and anhedonia in major depression.** *Arch Gen Psychiatry* 2009, **66**:478–486.
153. Kring AM, Sloan DM: *Emotion Regulation and Psychopathology: a Transdiagnostic Approach to Etiology and Treatment.* New York, NY: The Guilford Press; 2010.
154. Tremblay LK, Naranjo CA, Cardenas L, Herrmann N, Busto UE: **Probing brain reward system function in major depressive disorder: altered response to dextroamphetamine.** *Arch Gen Psychiatry* 2002, **59**:409–416.
155. Tremblay LK, Naranjo CA, Graham SJ, Herrmann N, Mayberg HS, Hevenor S, Busto UE: **Functional neuroanatomical substrates of altered reward processing in major depressive disorder revealed by a dopaminergic probe.** *Arch Gen Psychiatry* 2005, **62**:1228–1236.
156. Kahneman D, Riis J: **Living, and thinking about it: two perspectives on life.** In *The science of well-being.* Edited by Huppert FA, Baylis N, Keverne B. New York, NY: Oxford University Press; 2005.
157. Conner TS, Barrett LF: **Trends in ambulatory self-report: the role of momentary experience in psychosomatic medicine.** *Psychosom Med* 2012, **74**:327–337.
158. Kahneman D, Krueger AB, Schkade D, Schwarz N, Stone AA: **Would you be happier if you were richer? A focusing illusion.** *Science* 2006, **312**:1908–1910.
159. Kahneman D, Deaton A: **High income improves evaluation of life but not emotional well-being.** *Proc Natl Acad Sci* 2010, **107**:16489–16493.
160. Schwarz N: **Retrospective and concurrent self-reports: the rationale for real-time data capture.** In *The Science of Real-Time Data Caputre: Self-Reports in Health Research.* Google e-book; 2007:11–26.
161. Strauss GP, Gold JM: **A new perspective on anhedonia in schizophrenia.** *Am J Psychiatry* 2012.
162. Kagan J: **A trio of concerns.** *Perspect Psychol Sci* 2007, **2**:361–376.
163. Beck AT, Haigh E: **The generic cognitive model.** *Annu Rev Clin Psychol* 2013, **10**.

Increased ratio of anti-apoptotic to pro-apoptotic Bcl2 gene-family members in lithium-responders one month after treatment initiation

Lori Lowthert[1], Janine Leffert[1], Aiping Lin[2], Sheila Umlauf[3], Kathleen Maloney[1], Anjana Muralidharan[1], Boris Lorberg[1], Shrikant Mane[3], Hongyu Zhao[4], Rajita Sinha[1], Zubin Bhagwagar[1,5] and Robert Beech[1*]

Abstract

Background: Lithium is considered by many as the gold standard medication in the management of bipolar disorder (BD). However, the clinical response to lithium is heterogeneous, and the molecular basis for this difference in response is unknown. In the present study, we sought to determine how the peripheral blood gene expression profiles of patients with bipolar disorder (BD) changed over time following intitiation of treatment with lithium, and whether differences in those profiles over time were related to the clinical response.

Methods: Illumina Sentrix Beadchip (Human-6v2) microarrays containing > 48,000 transcript probes were used to measure levels of expression of gene-expression in peripheral blood from 20 depressed subjects with BD prior to and every two weeks during 8 weeks of open-label treatment with lithium.
Changes in gene-expression were compared between treatment responders (defined as a decrease in the Hamilton Depression Rating Scale of 50% or more) and non-responders. Pathway analysis was conducted using GeneGO Metacore software.

Results: 127 genes showed a differential response in responders vs. non-responders. Pathway analysis showed that regulation of apoptosis was the most significantly affected pathway among these genes. Closer examination of the time-course of changes among BCL2 related genes showed that in lithium-responders, one month after starting treatment with lithium, several anti-apoptotic genes including Bcl2 and insulin receptor substrate 2 (IRS2) were up-regulated, while pro-apoptotic genes, including BCL2-antagonist/killer 1 (BAK1) and BCL2-associated agonist of cell death (BAD), were down-regulated. In contrast, in lithium non-responders, BCL2 and IRS2 were down-regulated, while BAK1 and BAD up-regulated at the one-month time-point.

Conclusions: These results suggest that differential changes in the balance of pro- and anti- apoptotic gene-expression following treatment with lithium may explain some of the heterogeneity in clinical response in BD patients.

Keywords: Bipolar disorder, Microarray, Lithium-response, Gene expression, BCL2, Apoptosis, Mitochondria

* Correspondence: robert.beech@yale.edu
[1]Department of Psychiatry, New Haven, CT 06511, USA
Full list of author information is available at the end of the article

Background

Bipolar disorder (BD) is a devastating neurobiological illness, affecting from 0.8% to 1.2% of the population [1-3]. Clinically, the disorder is characterized by episodes of mania and major depression. However, as with the vast majority of psychiatric illnesses, the nature of the underlying pathophysiology remains poorly understood [4]. Lithium is considered by many as the gold standard medication in the management of bipolar disorder (BD). It was the first treatment with demonstrated efficacy in BD [5] and it is still considered first line treatment for acute mania, acute bipolar depression, and maintenance treatment [6-8]. It is also the only medication to be consistently associated with a reduction in suicidal ideation or attempts in patients with BD [9-11].

Previous studies have investigated polymorphisms in a variety of genes including serotonin transporter, glycogen synthase kinase-3beta, inositol polyphosphatase 1-phosphate, brain-derived neurotrophic factor and activator protein 2beta, and found that these variants are not predictive factors for response to lithium [12,13]. Genome-wide association studies have also been conducted to identify common gene variants that may be associated with lithium response [14,15]. While some loci with suggestive evidence for linkage have been found [14], to date no SNPs have met the threshold for genome-wide significance. Thus, despite decades of work related to this topic, the molecular basis for the heterogeneity in response to treatment with lithium remains unknown [16].

Previous studies have shown that chronic treatment of animals [17,18] with lithium increases expression of the anti-apoptotic gene BCL2 and decreases the expression of the pro-apoptotic gene BAX. Treatment with lithium has also been shown to block the reduction of the BCL2/BAX ratio in animals treated with methamphetamine [19]. These findings have led to the suggestion that changes in the expression of BCL2 and related genes may be responsible for some or all of the therapeutic effects of lithium [17,20,21]. However, with current technologies it is impossible to assess the time-course of such changes in the brains of living subjects. Thus, whether such changes occur in human patients treated with lithium, and, if so, how they are related to differences in treatment outcome among patients remains unknown.

In a recently completed study conducted by our laboratory [22], we compared gene-expression profiles in whole blood of depressed subjects with BD to that of healthy controls. We identified a large number of genes whose expression was altered in the blood of depressed BD subjects. Strikingly, in that study, all of the top 10 functional pathways identified were interconnected, and related directly or indirectly to mitochondrial functions including energy metabolism and the regulation of apoptosis by mitochondrial proteins. One advantage of studying peripheral markers, including peripheral blood gene-expression, is that they can be assessed repeatedly over time, and thus compared directly to changes in clinical status. In the present study, we sought to determine how the peripheral blood gene expression profiles of patients with BD changed over time when they were treated with the mood stabilizer lithium, and whether differences in those profiles over time were related to the clinical response to lithium.

Methods

Subjects

Subjects included in this study are identical to those included in our previous publication [22]. All procedures involving human subjects were approved by the Yale Human Investigation Committee and are in accordance with the Helsinki declaration of 1975. All subjects provided written informed consent at the time of enrollment in the study. Inclusion criteria for subjects with BD included age between 18 and 65 years, diagnosis of bipolar disorder (bipolar type I or II), currently depressed as defined by Diagnostic and Statistical Manual of Mental Disorders, fourth edition text revision (DSM-IV- TR) [23], and not being treated with lithium at the time of study entry. Diagnosis was determined by consensus of clinical interview by a Board Certified Psychiatrist (RDB or ZB) and the Structured Clinical Interview for DSM-IV Axis I Disorders [24] (performed by KM, AM, or BL). Exclusion criteria included DSM-IV-TR diagnoses other than bipolar I or II, current or recent (past 30 days) abuse of illicit substances (verified by urine toxicology screening), pre-existing thyroid pathology (e.g. hypothyroidism or hyperthyroidism) as evidenced by an abnormal thyroid function test at screening, or history or evidence of a medical condition that would expose them to an undue risk of a significant adverse event or interfere with assessments of safety or efficacy during the course of the trial, including but not limited to hepatic, renal, respiratory, cardiovascular, endocrine, neurological, or hematological disease.

A total of 26 subjects with BD were recruited for this study. To ensure that only BD subjects who had been exposed to lithium for a period of time sufficient to assess response were included in the gene-expression analysis, an *a priori* decision was made to include only those subjects who completed at least one month of treatment. A total of 20 subjects were included; one subject was withdrawn due to previously undiagnosed hypothyroidism, and five subjects dropped out of treatment without completing one month of treatment. Demographic and clinical information for the 20 subjects included in the study is summarized in Table 1.

Table 1 Study Participants- summary of demographic and clinical information

Gender	Lithium Responders	Lithium Non-Responders
	N (%)	N (%)
Male	2 (20)	4 (40)
Female	8 (80)	6 (60)
Ethnicity		
Caucasian	7 (70)	9 (90)
Non-caucasian	3 (30)	1 (10)
Bipolar I disorder	7 (70)	10 (100)
	Mean ± SD	Mean ± SD
Age	34.5 ± 10.6	42.0 ± 6.6
HAM-D (at entry)	26.2 ± 15.9	29.1 ± 14.8
HAM-A (at entry)	14.4 ± 8.6	14.7 ± 7.0
MADRS (at entry)	17.9 ± 11.6	20.7 ± 11.5
YMRS (at entry)	6.3 ± 5.8	5.9 ± 4.3
Lithium Level (average)	0.63 ± 0.14	0.65 ± 0.28

HAM-D = Hamilton Depression Rating Scale, HAM-A = Hamilton Anxiety Rating Scale, MADRS = Montgomery-Asberg Depression Rating Scale, YMRS = Young Mania Rating Scale.

An additional group of 15 healthy control subjects (5 male, 10 female) was recruited through advertising. None of the control subjects met criteria for any DSM-IV-TR axis I diagnosis as determined by the Structured Clinical Interview for DSM-IV Axis I Disorders [24] or current or recent abuse of illicit substances.

Treatments

All subjects received open label treatment with Lithium carbonate in addition to their previous psychiatric medications. Lithium was started at an initial dose of 300 mg p.o. BID. Doses were adjusted weekly based on lithium trough levels until a target level of 0.6 to 1.2 mEq/L was achieved or patients were unable to tolerate side effects. Of the 20 subjects included in the microarray analysis, there were 9 patients who were initially receiving no medication and 11 who were receiving one or more atypical antipsychotic medications (olanzapine, quietapine, risperidone, or ziprasidone). Two subjects were taking valproic acid in addition to an atypical antipsychotic and one subject each was taking carbamazepine, oxcarbazepine or topiramate in addition to an atypical antipsychotic. Mood ratings for BD subjects were performed using Hamilton Depression Rating Scale (HAM-D) [25,26], the Montgomery-Asberg Depression Rating Scale (MADRS) [27], Hamilton Anxiety Rating Scale [28], and the Young Mania Rating Scale (YMRS) [29].

Sample Preparation and Microarray Analysis

Blood draws for RNA isolation were done prior to initiation of treatment with lithium and every two weeks during 8-weeks of open label treatment with lithium for subjects with BD (five blood draws total). Blood draws for RNA isolation were done at the same time as those used to assess lithium trough levels, approximately 12 hours after the evening dose of lithium, and before the morning dose was taken. Total RNA was isolated from 10 cc whole blood using the PAXgene Blood RNA Isolation kit (QIAGEN, Valencia, CA) per the manufacturer's instructions, and depleted of globin mRNA message using GLOBINclear hybridization capture technology (Ambion, Austin, TX). Globin-reduced total RNA underwent cDNA synthesis and overnight *in vitro transcription* utilizing the Illumina TotalPrep RNA Amplification Kit (Ambion). Biotinylated cRNA (1.5 μg) was hybridized onto an Illumina Sentrix Beadchip (Human-6v2) then scanned on a BeadArray Reader. Microarray hybridization and scanning were carried out at the NIH Neuroscience Microarray Center at Yale (http:/info.med.yale.edu/neuromicroarray). Per the policies of the NIH microarray consortium, the complete project annotation in MAGE-ML, image files, as well as raw data files will be available for download. At the time of publication, all data will be deposited into the NCBI-GEO repository, while retaining links to the microarray consortium relational data warehouse.

Data Analysis

BD subjects were divided into lithium-responders and non-responders based on the *a priori* defined change from their initial HAM-D scores. Lithium-responders were defined as those having a >50% reduction in initial HAM-D at the time of the last assessment. BD subjects who did not meet these criteria were classified as "non-responders". Subjects who dropped out during weeks 4–8 were classified as lithium-responders or non-responders using an intent-to-treat analysis based on the last observation carried forward. Classification of BD subjects as lithium-responders vs. non-responders did not change if the MADRS was used instead of the HAM-D to classify subjects.

Statistical analysis of microarray data was carried out at the Keck Foundation Biotechnology Biostatistics Resource (http://keck.med.yale.edu/biostats). Illumina BeadStudio software was used to generate probe and gene expression profiles of each sample. Quantile normalization was carried out using the package incorporated in the Illumina BeadStudio software package [30]. Further statistical analysis was carried out on genes with a detection p-value <0.01 as determined using the Illumina BeadStudio software (i.e. a 99% probability that expression was above background) in 90% of the samples. A total of 17,240 genes on the array met these criteria. This is similar to the detection sensitivity seen in other studies of whole blood using the Illumina Sentrix Beadchip platform [31].

Baseline differences in gene-expression between lithium-responders and non-responders were assessed using t-tests as well as ANOVA analysis co-varied for age, sex, and co-administered medications. To identify genes whose expression changed differentially in lithium responders and non-responders after initiation of treatment, we performed a mixed model ANOVA of the complete microarray data set with group (responder or non-responder) as a between subjects factor, and time as a within subjects factor. Correction for multiple testing was done using estimated group-wise false discovery rates (FDR) [32,33].

Network analysis to identify the most significant pathways among genes identified by the ANOVA analysis (above) was carried out using GeneGO Metacore® software (GeneGO Inc., Encinitas, CA).

qRT-PCR analysis

qRT-PCR was carried out using the TaqMan® "Universal PCR Master Mix" Protocol (Applied Biosystems) and Real-Time PCR probes listed on the NCBI Probe Database (http://www.ncbi.nlm.nih.gov/sites/entrez?db=probe). Relative quantitation of gene-expression was done by comparing the efficiency of amplification of each gene of interest using the ΔΔCt method, as described in User Bulletin#2 for the ABI Prism 7700 Sequence Detection System (Applied Biosystems, available online at http://keck.med.yale.edu/affymetrix/rtpcr/index.htm).

Results

Lithium responders did not differ significantly from non-responders in their initial HAM-D, HAM-A, MADRS or YMRS scores, age, sex, ethnicity, or use of concomitant antipsychotic medication, however there was a non-significant trend for greater use of antipsychotic medications among the lithium non-responders. Average serum levels of lithium over the eight weeks of treatment did not differ significantly between responders and non-responders (responders: 0.63 ± 0.14; non-responders: 0.66 ± 0.28). Comparison of baseline (pre-treatment) expression profiles between lithium responders and non-responders using t-tests identified 606 genes, whose expression differed by ≥ 1.3 fold with a nominal p-value <0.05. However, when other factors such as age, sex, and use of co-administered medications were included as co-variates in an ANOVA model, none of these differences were significant after correction for multiple testing (FDR <0.05) (data not shown). Thus, it is unclear whether any of these pre-treatment differences are specifically associated with the subsequent response to lithium.

Next, to identify genes whose expression changed differentially in lithium responders and non-responders after initiation of treatment, we performed a mixed model ANOVA of the complete microarray data set with group (responder or non-responder) as a between subjects factor, and time (in weeks, after starting treatment with lithium) as a within subjects factor. There were 127 genes that showed a significant group x time interaction (i.e. difference in degree or direction of change between lithium-responders and non-responders) after FDR correction for multiple testing, and a fold-difference ≥ 1.3 between lithium responders and non-responders at least one time-point after treatment initiation. Interestingly, all of the significant differences between responders and non-responders occurred during the period from 4–6 weeks after initiation of treatment with lithium. This time period corresponds well with the typical 6–8-week delay in the acute antidepressant effect of lithium in the treatment of bipolar depression [34]. At week 4 there were 37 differentially expressed genes (22 up-regulated in responders vs. non-responders and 15 down-regulated) and at week 6 there were 90 differentially expressed genes (51 up-regulated and 39 down-regulated). The complete list of genes showing a significant group x time interaction is listed in Additional file 1 Table S1.

To better understand the functional implications of these differences, we conducted pathway analysis using GeneGO Metacore software for each of these clusters separately, and for the group of 127 genes as a whole. As seen in Table 2, 4 of the top 10 GeneGO Process Networks associated with the group as a whole are related to the regulation of apoptosis, although most of these pathways did not reach statistical significance. Moreover, when considered separately, each of the clusters of differentially expressed genes was related to one or more apoptotic pathways, although again, many of these pathways did not reach statistical significance. Notably, at 4 weeks after treatment initiation, pro-apoptotic mitochondrial genes appears to be down-regulated, while anti-apoptosis pathways regulated by external signals via PI3K/AKT appeared to be up-regulated in lithium-responders vs. non-responders. Based on these findings, as well as previous work implicating the Bcl2 family of proteins in the mechanism of action of lithium [17,18], we decided to examine the pattern of expression of various Bcl2 gene family members over time in lithium-responders and non-responders more closely.

Table 3 shows the expression level of various pro- and anti-apoptotic Bcl2 gene family member expression in lithium-responders and non-responders (normalized to healthy controls) as well as the ratio between responders and non-responders over the course of eight weeks following initiation of treatment with lithium. Strikingly, following initiation of treatment with lithium, all of the anti-apoptotic genes examined (BCL2, BCL2L1-tx var. 1, IRS2, and MCL1- tx. var. 1), showed an increase in relative expression in lithium responders compared to

Table 2 Biological pathways identified by GeneGO metacore pathway analysis as differing over time between BD subjects who responded or failed to respond to treatment with lithium

GeneGO Process Networks for genes showing significant group x time interaction		
Overall		**p-Value**
1	Apoptosis_Anti-Apoptosis mediated by external signals	0.013
2	Apoptosis_Apoptotic mitochondria	0.055
3	Cytoskeleton_Actin filaments	0.055
4	Apoptosis_Endoplasmic reticulum stress pathway	0.068
5	Cell cycle_Core	0.110
6	Protein folding_Folding in normal condition	0.117
7	Cell cycle_G1-S Interleukin regulation	0.123
8	Development_Hemopoiesis, Erythropoietin pathway	0.143
9	Immune response_BCR pathway	0.147
10	Apoptosis_Apoptosis stimulation by external signals	0.159
Week 4: down-regulated genes in Lithium responders vs. non-responders		
1	Apoptosis_Apoptotic mitochondria	0.053
2	Apoptosis_Endoplasmic reticulum stress pathway	0.060
3	Signal transduction_Nitric oxide signaling	0.061
4	Apoptosis_Anti-Apoptosis mediated by external signals by Estrogen	0.068
5	Protein folding_Folding in normal condition	0.081
6	Proteolysis_Proteolysis in cell cycle and apoptosis	0.085
7	Development_Hemopoiesis, Erythropoietin pathway	0.092
8	Apoptosis_Apoptosis stimulation by external signals	0.098
9	Proliferation_Negative regulation of cell proliferation	0.123
10	Cell adhesion_Amyloid proteins	0.127
Week 4: up-regulated genes in Lithium responders vs. non-responders		
1	Cell adhesion_Glycoconjugates	0.010
2	Apoptosis_Anti-Apoptosis mediated by external signals via PI3K/AKT	0.017
3	Autophagy_Autophagy	0.053
4	Signal transduction_Androgen receptor signaling cross-talk	0.069
5	Signal transduction_ERBB-family signaling	0.072
6	Cytoskeleton_Macropinocytosis and its regulation	0.081
7	Inflammation_IL-13 signaling pathway	0.087
8	Signal transduction_Leptin signaling	0.098
9	Signal Transduction_Cholecystokinin signaling	0.100
10	Inflammation_IL-4 signaling	0.108
Week 6: down-regulated genes in Lithium responders vs. non-responders		
1	Cell cycle_Core	0.027
2	Development_Hemopoiesis, Erythropoietin pathway	0.036
3	Response to hypoxia and oxidative stress	0.053
4	Transport_Synaptic vesicle exocytosis	0.059
5	Cell cycle_G0-G1	0.149
6	Neurophysiological process_Long-term potentiation	0.170
7	Blood coagulation	0.193
8	Apoptosis_Anti-Apoptosis mediated by external signals by Estrogen	0.202
9	Inflammation_IL-6 signaling	0.238
10	Cell cycle_G1-S Interleukin regulation	0.245

Table 2 Biological pathways identified by GeneGO metacore pathway analysis as differing over time between BD subjects who responded or failed to respond to treatment with lithium *(Continued)*

Week 6: up-regulated genes in Lithium responders vs. non-responders		
1	Development_Skeletal muscle development	0.024
2	Cell adhesion_Attractive and repulsive receptors	0.034
3	Cytoskeleton_Actin filaments	0.034
4	Development_Neurogenesis:Axonal guidance	0.056
5	Protein folding_ER and cytoplasm	0.074
6	Protein folding_Response to unfolded proteins	0.111
7	Apoptosis_Apoptotic mitochondria	0.123
8	Apoptosis_Endoplasmic reticulum stress pathway	0.138
9	Apoptosis_Anti-Apoptosis mediated by external signals by Estrogen	0.156
10	Protein folding_Folding in normal condition	0.184

Pathway analysis was conducted for the entire group of 127 genes showing a significant group x time interaction, as well as for up-regulated and down-regulated genes separately at each of the time-points where significant differences were seen (4 weeks and 6 weeks after treatment initiation).

non-responders during the first month of treatment. For BCL2L1, this increase peaked at 2 weeks after treatment initiation, while for the other genes the highest relative expression occurred at 4 weeks. Among the pro-apoptotic genes, BAD, BAK, BAX, and BMF showed a decrease in the relative expression in lithium responders, while BCL2L13, BCL2L1-tx. var. 2, BID, BNIP3, and MCL1, tx. var. 2, showed no change or inconsistent change over this time period. Thus, overall there appeared to be an increase in the relative expression of anti-apoptotic genes and a decrease in the expression of pro-apoptotic genes in lithium responders during the first month of treatment, while the opposite pattern was seen in lithium non-responders. This pattern was even more marked when the ratios of specific anti- and pro-apoptotic genes were compared in lithium responders and non-responders over time. Figure 1 shows the ratios of BCL2/ BAD (panel **A**), BCL2/BAK1 (panel **B**), IRS2/ BAD (panel **C**) and IRS2/BAK1 (panel **D**) in lithium responders and non-responders over the 8 weeks of the study. In each case, the ratio of anti- to pro-apoptotic genes increased in lithium responders over the first month of treatment and then returned to baseline, while the opposite pattern was observed in lithium non-responders. When the ratios of alternatively spliced versions of the same gene with either anti- or pro- apoptotic functions (e.g. BCL2L1 tx. variants 1 and 2, or MCL1 tx. variants 1 and 2) were compared, there was no significant group x time interaction, indicating that alternative splicing was not responsible for these effects.

We also performed qRT-PCR analysis of the 4 genes shown in Figure 1: BCL2, IRS2, BAK1 and BAD, and compared the ratio of anti-apoptotic to pro-apoptotic gene expression in lithium responders and non-responders 4 weeks after treatment initiation. In general, the results of the qRT-PCR analysis were similar to those obtained by microarray hybridization, with lithium-responders showing greater relative expression of anti-apoptotic genes than non-responders (BCL2/BAK1: 1.37 fold higher in responders vs. non-responders, BLC2/BAD: 1.69 fold higher in responders vs. non-responders, IRS2/BAK1: 1.04 fold higher in responders vs. non-responders, IRS2/BAD: 1.29 fold higher in responders vs. non-responders). However, due to the greater variability in the qRT-PCR results, none of these differences was statistically significant.

Discussion

In this study, we compared changes in gene-expression in peripheral blood among a group of depressed subjects with BD over a period of eight weeks following the initiation of treatment with lithium. We identified 127 genes whose expression changed differentially in lithium responders and non-responders. Pathway analysis of the differentially expressed genes using GeneGO Metacore software showed that regulation of apoptosis was the most significantly affected pathway among these genes. Strikingly, among lithium responders, several anti-apoptotic genes including BCL2 and insulin receptor substrate 2 (IRS2) were up-regulated, while pro-apoptotic genes, including BCL2-antagonist/killer 1 (BAK1) and BCL2-associated agonist of cell death (BAD), were down-regulated. In contrast, in lithium non-responders, BCL2 and IRS2 were down-regulated, while BAK1 and BAD up-regulated at the one-month time-point.

BCL2 gene family members are key regulators of apoptotic cell death and include both pro- and anti-apoptotic genes [35,36]. Collectively, the expression levels of the various BCL2 family members define thresholds for apoptosis in a given cell. The two pro-apoptotic proteins, BAX and BAK1 promote apoptosis by binding to the mitochondrial voltage-dependent anion channel (VDAC), and accelerating its opening,

Table 3 Expression of anti- and pro-apoptotic Bcl2-related genes in lithium responders and non-responders (normalized to expression levels in untreated healthy controls subjects) at each of the time points tested (baseline, 2,4,6, and 8 weeks after treatment initiation)

Normalized Expression Levels	Time (in weeks) since starting lithium				
Anti-Apoptotic Genes	**Baseline**	**2 weeks**	**4 weeks**	**6 weeks**	**8 weeks**
BCL2					
Lithium Responders	0.96	0.89	1.08	0.86	0.83
Non-Responders	0.94	0.90	0.78	0.88	0.93
Ratio	1.0	1.0	*1.4	1.0	0.9
BCL2L1 (tx var. 1) (aka BCL-xL)					
Lithium Responders	2.30	4.69	2.38	2.49	5.84
Non-Responders	3.04	3.49	2.08	3.13	1.85
Ratio	0.8	1.3	1.1	0.8	3.2
IRS2					
Lithium Responders	0.78	1.12	1.51	0.84	1.35
Non-Responders	1.22	0.99	0.68	1.00	1.13
Ratio	0.6	1.1	***2.2	0.8	1.2
MCL1 (tx. Var. 1)					
Lithium Responders	0.56	0.81	0.91	0.74	0.98
Non-Responders	1.18	1.00	0.79	1.02	1.05
Ratio	**0.5	0.8	1.1	0.7	0.9
Pro-Apoptotic Genes					
BAD					
Lithium Responders	1.54	1.49	1.29	1.44	1.32
Non-Responders	1.39	1.39	1.48	1.33	1.41
Ratio	1.1	1.1	0.9	1.1	0.9
BAK1					
Lithium Responders	1.47	0.92	0.80	0.89	0.76
Non-Responders	1.29	1.08	1.23	1.24	1.29
Ratio	1.1	0.9	***0.6	**0.7	0.6
BAX					
Lithium Responders	1.69	1.73	1.55	1.58	1.18
Non-Responders	1.14	1.39	1.25	1.42	1.53
Ratio	**1.5	1.2	1.2	1.1	0.8
BCL2L13 (aka BCL-Rambo)					
Lithium Responders	0.86	0.98	0.96	0.82	0.96
Non-Responders	0.96	1.03	0.86	0.97	0.85
Ratio	0.9	0.9	1.1	0.8	1.1
BCL2L1 (tx var. 2)(aka BCL-xL)					
Lithium Responders	1.58	2.34	1.54	1.42	1.54
Non-Responders	1.58	1.98	1.59	1.96	1.36
Ratio	1.0	1.2	1.0	0.7	1.1
BID					
Lithium Responders	1.03	1.06	1.09	0.98	1.01
Non-Responders	1.04	0.99	1.02	1.12	0.97
Ratio	1.0	1.1	1.1	0.9	1.0

Table 3 Expression of anti- and pro-apoptotic Bcl2-related genes in lithium responders and non-responders (normalized to expression levels in untreated healthy controls subjects) at each of the time points tested (baseline, 2,4,6, and 8 weeks after treatment initiation) *(Continued)*

BMF					
Lithium Responders	1.09	1.05	1.06	1.06	0.96
Non-Responders	0.91	0.97	1.10	0.82	1.06
Ratio	1.2	1.1	1.0	*1.3	0.9
BNIP3					
Lithium Responders	1.02	0.74	0.89	0.78	0.78
Non-Responders	0.81	0.84	0.77	0.82	0.91
Ratio	**1.3	0.9	1.2	0.9	0.9
MCL1 (tx. var. 2)					
Lithium Responders	1.08	1.21	1.14	1.10	1.34
Non-Responders	1.11	1.24	1.10	1.19	1.02
Ratio	1.0	1.0	1.0	0.9	*1.3

Following initiation of treatment with lithium, all of the anti-apoptotic genes examined (BCL2, BCL2L1-tx var. 1, IRS2, and MCL1- tx. var. 1), showed an increase in the relative expression in lithium responders compared to non-responders during the first month of treatment. Among the pro-apoptotic genes, BAD, BAK, BAX, and BMF showed a decrease in the relative expression in lithium responders, while BCL2L13, BCL2L1-tx. var. 2, BID, BNIP3, and MCL1, tx. var. 2, showed no change or inconsistent change over this time period.
Significant differences are marked with asterisks (* $p < 0.10$, ** $p < 0.05$, and *** $P < .01$).

leading to a loss in membrane potential, the release of cytochrome c, and subsequent activation of the intrinsic caspase pathway. Anti-apoptotic members of the BCL2 family, including BCL2 itself, the related protein BCL-xL (encoded by the BLCL1 gene) and MCL-1, prevent apoptosis by binding to BAX and BAK1, preventing their interaction with VDAC. Other pro-apoptotic BCL2 family members, termed the 'BH3-only' proteins, including BAD, BID, and BMF, are thought to indirectly promote apoptosis by binding to anti-apoptotic family members and preventing their interaction with BAX and BAK1 [35,36]. IRS2 is a cytoplasmic signaling molecule that mediates effects of insulin, insulin-like growth factor 1, and other cytokines by acting as a molecular adaptor between diverse receptor tyrosine kinases and downstream effectors. In addition, IRS2 has been shown to bind to the Bcl2 protein and block phosphorylation of Bcl2 induced by insulin and suppress apoptotic cell death [37]. Thus, our finding that BCL2 and IRS2 are both increased in lithium responders at the one month time point, while BAK1 and BAD were down-regulated, suggests that in lithium responders there was a shift in the balance of expression among pro- and anti- apoptotic members of the BCL2 family favoring the anti-apoptotic genes. Conversely, in lithium non-responders there was a decrease in BCL2 and IRS2 and an increase BAK1 and BAD, suggesting that there was a shift in the opposite direction, favoring the pro-apoptotic members of the BCL2 family. Intriguingly, changes in the ratio of anti- to pro-apoptotic gene expression among both lithium responders and non-responders appeared to return to baseline by the 8-week time-point, although differences in clinical status were more marked at this point than at 4 weeks. This suggests that transient changes in gene-expression can have enduring effects on the state of the organism, even when those differences can no longer be directly observed. Additional studies will be required to determine if there are changes in the level or function of the proteins encoded by these genes that are longer lasting and perhaps more directly related to the clinical status of the patients.

While changes in the expression of BCL2 family genes in peripheral blood are unlikely to be directly related to the changes in mood symptoms, systemic differences in the way subjects with different genetic and epigenetic backgrounds respond at the biochemical level to treatment with lithium may underlie some of the heterogeneity in clinical response to lithium.

Studies of post-mortem tissue from human subjects has shown that activity of mitochondrial complex I is decreased, and oxidative damage is increased in the prefrontal cortex of patients with BD [38]. Lithium has been shown to increase the activity of mitochondrial ETC. complexes in extracts from human post-mortem brain tissue at therapeutically relevant concentrations [39], while rats subjected to an experimental model of depression showed impaired mitochondrial function [40]. Conversely, transgenic mice expressing the anti-apoptotic protein Bax Inhibitor 1, showed protection in the learned helplessness model of depression [41]. These results have been interpreted in the context of a neurotrophic hypothesis of mood disorders [42,43], indicating that increased expression of BCL2 and related genes is necessary for the therapeutic effects of lithium and other

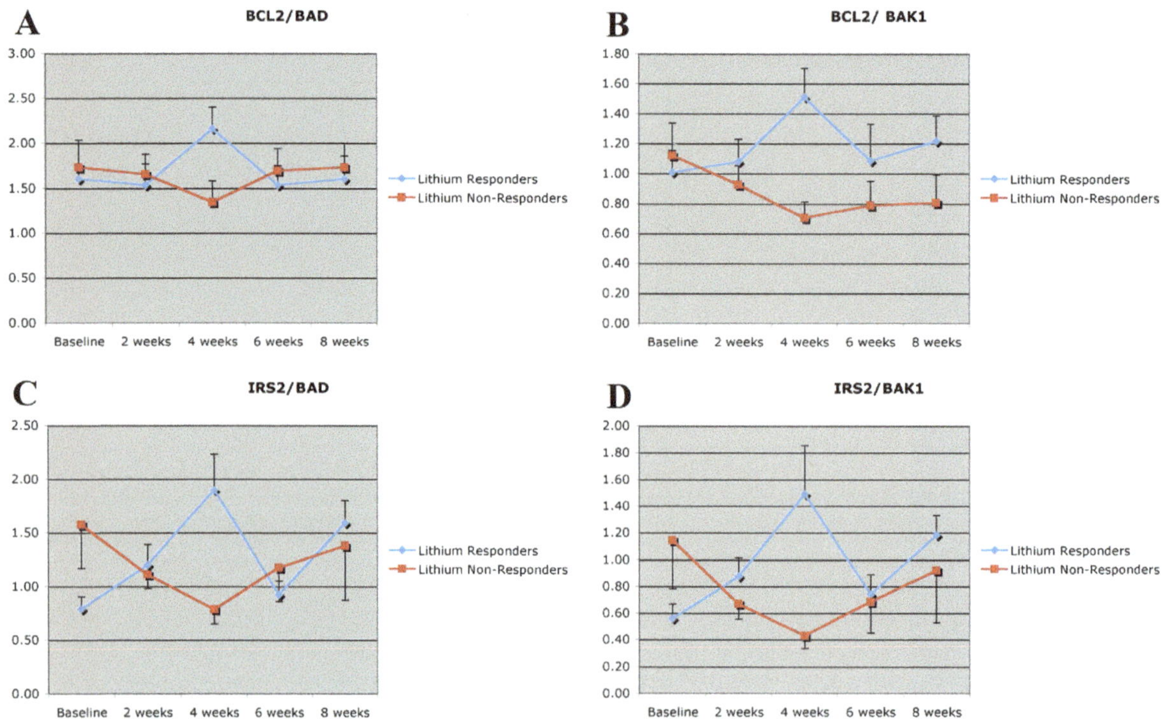

Figure 1 Ratios of BCL2/ BAD (panel A), BCL2/BAK1 (panel B), IRS2/BAD (panel C) and IRS2/BAK1 (panel D) in lithium responders and non-responders over the 8 weeks of the study. In each case, the ratio of anti- to pro-apoptotic genes increased in lithium responders over the first month of treatment and then returned to baseline, while the opposite pattern was observed in lithium non-responders.

mood stabilizers. Our results indicate that in a substantial group of patients, this effect does not occur, and in fact the opposite effect was seen in patients who did not respond to lithium. Better understanding of the mechanisms underlying this difference may lead to improved methods for personalizing treatment for bipolar disorder in the future.

Limitations of this study include a relatively small sample-size, admixture of subjects with BD I and BD II, and the fact that BCL2 family members were assayed at the level of gene-expression rather than protein or functional assays. A further caveat is that while the average Li level in both groups was similar, and was within our target range of 0.6 to 1.2 mEq/L, there were several subjects in both groups whose levels were outside of that range, which may have affected both their response to treatment and the patterns of gene-induction observed in these subjects. In addition, these studies address only the acute anti-depressant properties of lithium, and do not address changes in gene-expression that may be related to lithium's anti-manic, prophylactic or anti-suicide properties, each of which may be associated with a unique molecular profile. Due to the small sample size and limited information that was collected regarding prior episodes, we are unable to address the relationship, if any, between these molecular changes and the proposed specificity of lithium for "classic bipolar disorder" as opposed to the broader spectrum of bipolar illnesses [8]. Future studies will be needed to confirm these findings in a larger cohort of patients and to determine the relevancy of these changes to other aspects of lithium's clinical effects in patients with BD.

Conclusions

In this study, we compared changes in gene-expression in peripheral blood among a group of depressed subjects with BD over a period of eight weeks following the initiation of treatment with lithium. We found that the ratio of anti- to pro-apoptotic gene expression increased in lithium responders over the first month of treatment and then returned to baseline, while the opposite pattern was observed in lithium non-responders. These results suggest that individual differences in the response to treatment with lithium occur at the level of gene-induction, and are clinically relevant. If validated in larger studies, such changes could be useful clinically as surrogate outcome markers allowing treatment decisions (including whether to continue or discontinue treatment with lithium) to be made earlier, and thus facilitate recovery in patients with BD.

Additional file

Additional file 1: Table S1. Fold difference and p-value for each of 127 genes, grouped by cluster, that showed a significant group x time interaction (i.e. difference in degree or direction of change between lithium-responders and non-responders) after FDR correction for multiple testing, and a fold-difference ≥ 1.3 between lithium responders and non-responders at least one time-point after treatment initiation.

Competing interests

The authors declare that they have no competing interests.

Authors' contributions

LL participated in the design of the study, carried out RT-PCR analyses of candidate mRNAs and wrote the initial draft of the manuscript. JL performed RNA isolation from blood samples and maintained the laboratory database of samples. AL carried out statistical analyses of microarray and clinical data. SU carried out quality control on RNA samples and performed microarray hybridizations. KM carried out subject recruitment and assessment. AM carried out subject recruitment and assessment. BL carried out subject recruitment and assessment. SM participated in the design of the study and supervised microarray hybridizations. HZ participated in the design of the study and supervised the statistical analysis. RS participated in the design of the study, supervised recruitment and assessment of healthy controls. ZB participated in the design of the study, supervised subject recruitment and assessment, performed diagnostic interviews, and helped to draft the manuscript. RB conceived of the study, participated in its design and coordination, carried out diagnostic interviews and subjects assessments, and wrote the final draft of the mancuscript. All authors read and approved the final manuscript.

Acknowledgements

This work was supported by grants from the California Bipolar Foundation (RDB), Donaghue Foundation Grant # DF08-009 (RDB), Stanley Medical Research Institute Grants # 05R-864 (RDB) and #05 T-68 (ZB), NIH/NIDA K12 DA-00167(RDB), 1K23MH077914-01A1 (ZB), NARSAD (ZB) CTSA Grant Number UL1 RR024139 from the National Center for Research Resources to Yale University (ZB), R01-AA013892 (RS), RO1- AA013892 (RS), UL1-DE019586 (RS) and PL1-DA024859 (RS).

Author details

[1]Department of Psychiatry, New Haven, CT 06511, USA. [2]Keck Foundation Biotechnology Biostatistics Resource, New Haven, CT 06511, USA. [3]Center for Genome Analysis, New Haven, CT 06511, USA. [4]Department of Epidemiology and Public Health, Yale University School of Medicine, New Haven, CT 06511, USA. [5]Neuroscience Global Clinical Research, Bristol-Myers Squibb, Wallingford, CT 06492-1996, USA.

References

1. Merikangas KR, Akiskal HS, Angst J, Greenberg PE, Hirschfeld RM, Petukhova M, Kessler RC: **Lifetime and 12-month prevalence of bipolar spectrum disorder in the National Comorbidity Survey replication.** *Arch Gen Psychiatry* 2007, **64:**543–552.
2. Kessler RC, Berglund P, Demler O, Jin R, Merikangas KR, Walters EE: **Lifetime prevalence and age-of-onset distributions of DSM-IV disorders in the National Comorbidity Survey Replication.** *Arch Gen Psychiatry* 2005, **62:**593–602.
3. Waraich P, Goldner EM, Somers JM, Hsu L: **Prevalence and incidence studies of mood disorders: a systematic review of the literature.** *Can J Psychiatry* 2004, **49:**124–138.
4. Martinowich K, Schloesser RJ, Manji HK: **Bipolar disorder: from genes to behavior pathways.** *J Clin Invest* 2009, **119:**726–736.
5. Cade JF: **Lithium salts in the treatment of psychotic excitement.** *Med J Aust* 1949, **2:**349–352.
6. APA: **Practice guideline for the treatment of patients with bipolar disorder (revision).** *Am J Psychiatry* 2002, **159:**1–50.
7. Grof P, Muller-Oerlinghausen B: **A critical appraisal of lithium's efficacy and effectiveness: the last 60 years.** *Bipolar Disorders* 2009, **11:**10–19.
8. Gershon S, Chengappa KN, Malhi GS: **Lithium specificity in bipolar illness: a classic agent for the classic disorder.** *Bipolar Disord* 2009, **11**(Suppl 2):34–44.
9. Tondo L, Hennen J, Baldessarini RJ: **Lower suicide risk with long-term lithium treatment in major affective illness: a meta-analysis.** *Acta Psychiatr Scand* 2001, **104:**163–172.
10. Ernst CL, Goldberg JF: **Antisuicide properties of psychotropic drugs: a critical review.** *Harv Rev Psychiatry* 2004, **12:**14–41.
11. Goodwin FK, Fireman B, Simon GE, Hunkeler EM, Lee J, Revicki D: **Suicide risk in bipolar disorder during treatment with lithium and divalproex.** *JAMA* 2003, **290:**1467–1473.
12. Michelon L, Meira-Lima I, Cordeiro Q, Miguita K, Breen G, Collier D, Vallada H: **Association study of the INPP1, 5HTT, BDNF, AP-2beta and GSK-3beta GENE variants and restrospectively scored response to lithium prophylaxis in bipolar disorder.** *Neurosci Lett* 2006, **403:**288–293.
13. Bremer T, Diamond C, McKinney R, Shehktman T, Barrett TB, Herold C, Kelsoe JR: **The pharmacogenetics of lithium response depends upon clinical co-morbidity.** *Mol Diagn Ther* 2007, **11:**161–170.
14. Perlis RH, Smoller JW, Ferreira MA, McQuillin A, Bass N, Lawrence J, Sachs GS, Nimgaonkar V, Scolnick EM, Gurling H, *et al*: **A genomewide association study of response to lithium for prevention of recurrence in bipolar disorder.** *Am J Psychiatry* 2009, **166:**718–725.
15. Schulze TG, Alda M, Adli M, Akula N, Ardau R, Bui ET, Chillotti C, Cichon S, Czerski P, Del Zompo M, *et al*: **The International Consortium on Lithium Genetics (ConLiGen): an initiative by the NIMH and IGSLI to study the genetic basis of response to lithium treatment.** *Neuropsychobiology* 2010, **62:**72–78.
16. Belmaker RH, Agam G: **Bipolar disorder: Neurochemistry and drug mechanisms.** *Discov Med* 2005, **5:**191–198.
17. Chen G, Zeng WZ, Yuan PX, Huang LD, Jiang YM, Zhao ZH, Manji HK: **The mood-stabilizing agents lithium and valproate robustly increase the levels of the neuroprotective protein bcl-2 in the CNS.** *J Neurochem* 1999, **72:**879–882.
18. Manji HK, Moore GJ, Chen G: **Lithium up-regulates the cytoprotective protein Bcl-2 in the CNS in vivo: a role for neurotrophic and neuroprotective effects in manic depressive illness.** *J Clin Psychiatry* 2000, **61**(Suppl 9):82–96.
19. Bachmann RF, Wang Y, Yuan P, Zhou R, Li X, Alesci S, Du J, Manji HK: **Common effects of lithium and valproate on mitochondrial functions: protection against methamphetamine-induced mitochondrial damage.** *Int J Neuropsychopharmacol* 2009, **12:**1–18.
20. Manji HK, Moore GJ, Chen G: **Clinical and preclinical evidence for the neurotrophic effects of mood stabilizers: implications for the pathophysiology and treatment of manic-depressive illness.** *Biol Psychiatry* 2000, **48:**740–754.
21. Einat H, Manji HK: **Cellular Plasticity Cascades: Genes-To-Behavior Pathways in Animal Models of Bipolar Disorder.** *Biol Psychiatry* 2006, **59:**1160–1171.
22. Beech RD, Lowthert L, Leffert JJ, Mason PN, Taylor MM, Umlauf S, Lin A, Lee JY, Maloney K, Muralidharan A, *et al*: **Increased peripheral blood expression of electron transport chain genes in bipolar depression.** *Bipolar Disord* 2010, **12:**813–824.
23. APA: *Diagnostic and Statistical Manual of Mental Disorders, Fourth Edition, Text Revision (DSM-IV-TR).* Washington, DC: American Psychiatric Association; 2000.
24. First MB, Spitzer RL, Gibbon M, Williams J: *Structured Clinical Interview for DSM-IV Axis I Disorders — Patient Edition (SCID-I/P, Version 2.0).* New York: Biometrics Research Department, New York State Psychiatric Institute; 1996.
25. Hamilton M: **A rating scale for depression.** *J Neurol Neurosurg Psychiatry* 1960, **23:**56–62.
26. Mazure C, Nelson JC, Price LH: **Reliability and validity of the symptoms of major depressive illness.** *Arch Gen Psychiatry* 1986, **43:**451–456.
27. Montgomery SA, Asberg M: **A new depression scale designed to be sensitive to change.** *Br J Psychiatry* 1979, **134:**382–389.
28. Hamilton M: **The assessment of anxiety states by ratings.** *Br J Med Psychol* 1959, **32:**50–55.
29. Young RC, Biggs JT, Ziegler VE, Meyer DA: **A rating scale for mania: reliability, validity and sensitivity.** *Br J Psychiatry* 1978, **133:**429–435.

30. Illumina: **BeadStudio Gene Expression Module v32 User Guide.** In *Chapter 4: Normalization and Differential Analysis.* 2009th edition. San Diego, CA: Illumina Technical Support; 2009.
31. Barnes M, Freudenberg J, Thompson S, Aronow B, Pavlidis P: **Experimental comparison and cross-validation of the Affymetrix and Illumina gene expression analysis platforms.** *Nucleic Acids Res* 2005, **33:**5914–5923.
32. Reiner A, Yekutieli D, Benjamini Y: **Identifying differentially expressed genes using false discovery rate controlling procedures.** *Bioinformatics* 2003, **19:**368–375.
33. Storey JD, Xiao W, Leek JT, Tompkins RG, Davis RW: **Significance analysis of time course microarray experiments.** *Proc Natl Acad Sci U S A* 2005, **102:**12837–12842.
34. Malhi GS, Adams D, Berk M: **Medicating mood with maintenance in mind: bipolar depression pharmacotherapy.** *Bipolar Disord* 2009, **11**(Suppl 2):55–76.
35. Danial NN, Korsmeyer SJ: **Cell death: critical control points.** *Cell* 2004, **116:**205–219.
36. Adams JM, Cory S: **Bcl-2-regulated apoptosis: mechanism and therapeutic potential.** *Curr Opin Immunol* 2007, **19:**488–496.
37. Ueno H, Kondo E, Yamamoto-Honda R, Tobe K, Nakamoto T, Sasaki K, Mitani K, Furusaka A, Tanaka T, Tsujimoto Y, *et al*: **Association of insulin receptor substrate proteins with Bcl-2 and their effects on its phosphorylation and antiapoptotic function.** *Mol Biol Cell* 2000, **11:**735–746.
38. Andreazza AC, Shao L, Wang JF, Young LT: **Mitochondrial complex I activity and oxidative damage to mitochondrial proteins in the prefrontal cortex of patients with bipolar disorder.** *Arch Gen Psychiatry* 2010, **67:**360–368.
39. Maurer IC, Schippel P, Volz HP: **Lithium-induced enhancement of mitochondrial oxidative phosphorylation in human brain tissue.** *Bipolar Disord* 2009, **11:**515–522.
40. Rezin GT, Cardoso MR, Goncalves CL, Scaini G, Fraga DB, Riegel RE, Comim CM, Quevedo J, Streck EL: **Inhibition of mitochondrial respiratory chain in brain of rats subjected to an experimental model of depression.** *Neurochem Int* 2008, **53:**395–400.
41. Hunsberger JG, Machado-Vieira R, Austin DR, Zarate C, Chuang DM, Chen G, Reed JC, Manji HK: **Bax inhibitor 1, a modulator of calcium homeostasis, confers affective resilience.** *Brain Res* 2011, **1403:**19–27.
42. Shaltiel G, Chen G, Manji HK: **Neurotrophic signaling cascades in the pathophysiology and treatment of bipolar disorder.** *Curr Opin Pharmacol* 2007, **7:**22–26.
43. Hunsberger JG, Austin DR, Chen G, Manji HK: **Cellular mechanisms underlying affective resiliency: the role of glucocorticoid receptor- and mitochondrially-mediated plasticity.** *Brain Res* 2009, **1293:**76–84.

11

Habenula volume in post-traumatic stress disorder measured with high-resolution MRI

Jonathan B Savitz[1,2*], Omer Bonne[3], Allison C Nugent[1,4], Meena Vythilingam[1,5], Wendy Bogers[1], Dennis S Charney[6] and Wayne C Drevets[1,2]

Abstract

Background: The habenula plays an important role in regulating behavioral responses to stress and shows increased cerebral blood flow and decreased gray matter volume in patients with mood disorders. Here, we compare the volume of the habenula in unmedicated patients with post-traumatic stress disorder (PTSD) and healthy controls (HC) using MRI.

Findings: High-resolution images (resolution of approximately 0.4 mm^3) were acquired using a 3T scanner and a pulse sequence optimized for tissue contrast resolution. The habenula was manually segmented by one rater blind to diagnosis. PTSD and HC participants did not differ significantly in absolute or normalized habenula volume. Post hoc analyses controlling for the effects of comorbid major depressive disorder (MDD) and type and age of trauma exposure were not significant. Further, there was no association between PTSD severity and habenula volume.

Conclusions: Our data suggest that PTSD is not associated with robust structural changes in the habenula. The modest size of the PTSD sample may have reduced statistical power thereby accounting for the negative results obtained.

Introduction

Post-traumatic stress disorder (PTSD) is associated with an impaired ability to extinguish conditioned fear responses to threatening stimuli. This deficit attributed is hypothesized to reflect deficient inhibition of the amygdala by the ventromedial prefrontal cortex (vmPFC) [1-3]. Nevertheless, additional neurocircuitry likely is involved in the pathophysiology of PTSD. The habenula receives projections from limbic regions, including the vmPFC, and modulates cortical function via its projections to the raphe and ventral tegmental area (VTA) [4]. Conditioned aversive stimuli have been shown to activate the habenula, inhibiting VTA-mediated dopamine release and potentially both inhibiting and facilitating raphe-mediated serotonin release [4]. Conceivably, therefore, the habenula may a key role in the inhibition of conditioned fear, and by extension, PTSD.

The extant preclinical data appear consistent with this hypothesis. Rats exposed to chronic stress or undergoing dopamine depletion showed elevated glucose metabolism in the lateral habenula that was prevented by administration of an antidepressant [5]. Similarly, rats exposed to inescapable shock no longer developed learned helplessness after lesioning of the habenula [6], a finding that receives support from a more recent study demonstrating that lesioning of the lateral habenula results in increased serotonin turnover in the dorsal raphe concomitant with decreased immobility time in the forced-swim test [7]. The potential relationship between habenula function and stress is supported by the finding that congenitally helpless rats show a 64% to 71% elevation in habenula metabolism compared with non-helpless strains [8], which is reduced, together with immobility in the forced swim test, by fluoxetine [9].

In humans, using arterial spin labeling and an emotional word processing paradigm we have previously shown that remitted major depressive disorder (MDD) patients had greater blood flow to the habenula than healthy controls after acute tryptophan depletion [10]. A recent postmortem study reported a reduction in volume, neuronal numbers and neuronal cell area of the medial habenula in patients with affective illness [11]. Consistent with these

* Correspondence: jsavitz@laureateinstitute.org
[1]Section on Neuroimaging in Mood and Anxiety Disorders, NIH/NIMH, Bethesda, MD, USA
Full list of author information is available at the end of the article

data, we recently reported a decrease in the habenula volume of unmedicated patients with bipolar disorder (BD) and female patients with MDD [12]. Elucidation of the role of the habenula in stress and depression may have future clinical applications; deep brain stimulation of the lateral habenula was found to induce remission of symptoms in a patient with treatment refractory MDD [13].

Here, using high-resolution imaging, we conduct the first MRI study of habenula volume in PTSD. Based on the literature and our findings in patients with affective illness, which indicate elevated activity of the habenula during stress (possibly leading to excitotoxicity), we hypothesized that patients with PTSD would show smaller habenula volumes than healthy subjects.

Methods

Subjects gave written informed consent to participate, as approved by the National Institutes of Mental Health Institutional Review Board (NIMH IRB). Patients (n = 22) met *Diagnostic and Statistical Manual of Mental Disorders*, fourth edition (DSM-IV) criteria for chronic PTSD based upon the Structured Clinical Interview for the DSM-IV (SCID-IV), and the Clinician-Administered PTSD Scale (CAPS) [14]. All patients were medication free for at least 3 weeks (6 weeks for fluoxetine) prior to scanning. A total of 15 patients were medication naïve. Seven patients were previously been treated with medication, six with antidepressants (mostly selective serotonin reuptake inhibitors (SSRIs), three combined with a benzodiazepine), and one with a benzodiazepine, alone. The sample was evenly divided into currently depressed and non-depressed patients. One patient had generalized anxiety, and another had a specific phobia. No patients had comorbid BD. Symptoms of depression and anxiety were rated using the Inventory of Depressive Symptomatology (IDS) [15] and Hamilton Rating Scale for Anxiety (HAM-A) [16], respectively.

A total of 11 PTSD subjects experienced prolonged prepubertal trauma: sexual (N = 6) or physical/emotional (N = 5) abuse. A total of 11 PTSD subjects were exposed to a single traumatic event in adulthood: sexual assault (N = 4), motor vehicle accident (N = 4), and assault/robbery (N = 3). The time elapsed from exposure to trauma (mean ± SD) was 9.3 ± 8.0 years in the adult single trauma group and 26.0 ± 4.0 years in patients who underwent prolonged prepubertal trauma. The Early Trauma Inventory (ETI) [17] was used to document childhood trauma.

The following exclusion criteria applied: a CAPS score of less than 50, significant medical disorders, past head injury with loss of consciousness, significant risk of suicide, meeting DSM-IV criteria for substance abuse or dependence within the previous 6 months, general MRI exclusion criteria or positive illicit drug or HIV screen. Healthy control (HC) subjects (n = 75) met the same exclusion criteria, had no current or lifetime history of a psychiatric disorder or exposure to trauma, and no first degree relative with a mood or anxiety disorder, as established using the Family Interview for Genetic Studies (FIGS) [18]. The HC data were used in a previous study of habenula volume in mood disorders [12].

High-resolution anatomical images were acquired using a GE, Waukesha, WI, USA 3T MRI scanner, a standard head radiofrequency coil, and a magnetization-prepared, rapid gradient echo (MP-RAGE) pulse sequence: (echo time (TE) = 2.1 ms, repetition time (TR) = 7.8 ms, flip angle = 6°). In all, 124 coronal slices (slice thickness = 0.6 mm) were acquired with a 14 cm field-of-view and in-plane resolution of 224 × 224 voxels, resampled to 256 × 256 × 124 voxels for reconstruction, resulting in a displayed resolution of 0.55 × 0.55 × 0.6 mm. Three to four 13-min scans were consecutively acquired, coregistered, and summed to increase signal-to-noise ratio. Prior to analysis the signal-to-noise ratio was increased by summing each of two consecutive coronal planes to enhance the accuracy of manual segmentation. Thus the in-plane voxel size remained at 0.55 × 0.55 mm while the coronal slice thickness increased to 1.2 mm for segmentation (three-dimensional volumetric resolution approximately 0.4 mm^3).

A second MP-RAGE image of the entire brain also was acquired to measure whole brain volume (WBV) (TE = 4.94 ms; TR = 11.6 ms, preparation time = 725 ms; delay time = 1400 ms; voxel size = 0.85 × 0.85 × 1.2 mm).

The habenula was segmented by one rater (WB), blind to diagnosis, in each coronal plane in which this structure was seen bulging into the third ventricle along the ventromedial aspect of the thalamus or lying ventral and medial to the stria medullaris of the thalamus. The medial boundary was formed by the cerebrospinal fluid of the third ventricle, and the ventral boundary by the white matter of the posterior commissure. The dorsal and lateral borders were defined by the white matter of the stria medullaris of the thalamus in anterior planes or the mediodorsal thalamic nucleus, limitans nucleus or pretectal area in posterior planes (Figure 1). Using this method, we have previously obtained an inter-rater reliability coefficient for segmentation of 0.97 for the left habenula and 0.95 for the right habenula [12].

WBV was measured using the FSL tool, FAST [19]. The whole brain image was segmented into gray matter, white matter and cerebrospinal fluid images, after correcting for intensity non-uniformity using the MINC tool, N3. The gray and white matter components then were summed to generate the WBV.

Independent sample t tests (two-tailed, $\alpha = 0.05$) were used to compare the groups on clinical and demographic variables. There was no significant difference between

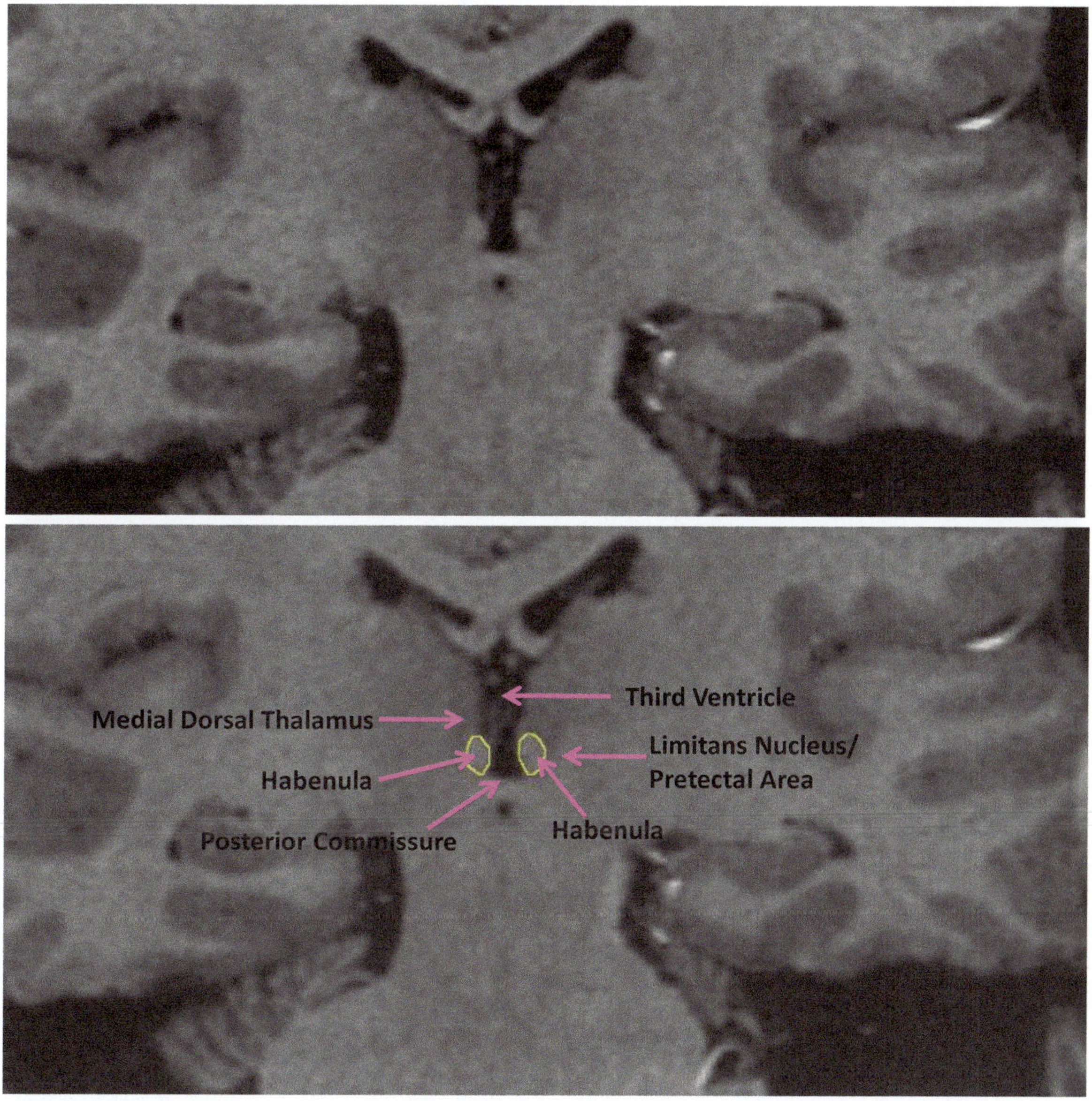

Figure 1 Coronal MRI sections showing the habenula and the local anatomical landmarks that enabled its segmentation. Because the habenular nuclei contain relatively dense white matter plexuses they can be delimited from the gray matter of the adjacent thalamus dorsolaterally, and by the limitans nucleus and pretectal area ventrolaterally [23]. Moreover, in posterior planes the habenula is clearly evident as a pyramidal-shaped structure that bulges into the third ventricle along the ventromedial aspect of the thalamus, whereas in anterior planes it can be delimited ventrally and medially from the thalamus by the stria medullaris of thalamus (the white matter track that delimits the ventromedial aspect of the medial thalamus). In the image shown the habenular location shows sufficient asymmetry that the typical view of the posterior aspect is illustrated by the habenular nuclear complex located on the reader's left, while the latter case is illustrated by the habenular complex on the reader's right. Finally, the habenular nuclei are delimited ventrally by the white matter of the posterior commissure. The medial and lateral habenular nuclei could not be resolved specifically, so were combined within a single habenular volume-of-interest. The upper and lower panels are identical images. The tracing of the habenula is shown in yellow in the lower panel.

the control and PTSD groups in gender distribution or age (Table 1). However, more PTSD subjects than controls were left handed and therefore a general linear model (two-tailed, $\alpha = 0.05$) with handedness as a covariate was used to test our *a priori* hypothesis that habenula volume would differ between groups.

Table 1 Clinical and volumetric data and statistical differences between the post-traumatic stress disorder (PTSD) and healthy control groups

	PTSD	Healthy controls	Comparison (statistic, df, *P* value)
N	22	75	-
Age	34.8 ± 10.4	36.9 ± 11.9	t = 0.7, 95, 0.472
Gender (% female)	77%	61%	χ^2 = 1.9, 1, 0.168
Handedness (r/l)	18/4	72/3	χ^2 = 5.1, 1, 0.024*
Trauma exposure (childhood/adult)	9/13	NA	-
Type of trauma (sexual abuse/physical abuse/other)	10/6/6	NA	-
Concurrent MDD episode (yes/no)	11/11	NA	-
History of substance abuse (yes/no)	2/20	NA	-
IDS score	21.4 ± 14.1	0.7 ± 1.3	t = 8.9, 57, < 0.001**
CAPS score	76.4 ± 16.6	NA	-
HAM-A score	10.3 ± 6.1	0.4 ± 0.8	t = 12.0, 75, < 0.001**
Total brain volume (mm^3)	1 144 067 ± 94962	1 174 544 ± 118 902	F = 1.2, 1, 0.278
Left habenula volume (mm^3)	18.8 ± 3.6	19.8 ± 5.1	F = 0.8, 1, 0.384
Normalized left habenula volume	0.000016 ± 0.0000036	0.000017 ± 0.0000052	F = 0.1, 1, 0.999
Right habenula volume (mm^3)	16.4 ± 3.7	17.1 ± 4.6	F = 0.2, 1, 0.688
Normalized right habenula volume	0.000014 ± 0.0000032	0.000015 ± 0.0000044	F = 0.1, 1, 0.999
Total habenula volume (mm^3)	35.2 ± 6.7	36.9 ± 8.5	F = 0.7, 1, 0.403
Normalized total habenula volume	0.000031 ± 0.0000062	0.000032 ± 0.0000094	F = 0.3, 1, 0.589

CAPS = Clinician-Administered PTSD Scale; IDS = Inventory of Depressive Symptomatology; HAM-A = Hamilton Anxiety Rating scale; MDD = major depressive disorder; NA = not applicable.

* p < 0.05

** p < 0.01

Results

No significant volumetric difference was found between groups (Table 1). The difference in habenula volume between the groups remained non-significant when the analysis was limited to females or right-handed individuals. Post hoc tests were also carried out to evaluate whether PTSD patients with concurrent MDD differed in total habenula volume from PTSD patients without MDD or HC subjects. We also tested whether PTSD patients with prepubertal trauma differed in total habenula volume from PTSD patients with adult-onset trauma or HC subjects, and whether the type of PTSD-inducing trauma impacted habenula volumes. The mean absolute and normalized volumes did not differ significantly between groups (all *P* values > 0.3). Further, there was no significant correlation between total habenula volume and the CAPS, IDS, or HAM-A scores of the PTSD group (CAPS: r = 0.103, *P* = 0.716; IDS: r = 0.22, *P* = 0.318; HAM-A: r = 0.08, *P* = 0.745). CAPS subscale scores also did not correlate significantly with habenula volume in the PTSD group: CAPS-A (r = 0.042, *P* = 0.881), CAPS-B (r = 0.343, *P* = 0.211), and CAPS-C (r = -0.205, *P* = 0.463). Similarly, there was no significant association between total ETI score and total habenula volume (r = -0.237, *P* = 0.415).

Discussion

Theoretically, the negative results reported here could be due to the modest PTSD sample size. Neverthless, we note that we found significant habenula volume reductions in a sample of 22 patients with BD (Cohen's f^2 = 0.12) and 15 female patients with MDD (f^2 = 0.11) [12]. (By convention, effect sizes of 0.02, 0.15, and 0.35 are termed small, medium, and large, respectively [20].) Thus our study may have been adequately powered to detect habenula volume changes of a moderate effect size. Nevertheless, it is possible that habenula abnormalities are only present in particular subtypes of PTSD patients that would yield a small effect size across a heterogeneous patient sample. In this case our study may not have been adequately powered to detect such a structural effect.

Several limitations of our study design merit comment. Even with high-resolution images, it remains difficult to accurately segment the habenula from adjacent tissues. However, there is no reason to expect that the extent of any errors would differ systematically between PTSD patients and controls since segmentation was performed blind to subject identity/diagnosis. Further, current MRI technology does not allow the lateral and medial habenula to be distinguished from each other.

Thus, it is possible that PTSD patients would have displayed structural changes in either the medial or lateral habenula were these regions measured separately.

In summary, although we found no significant differences between groups, given the habenula's central role in adaptation to stressful events [6,21,22], future, better-powered studies are needed to definitively establish the presence or absence of structural habenula effects in PTSD. For example, based upon the mean group difference and variance in habenula volumes measured herein (Cohen's d = 0.2), a future study would have 80% power to detect a difference in mean habenula volumes between PTSD and HC samples using a one-tailed t test with an approximate sample size of 300 cases and 300 controls.

Acknowledgements

We gratefully acknowledge the individuals who participated in the study as well as the outstanding support provided by our clinical staff and post-baccalaureate research assistants at the NIMH. The National Institute of Mental Health Intramural Research Program is acknowledged as the funding source for this work.

Author details

[1]Section on Neuroimaging in Mood and Anxiety Disorders, NIH/NIMH, Bethesda, MD, USA. [2]Laureate Institute for Brain Research, Tulsa University, and University of Oklahoma, Tulsa, OK, USA. [3]Department of Psychiatry, Hadassah-Hebrew University Medical Center, Jerusalem, Israel. [4]Experimental Therapeutics and Pathophysiology Branch, NIH/NIMH, Bethesda, MD, USA. [5]Psychological Health Strategic Operations, Force Health Protection & Readiness, Office of the Assistant Secretary of Defense, Falls Church, VA, USA. [6]Mount Sinai School of Medicine, New York, NY, USA.

Authors' contributions

JS conducted the statistical analyses and wrote the paper, OB interviewed patients, recruited patients, and revised the paper, AN contributed to the analysis of the imaging data, MV interviewed and recruited patients, WB segmented the habenula, DC contributed to the study design and the provision of resources, WD designed the study, revised the paper, and provided the resources required for the study. All authors provided intellectual input into the final draft of the paper and read and approved the final manuscript.

Competing interests

In 2006 and 2007, DC consulted for Astra Zeneca, Bristol Myers Squibb Company, Cyberonics, Neurogen, Neuroscience Education Institute, Novartis Pharmaceuticals Corporation, Orexin, and Unilever UK Central Resources Limited. DC also has a patent pending for the use of ketamine in the treatment of depression. WD has consulted for Pfizer Pharmaceuticals, Johnson & Johnson, Rules Based Medicine, and Eisai. The other authors have no disclosures to make.

References

1. Shin LM, Rauch SL, Pitman RK: **Amygdala, medial prefrontal cortex, and hippocampal function in PTSD.** *Ann NY Acad Sci* 2006, **1071**:67-79.
2. Lanius RA, Vermetten E, Loewenstein RJ, Brand B, Schmahl C, Bremner JD, Spiegel D: **Emotion modulation in PTSD: clinical and neurobiological evidence for a dissociative subtype.** *Am J Psychiatry* 2010, **167**:640-647.
3. Jovanovic T, Ressler KJ: **How the neurocircuitry and genetics of fear inhibition may inform our understanding of PTSD.** *Am J Psychiatry* 2010, **167**:648-662.
4. Hikosaka O: **The habenula: from stress evasion to value-based decision-making.** *Nat Rev Neurosci* 2010, **11**:503-513.
5. Caldecott-Hazard S, Mazziotta J, Phelps M: **Cerebral correlates of depressed behavior in rats, visualized using 14C-2-deoxyglucose autoradiography.** *J Neurosci* 1988, **8**:1951-1961.
6. Amat J, Sparks PD, Matus-Amat P, Griggs J, Watkins LR, Maier SF: **The role of the habenular complex in the elevation of dorsal raphe nucleus serotonin and the changes in the behavioral responses produced by uncontrollable stress.** *Brain Res* 2001, **917**:118-126.
7. Yang LM, Hu B, Xia YH, Zhang BL, Zhao H: **Lateral habenula lesions improve the behavioral response in depressed rats via increasing the serotonin level in dorsal raphe nucleus.** *Behav Brain Res* 2008, **188**:84-90.
8. Shumake J, Edwards E, Gonzalez-Lima F: **Opposite metabolic changes in the habenula and ventral tegmental area of a genetic model of helpless behavior.** *Brain Res* 2003, **963**:274-281.
9. Shumake J, Colorado RA, Barrett DW, Gonzalez-Lima F: **Metabolic mapping of the effects of the antidepressant fluoxetine on the brains of congenitally helpless rats.** *Brain Res* 2010, **1343**:218-225.
10. Roiser JP, Levy J, Fromm SJ, Nugent AC, Talagala SL, Hasler G, Henn FA, Sahakian BJ, Drevets WC: **The effects of tryptophan depletion on neural responses to emotional words in remitted depression.** *Biol Psychiatry* 2009, **66**:441-450.
11. Ranft K, Dobrowolny H, Krell D, Bielau H, Bogerts B, Bernstein HG: **Evidence for structural abnormalities of the human habenular complex in affective disorders but not in schizophrenia.** *Psychol Med* 2009, **40**:557-67.
12. Savitz JB, Nugent AC, Bogers W, Roiser JP, Bain EE, Neumeister A, Zarate CA Jr, Manji HK, Cannon DM, Marrett S, Henn F, Charney DS, Drevets WC: **Habenula volume in bipolar disorder and major depressive disorder: a high-resolution magnetic resonance imaging study.** *Biol Psychiatry* 2011, **69**:336-343.
13. Sartorius A, Kiening KL, Kirsch P, von Gall CC, Haberkorn U, Unterberg AW, Henn FA, Meyer-Lindenberg A: **Remission of major depression under deep brain stimulation of the lateral habenula in a therapy-refractory patient.** *Biol Psychiatry* 2010, **67**:e9-e11.
14. Blake DD, Weathers FW, Nagy LM, Kaloupek DG, Gusman FD, Charney DS, Keane TM: **The development of a clinician-administered PTSD scale.** *J Trauma Stress* 1995, **8**:75-90.
15. Rush AJ, Gullion CM, Basco MR, Jarrett RB, Trivedi MH: **The Inventory of Depressive Symptomatology (IDS): psychometric properties.** *Psychol Med* 1996, **26**:477-486.
16. Hamilton M: **The assessment of anxiety states by rating.** *Br J Med Psychol* 1959, **32**:50-55.
17. Bremner JD, Vermetten E, Mazure CM: **Development and preliminary psychometric properties of an instrument for the measurement of childhood trauma: the early trauma inventory.** *Depress Anxiety* 2000, **12**:1-12.
18. Maxwell M: *Family Interview for Genetic Studies (FIGS): Manual for FIGS* Bethesda, MD: Clinical Neurogenetics Branch, Intramural Research Program, National Institute of Mental Health; 1992.
19. Savitz J, Nugent AC, Bogers W, Liu A, Sills R, Luckenbaugh DA, Bain EE, Price JL, Zarate C, Manji HK, Cannon DM, Marrett S, Charney DS, Drevets WC: **Amygdala volume in depressed patients with bipolar disorder assessed using high resolution 3T MRI: the impact of medication.** *Neuroimage* 2010, **49**:2966-2976.
20. Cohen J: *Statistical Power Analysis for the Behavioral Sciences.* 2 edition. Hillsdale, NJ: Lawrence Erlbaum Associates; 1988.
21. Thornton EW, Bradbury GE: **Effort and stress influence the effect of lesion of the habenula complex in one-way active avoidance learning.** *Physiol Behav* 1989, **45**:929-935.
22. Wirtshafter D, Asin KE, Pitzer MR: **Dopamine agonists and stress produce different patterns of Fos-like immunoreactivity in the lateral habenula.** *Brain Res* 1994, **633**:21-26.
23. Mai JK, Assheuer J, Paxinos G: *Atlas of the Human Brain.* 2 edition. Amsterdam: Elsevier; 2004.

12

Increased default mode network activity in socially anxious individuals during reward processing

Erin L Maresh*, Joseph P Allen and James A Coan*

Abstract

Background: Social anxiety has been associated with potentiated negative affect and, more recently, with diminished positive affect. It is unclear how these alterations in negative and positive affect are represented neurally in socially anxious individuals and, further, whether they generalize to non-social stimuli. To explore this, we used a monetary incentive paradigm to explore the association between social anxiety and both the anticipation and consumption of non-social incentives. Eighty-four individuals from a longitudinal community sample underwent functional magnetic resonance imaging (fMRI) while participating in a monetary incentive delay (MID) task. The MID task consisted of alternating cues indicating the potential to win or prevent losing varying amounts of money based on the speed of the participant's response. We examined whether self-reported levels of social anxiety, averaged across approximately 7 years of data, moderated brain activity when contrasting gain or loss cues with neutral cues during the anticipation and outcome phases of incentive processing. Whole brain analyses and analyses restricted to the ventral striatum for the anticipation phase and the medial prefrontal cortex for the outcome phase were conducted.

Results: Social anxiety did not associate with differences in hit rates or reaction times when responding to cues. Further, socially anxious individuals did not exhibit decreased ventral striatum activity during anticipation of gains or decreased MPFC activity during the outcome of gain trials, contrary to expectations based on literature indicating blunted positive affect in social anxiety. Instead, social anxiety showed positive associations with extensive regions implicated in default mode network activity (for example, precuneus, posterior cingulate cortex, and parietal lobe) during anticipation and receipt of monetary gain. Social anxiety was further linked with decreased activity in the ventral striatum during anticipation of monetary loss.

Conclusions: Socially anxious individuals may increase default mode network activity during reward processing, suggesting high self-focused attention even in relation to potentially rewarding stimuli lacking explicit social connotations. Additionally, social anxiety may relate to decreased ventral striatum reactivity when anticipating potential losses.

Keywords: Social anxiety, Default mode network, Reward, Punishment, Anticipation, Consumption, fMRI

* Correspondence: elm2cg@virginia.edu; jcoan@virginia.edu
Department of Psychology, University of Virginia, 314 Gilmer Hall, P.O. Box 400400, Charlottesville, VA 22904, USA

Background

Although heterogeneous in presentation, anxiety disorders are in part classified based on the shared dimension of heightened negative affect. A stable, higher-order temperamental factor, negative affect encompasses a broad range of distressing emotions, including guilt, hostility, self-dissatisfaction, nervousness, and uneasiness [1,2], that motivate individuals to avoid punishing, threatening, or unfamiliar stimuli [3-5]. This manifests in risk-averse behaviors such as withdrawal and inhibition of behavioral impulses, particularly in the presence of approach/avoidance conflicts [5,6]. Accordingly, high trait levels of negative affect are related to avoidance of both social and non-social threats and may represent a general risk factor for the development and maintenance of anxiety disorders [7-9].

By contrast, there is relatively little work on the role of positive affect in anxiety disorders. Positive affect maintains rewarding, goal-directed behavior, which underlies approach-oriented, appetitive motivation [5,10]. Theoretical and empirical data suggest that anxiety is defined by higher levels of negative affect and withdrawal-related behaviors, while experiences of positive emotions and goal-directed behavior are generally unaffected [4,5,11-13]. Indeed, low positive, approach-related affect is posited to be a feature distinctive to depression [14-17]. Blunted positive emotionality presents as reduced reward-seeking behavior, as well as reduced appetitive and consummatory responses to rewarding stimuli, which characterizes the anhedonia that frequently accompanies depression [18,19].

Accumulating research suggests that social anxiety disorder is an exception to the view that positive affect and corresponding approach-oriented behavior are not altered in anxiety. In assessing associations between positive and negative affect in depression and anxiety diagnoses among 350 outpatients, Brown et al. [20] found low positive affect to associate solely with social anxiety disorder among the anxiety disorders and, further, to be approximately equally related to social anxiety disorder and depression. More recent research has examined how socially anxious individuals experience altered positive affect in daily life. Individuals with high social anxiety experience positive emotions and events both less intensely and less frequently than those with less social anxiety, particularly on days when they are feeling especially socially anxious [21,22]. It has been proposed that high levels of behavioral inhibition and low levels of approach motivation act as both distal and proximal causes for the development and maintenance of social anxiety [23,24].

Although altered experiences of positive and negative affect in social anxiety have primarily been observed in self-report and behavioral studies, less is known about how they may be represented on the neural level. Some research suggests altered striatal morphology and function in individuals with social anxiety disorder [25], yet how this interferes with behavior, particularly during situations not explicitly social in nature, is poorly understood. One way to address these issues is to examine how social anxiety interacts with neural responses during incentive processing using tasks developed for use in the functional magnetic resonance imaging (fMRI) environment. The monetary incentive delay (MID) task [26] uses visual cues to indicate the potential of winning or losing varying amounts of money based on speed in response to a subsequent target cue. This task allows for analysis of multiple phases of incentive processing, including the anticipation phase and the outcome phase. The MID task produces robust activity in basal ganglia during anticipation of incentives and in the orbital and medial prefrontal cortices (MPFC) during consumption of incentives [27-29].

Using the MID task, we sought to identify whether levels of social anxiety moderated the neural response to both the anticipation and consumption of reward and punishment. Due to reported differences in the experience of positive and negative affective states between social anxiety and other types of anxiety, we were additionally interested in comparing effects due to social anxiety with effects due to generalized trait anxiety on neural reward and punishment anticipation. To this end, we examined whether continuous levels of social and trait anxiety in a large, non-clinical community sample would be predictive of differences in reward and punishment sensitivity.

Because social anxiety is related to altered positive and negative affect, we expected to find associations between social anxiety and neural activity in response to processing monetary incentives. Specifically, we hypothesized that: (1) during the anticipation of monetary incentives, higher levels of social anxiety would associate with decreased activity in reward-related regions such as the ventral striatum, and (2) during monetary incentive outcomes, higher levels of social anxiety would associate with decreased activity in regions previously found to be related to reward consumption, such as the MPFC. These hypotheses were explored using both whole brain and region of interest (ROI) analyses targeted on the ventral striatum for the anticipation phase and the medial prefrontal cortex for the outcome phase.

Methods

Participants and questionnaire data

Participants from a larger longitudinal study on adolescent social development [30,31] were invited to participate in an fMRI study. This sample has been followed for over 12 years, beginning when participants were young teenagers. For the present study, participants were excluded if they were pregnant or exhibited risk for incident in the fMRI environment. The final sample consisted of

84 participants (42 women) who predominantly self-identified as Caucasian (n = 45) or African American (n = 33). Average age of participants at the time of the scan was 24.56 (SD = 1.17) years old. No participants reported having clinical social anxiety disorder, although two reported having bipolar disorder via self-report on the Medical Information Questionnaire. Excluding these two participants did not alter the results, so they are included in all analyses. No participants reported taking any psychiatric medications at the time of the study. All participants gave written consent and were provided monetary compensation for their time. The study was approved by the University of Virginia Institutional Review Board for Health Sciences Research (#12984).

During each wave of data collection, participants completed a battery of questionnaires on personality, attachment style, and relationships. Because the longitudinal study began when participants were adolescents, levels of social anxiety were measured using the Social Anxiety Scale for Adolescents (SAS-A) [32]. The SAS-A is a self-report questionnaire consisting of 22 questions (18 social anxiety-related questions and four filler questions) that participants answer using a five-point Likert scale to indicate how much the statement describes them. The SAS-A generally loads onto three factors: Fear of Negative Evaluation (FNE) (eight items, for example, 'I worry about what others think of me'), Social Avoidance and Distress in New Situations (SAD-New) (six items, for example, 'I get nervous when I meet new people'), and Social Avoidance and Distress in General Situations (SAD-General) (four items, for example, 'I feel shy even with people I know well') [33]. For most of our analyses, we used a total social anxiety score determined by summing these three subscales, resulting in a possible range of scores from 18 to 90. We also examined associations between individual subscales and neural activity. To assess levels of trait anxiety, we used scores on the Trait portion of the State-Trait Anxiety Inventory (STAI) [34], which has a possible range of scores from 20 to 80. Each scale, the SAS-A and STAI, had seven waves of data available in our longitudinal sample, dating from when participants were an average of 18.24 (SD = 1.05) years old to an average of 25.28 (SD = 0.88) years old. This last wave of data was collected an average of 295.30 (SD = 250.18) days after the fMRI scan. The SAS-A and STAI scales showed excellent test-retest reliability (SAS-A: Cronbach's alpha = 0.92; STAI: Cronbach's alpha = 0.90). Thus, we collapsed across the available waves for each participant, yielding an average SAS-A and STAI score across time, indicative of a stable trait for each participant.

Monetary incentive delay task

The monetary incentive delay (MID) task is designed to assess one's neural response to the anticipation and receipt of rewarding or punishing monetary stimuli [27]. Participants entered an fMRI scanner and underwent two runs of the MID task, each consisting of 72 trials for a total of 144 trials (Figure 1). During each trial, one of seven possible cue shapes was presented for 500 ms (anticipation phase). Three of the cue shapes indicated the potential to win varying amounts of money ('gain' cues, represented by circles, n = 54), three of the cue shapes indicated a potential to lose varying amounts of money ('loss' cues, represented by squares, n = 54), and one cue shape indicated no money would be won or lost ('neutral' cue, represented by a triangle, n = 36). Horizontal lines across each shape represented the amount of money one could potentially win or lose, with one line signifying the potential to win or lose \$0.20, two lines signifying \$1.00, and three lines signifying \$5.00. After presentation of the cue, a fixation cross was displayed for 2,000 to 2,500 ms, followed by presentation of a white

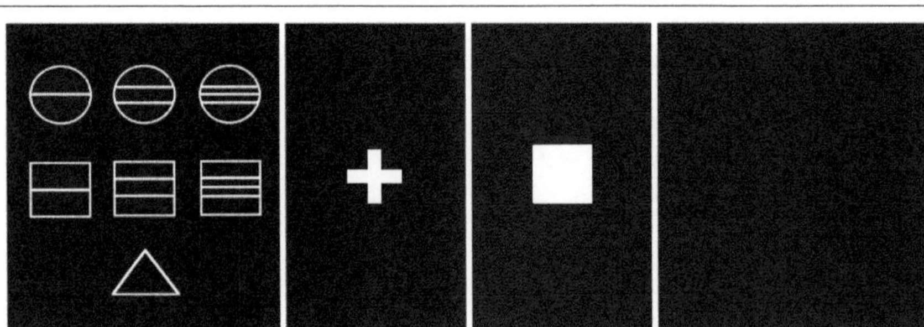

Figure 1 Monetary incentive delay (MID) task. Each run of the MID task consisted of 72 trials. The first box shows the cue types presented, with circles indicating the potential to win money (gain cue), squares indicating the potential to lose money (loss cue), and a triangle indicating no money will be won or lost (neutral cue). A cue was presented for 500 ms, followed by a fixation cross (2,000 to 2,500 ms) and then the target square (160 to 260 ms), during which the participant was instructed to press a button as quickly as possible to win or avoid losing money. A feedback screen (1,650 ms), in which the top number indicated the amount of money won or lost during that trial and the bottom number indicated the participant's total amount, was presented at the end of each trial.

target square for 160 to 260 ms. Participants were instructed that, upon seeing the target square, they were to press a button on a provided button box as quickly as possible to gain or avoid losing money. A practice trial before the two runs calibrated the length of time the target square was presented so that all participants accurately pressed the button approximately 80% of the time. Trial outcomes were based on actual performance. A feedback screen (outcome phase), presented for 1,650 ms, displayed whether they had won or lost money during that trial and their cumulative earnings. Each participant was initially given $40 and was paid the final amount of money earned based on their performance.

Image acquisition

Images were acquired using a Siemens 3.0 Tesla MAGNETOM Trio high-speed magnetic imaging device with a circular polarized transmit/receive head coil and integrated mirror. A total of 176 high-resolution T1-magnetization-prepared rapid-acquisition gradient echo images were collected to determine the localization of function (1-mm slices, repetition time = 1,900 ms, echo time = 2.53 ms, flip angle = 9°, field of view = 250 mm, voxel size = 1 × 1 × 1 mm). A total of 224 functional T2*-weighted echo planar images sensitive to blood oxygen level-dependent (BOLD) contrasts were collected per block in volumes of 28 3.5-mm transversal echo-planar slices covering the whole brain (1-mm slice gap, repetition time = 2,000 ms, echo time = 40 ms, flip angle = 90°, field of view = 192 mm, matrix = 64 × 64, voxel size = 3 × 3 × 3.5 mm).

Data were preprocessed using FMRIB Software Library (FSL) software (Version 5.0.5; www.fmrib.ox.ac.uk/fsl). Motion was corrected using FMRIB Linear Image Registration Tool (FLIRT), an intra-modal correction algorithm tool [35], with slice scan-time correction and a high-pass filtering cutoff point of 100 s, removing signals that were irrelevant to the stimuli. We used FSL's Brain Extraction Tool (BET) to eliminate unwanted, non-brain material voxels in the fMRI data. Spatial smoothing was conducted with a 5-mm full width at half minimum Gaussian kernel. Images were registered to the Montreal Neurological Institute (MNI) standard space by FLIRT [35].

Data analysis

Data analysis was conducted using fMRI Expert Analysis Tool (FEAT) Version 6.00 in the FSL software package. Both the anticipation and outcome phases of incentive processing are captured by the MID task, and similar analyses were conducted for each. At the first level of analysis, reward and punishment maps were created by subtracting the neural response to the neutral anticipation and outcome cues from the neural response to the gain or loss anticipation and outcome cues, respectively. We collapsed across all amounts of gain or loss ($0.20, $1.00, and $5.00) to examine overall neural activity attributable to each. At the second level of analysis, we combined data from the two runs of the MID task for each participant using a fixed effects model. At the third level of analysis, we ran our primary model of interest - a mixed effects model taking into account within-subject fixed effect variance and between-subject random effect variance - for reward and punishment contrasts in both the anticipation phase and the outcome phase, with total SAS-A scores entered as a covariate. This model was used to determine both main effects of gain and loss during the anticipation and outcome phases, as well as to determine regions differentially associated with social anxiety.

We conducted several complementary models for both gain and loss in the anticipation and outcome phases to examine nuances in the role of social anxiety in reward and punishment processing and to rule out alternative explanations. For example, to assess the degree to which social anxiety uniquely impacts incentive processing, we conducted a model in which both social anxiety and trait anxiety scores were entered as covariates. Detailed results of the following analyses can be found in the Additional file 1. First, to explore differences in neural reactivity based on incentive magnitude, we examined contrasts of large ($5.00) minus small ($0.20) incentives for gain and loss in the anticipation and outcome phases. Next, to determine which specific facets of the SAS-A relate to brain activity, we conducted separate models for each of the three individual subscale scores (FNE, SAD-New, and SAD-General). Following that, we sought to examine the degree to which trait anxiety corresponds with brain activity in regions implicated in our analyses. This was accomplished by assessing the impact - if any - of trait anxiety within clusters we found to co-vary with social anxiety scores. Finally, we explored differences related to social anxiety in gain *versus* loss contrasts for the anticipation and outcome phases. Because of previous findings suggesting gender differences in incentive processing [36], we compared analyses with gender entered as a covariate to those without. Including gender as a covariate yielded highly similar results; therefore, all analyses reported do not include gender.

To correct for multiple comparisons within models, we performed a whole brain, cluster-wise correction derived from Gaussian Random Field (GRF) theory (see [37]). To balance risk of type I and type II errors [38], a GRF-corrected maximum height threshold of $z > 1.96$ was used to define contiguous clusters [39]. Cluster significance levels were then compared with a family-wise error (FWE) corrected cluster-significance threshold of $P < 0.05$. For each cluster, we report the location of the peak voxel as well as five local maxima (voxels with surrounding voxels of lower intensities). Anatomical labels for cluster maxima were identified using the Harvard-

Oxford cortical and subcortical structural atlases or the Juelich histological atlas if no label was available in the Harvard-Oxford atlases. All coordinates are reported in MNI space.

Because our initial hypotheses involved reward-related regions, we additionally performed region-of-interest (ROI) analyses using a mask of the bilateral ventral striatum for the anticipation phase and a mask of the MPFC for the outcome phase, both thresholded at an uncorrected P value of $P < 0.005$ with total social anxiety scores entered as a covariate. These masks were derived from the nucleus accumbens structure and the frontal medial cortex structure in the Harvard-Oxford subcortical structural atlas. To further describe interactions between social anxiety and ventral striatum or MPFC activity, we examined complementary models for both the anticipation and outcome phases: one with both social and trait anxiety scores entered as covariates and three including each of the social anxiety subscales. Clusters were defined as areas of at least 10 contiguous significantly active voxels.

Results

Questionnaire results

Multiple waves of questionnaire data for social and trait anxiety scores were available for all 84 participants, with the number of available waves for each participant in the range of 3 to 7 ($M = 6.30$, SD = 0.95). Average total social anxiety scores on the SAS-A ranged from 18.43 to 63.14 ($M = 31.18$, SD = 9.49), and average trait anxiety scores from the STAI ranged from 22.33 to 56.86 ($M = 35.37$, SD = 7.48). Both SAS-A scores and STAI scores were slightly positively skewed (SAS-A skewness = 0.81, SE = 0.26; STAI skewness = 0.44, SE = 0.26). However, log-transforming the variables did not substantially change the results; therefore, untransformed data were used in all analyses. Social anxiety and trait anxiety scores were moderately correlated ($r = 0.58$, $P < 0.0001$). Social anxiety scores did not differ by gender ($P = 0.47$); however, trait anxiety scores showed a trend toward differing by gender ($P = 0.06$). Follow-up testing showed that women trended toward reporting higher trait anxiety scores ($M = 36.90$, SD = 7.70) than men ($M = 33.83$, SD = 7.01).

Behavioral data

Reaction times (RTs) significantly differed between gain and loss cue types, $F(1, 82) = 16.32$, $P < 0.0005$, $\eta_p^2 = 0.16$, such that participants were significantly faster reacting to gain cues ($M = 0.270$ s, SD = 0.04 s) than to loss cues ($M = 0.278$ s, SD = 0.04 s). Neither social anxiety nor trait anxiety had a significant effect on RTs by cue type, $F(1, 82) = 3.27$, $P = 0.07$, $\eta_p^2 = 0.04$ and $F(1, 82) = 0.56$, $P = 0.46$, $\eta_p^2 = 0.01$, respectively, although the nearly significant association between social anxiety and RT warranted a closer look. Follow-up analysis revealed that individuals higher in social anxiety trended toward greater reaction times to gain cues but not to loss cues. Neither social anxiety nor trait anxiety showed a significant effect on hit rate, $F(1, 82) = 0.34$, $P = 0.56$, $\eta_p^2 = 0.004$, and $F(1, 82) = 0.01$, $P = 0.93$, $\eta_p^2 < 0.0005$, respectively.

fMRI data

For quick reference, a summary of significant findings can be found in Table 1.

Anticipation phase

Main effects of gain anticipation

Anticipation of monetary reward was analyzed by contrasting neural activity during anticipation of gain cues with neural activity during anticipation of neutral cues. This contrast yielded extensive bilateral activations in regions previously found to be active in response to reward anticipation (for example, Knutson et al., 2001 [27,28]). These regions included the supplementary motor cortex, paracingulate cortex, ACC, superior frontal gyrus, precentral gyrus, postcentral gyrus, right supramarginal gyrus, angular gyrus, superior parietal lobule, precuneus, temporal occipital fusiform cortex, lateral occipital cortex,

Table 1 Significant associations between social anxiety and brain activity in whole brain and ROI analyses

	Anticipation		Outcome	
Whole brain	**Gain**	**Loss**	**Gain**	**Loss**
Total SA	+		+	
FNE	+		+	+
SAD-New	+		+	
SAD-Gen				-
SA with TA	+		+	
Ventral striatum				
Total SA		-		
FNE		-		
SAD-New		-		
SAD-Gen	-			
SA with TA		-		
MPFC				
Total SA				
FNE				
SAD-New				
SAD-Gen				
SA with TA				

Ventral striatum analyses were conducted for the anticipation phase only; MPFC analyses were conducted for the outcome phase only.
FNE = Fear of Negative Evaluation subscale; SA = social anxiety; SAD-Gen = Social Avoidance and Distress in General Situations subscale; SAD-New = Social Avoidance and Distress in New Situations subscale; TA = trait anxiety; + = positive association with brain activity; – = negative association with brain activity.

occipital pole, insula, putamen, caudate, nucleus accumbens, and brainstem (Additional file 2: Table S1, Figure 2A). The reverse contrast, neutral *versus* gain anticipation, is described in Additional file 1 and Additional file 2: Table S1.

Social anxiety and gain anticipation

Our primary research question was whether social anxiety was linked to altered neural reactivity during reward processing. Higher levels of social anxiety predicted increased gain anticipation activity in one main cluster (Figure 3A, Table 2). This cluster peaked in the right medial parietal lobe and extended to the right precuneus, posterior cingulate cortex, angular gyrus, superior parietal lobule, supramarginal gyrus, and lateral occipital cortex. Social anxiety was more strongly related to activity during anticipation of small compared to large rewards (Additional file 1 and Additional file 2: Table S2). Further, brain activity specifically associated with scores on the FNE and SAD-New subscales (Additional file 1 and Additional file 2: Table S3).

With trait anxiety

Due to conceptual overlap between social anxiety and trait anxiety, we investigated whether social anxiety made unique contributions to predicting neural responses to reward anticipation beyond that provided by trait anxiety. When including trait anxiety scores in the model, social anxiety remained predictive, associating with increased activity in two clusters (Figure 3B, Table 3). The first cluster peaked in the left frontal pole and extended to the left middle frontal gyrus and ACC. The second cluster peaked in the left precuneus and extended to the left PCC.

Ventral striatum ROI analysis

To directly assess our hypothesis that social anxiety would correspond with decreased activity in reward-related regions during reward processing, we used an ROI of the bilateral ventral striatum. Social anxiety, whether by itself or with trait anxiety included in the model, showed no association with activity in this region during anticipation of gain. However, when looking at subscales of the SAS-A, right ventral striatum activity showed a negative association with scores on the SAD-General subscale.

Main effects of loss anticipation

Anticipation of monetary loss was analyzed by contrasting neural activity during loss anticipation cues with neural activity during neutral anticipation cues. This contrast resulted in bilateral activations similar to those seen in anticipation during gain (Figure 2B, Additional file 2: Table S4). These activations were found in regions including the lateral occipital cortex, occipital pole, occipital fusiform gyrus, temporal occipital fusiform gyrus, superior parietal cortex, supramarginal gyrus, angular gyrus, middle frontal gyrus, superior frontal gyrus, precentral gyrus, paracingulate, ACC, and supplementary motor cortex. The reverse contrast, neutral *versus* loss anticipation, is described in Additional file 1 and Additional file 2: Table S4.

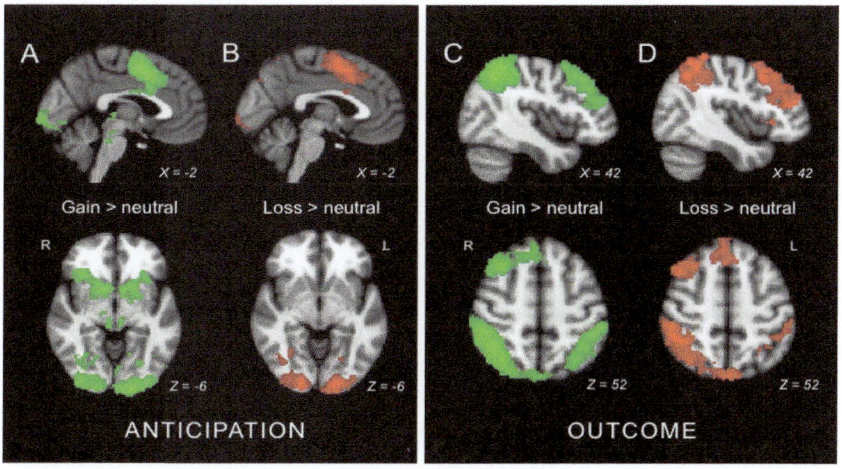

Figure 2 Main effects of reward and punishment in anticipation and outcome phases. Colored regions indicate clusters more active during **(A)** anticipation during gain *versus* neutral cues, **(B)** anticipation during loss *versus* neutral cues, **(C)** outcome after gain *versus* neutral cues, and **(D)** outcome after loss *versus* neutral cues. Clusters were identified using whole brain, cluster-wise correction with a z threshold of 1.96 and a corrected cluster significance threshold of $P < 0.05$.

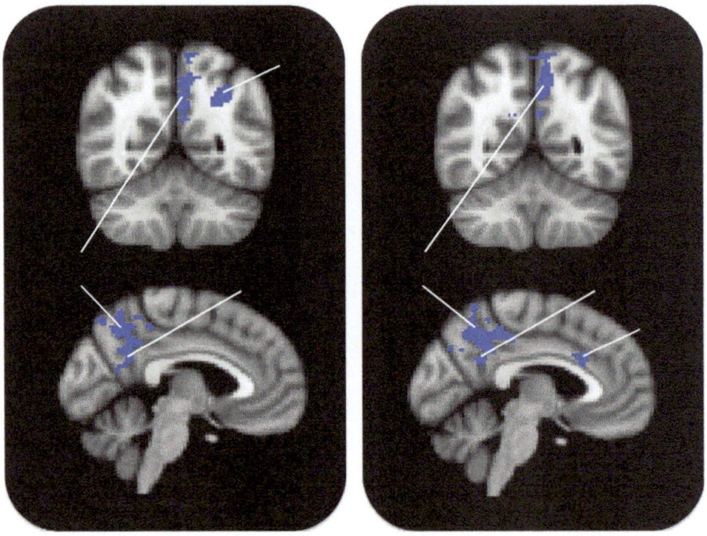

Figure 3 Clusters related to social anxiety during reward anticipation. Colored regions indicate clusters positively associated with social anxiety in the gain anticipation > neutral anticipation contrast. Shown are models **(A)** with social anxiety alone, and **(B)** with both social and trait anxiety included. For top row, Y = −56; for bottom row, X = −4. ACC = anterior cingulate cortex; PCC = posterior cingulate cortex.

Table 2 Positive associations with social anxiety in gain > neutral anticipation contrast using whole brain analysis

Cluster *P* value	Cluster size	Peak Z	x	y	z	Region	R/L
Model with SA only							
<0.01	966	3.21	−18	−40	36	Callosal body	L
		3.12	−30	−56	36	Intra-parietal sulcus	L
		3.12	−8	−54	48	Precuneus	L
		3.08	0	−78	52	Precuneus	R/L
		2.98	−34	−56	42	Superior parietal lobule	L
		2.97	−6	−54	36	Precuneus	L
Model with SA + TA							
<0.001	1,258	3.57	−20	44	18	Frontal pole	L
		3.56	−26	34	42	Middle frontal gyrus	L
		3.44	−20	42	10	Callosal body	L
		3.23	−28	56	12	Frontal pole	L
		3.15	−22	34	28	Middle frontal gyrus	L
		3.15	−22	16	36	Unclassified white matter	L
<0.01	1,085	3.48	−8	−56	48	Precuneus	L
		3.25	−10	−66	34	Precuneus	L
		3.15	−8	−42	48	Precuneus	L
		3.09	−6	−54	38	Precuneus	L
		2.89	−6	−50	34	Posterior cingulate cortex	L
		2.89	−10	−52	38	Precuneus	L

L = left hemisphere; R = right hemisphere; SA = social anxiety; TA = trait anxiety.

Table 3 Positive associations with social anxiety in gain > neutral outcome contrast using whole brain analysis

Cluster *P* value	Cluster size	Peak Z	x	Y	z	Region	R/L
Model with SA only							
<0.0001	2,152	3.82	−36	−42	54	Superior parietal lobule	L
		3.78	−52	−32	50	Supramarginal gyrus	L
		3.59	8	−48	60	Precuneus	R
		3.54	−36	−54	54	Superior parietal lobule	L
		3.50	−42	−48	56	Superior parietal lobule	L
		3.49	−10	−42	54	Postcentral gyrus	L
Model with SA + TA							
<0.0001	1,392	3.43	−54	−50	46	Supramarginal gyrus	L
		3.41	−54	−34	50	Supramarginal gyrus	L
		3.30	−36	−44	54	Superior parietal lobule	L
		3.27	−42	−48	56	Superior parietal lobule	L
		3.26	−46	−50	56	Supramarginal gyrus	L
		3.23	−50	−50	50	Supramarginal gyrus	L

L = left hemisphere; R = right hemisphere; SA = social anxiety; TA = trait anxiety.

Social anxiety and loss anticipation

Unlike anticipation during gain cues, anticipation during loss cues compared to anticipation during neutral cues did not reveal any clusters of activity significantly related to social anxiety. This remained after including trait anxiety scores in the model.

Ventral striatum ROI analysis

During anticipation of loss, a cluster in the right ventral striatum emerged as negatively related to social anxiety. This result remained after including trait anxiety in the model. In particular, ventral striatum activity was negatively related with scores on the FNE and SAD-New subscales.

Gain *versus* loss anticipation with social anxiety

To further explore the role of social anxiety in gain and loss anticipation, we examined gain *versus* loss anticipation with social anxiety entered as a covariate. Social anxiety was not significantly associated with neural activity in this contrast. This is not altogether surprising due to the similarity in brain activity during gain and loss anticipation trials. In other words, while there is a large difference between gain/loss anticipation and neutral anticipation, the variability between gain and loss anticipation may be too small to observe an effect associated with social anxiety.

Outcome phase

Main effects of gain outcome

Monetary reward outcome was analyzed by contrasting neural activity during gain outcome cues with neural activity during neutral outcome cues. Contrasting gain outcome cues with neutral outcome cues yielded activation in predictable regions including the bilateral angular gyrus, supramarginal gyrus, superior parietal lobule, precuneus, and lateral occipital cortex, and right middle and superior frontal gyri, dorsolateral prefrontal cortex, and paracingulate (Additional file 2: Table S5, Figure 2C). The reverse contrast, neutral *versus* gain outcome, is described in Additional file 1 and Additional file 2: Table S5.

Social anxiety and gain outcome

Contrasting gain outcome with neutral outcome yielded one cluster positively associated with social anxiety (Table 3, Figure 4A). This cluster peaked in the left superior parietal lobule and extended to bilateral lateral occipital cortex and right superior parietal lobule, precuneus, left supramarginal gyrus, precentral gyrus, and postcentral gyrus. Social anxiety associated with greater activity in large gain outcomes compared to small gain outcomes (Additional file 1 and Additional file 2: Table S6). Similarly to gain anticipation, the FNE and SAD-New subscales, but not SAD-General, showed a relationship with brain activity during gain outcome (Additional file 1 and Additional file 2: Table S7).

With trait anxiety

With both social and trait anxiety in the same model, social anxiety showed a positive association with activity in a cluster similar to that seen with social anxiety alone, although the cluster was less extensive and was confined to the left hemisphere (Table 3, Figure 4B). This cluster peaked in the left supramarginal gyrus and extended to the left superior parietal lobule, angular gyrus, and postcentral gyrus.

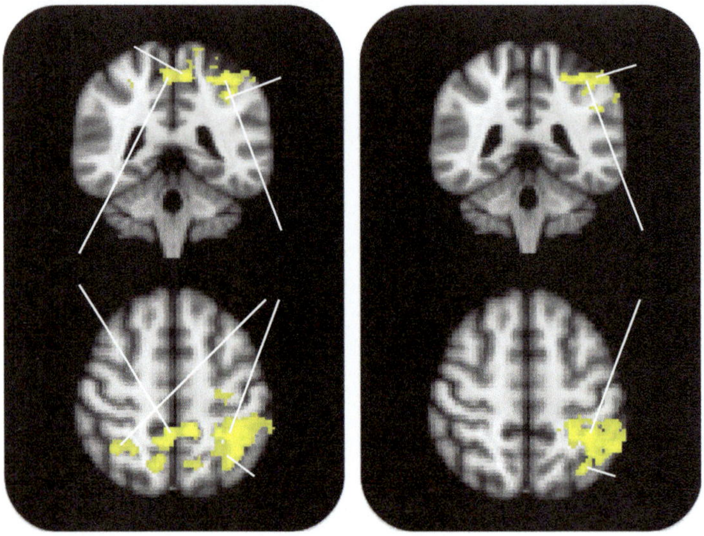

Figure 4 Clusters related to social anxiety during reward outcome. Colored regions indicate clusters positively associated with social anxiety in the gain outcome > neutral outcome contrast. Shown are models **(A)** with social anxiety alone, and **(B)** with both social and trait anxiety included. For top row, Y = −42; for bottom row, Z = 54.

MPFC ROI analysis

Using an ROI of the MPFC revealed no associations between social anxiety and brain activity during gain outcome. Subsequent analyses including trait anxiety or examining specific social anxiety subscales also showed no associations.

Main effects of loss outcome

Contrasting loss outcome cues with neutral outcome cues resulted in activations in areas including bilateral supramarginal gyrus, angular gyrus, superior parietal lobule, superior frontal gyrus, paracingulate, lateral occipital cortex, cuneus, precuneus, and right frontal pole, middle frontal gyrus, inferior frontal gyrus, and insula (Additional file 2: Table S8, Figure 3D). The reverse contrast, neutral *versus* loss, is described in Additional file 1 and Additional file 2: Table S8.

Social anxiety and loss outcome

Social anxiety, both by itself and with trait anxiety in the model, was not significantly associated with neural activity when contrasting loss outcome cues with neutral outcome cues. However, examining subscales revealed significant relationships: brain activity during gain outcome showed a positive association with the FNE subscale and a negative association with the SAD-General subscale (Additional file 1 and Additional file 2: Table S9).

MPFC ROI analysis

Examining loss outcome using an ROI of the MPFC yielded no relationship with social anxiety, whether using total scores, subscale scores, or adjusting for trait anxiety.

Gain *versus* loss outcomes with social anxiety

Contrasting activity during gain compared to loss outcomes yielded one cluster positively related to social anxiety that peaked in the left supramarginal gyrus and extended to the left angular gyrus, superior parietal lobule, and lateral occipital cortex (Additional file 2: Table S10). In other words, individuals higher in social anxiety showed greater activity in these areas during gain outcomes than during loss outcomes.

Discussion

Emerging evidence suggests that social anxiety disorder is unique among anxiety disorders in that it is characterized not only by increased experiences of negative affect but also by decreased experiences of positive affect. It is unclear how this may be reflected in the brain and whether this is seen solely in response to social cues. We used a well-known and much replicated fMRI paradigm, the monetary incentive delay (MID) task, to investigate how levels of social anxiety moderate brain activity during both the anticipation and receipt of non-social reward and punishment in a non-clinical community sample.

Our findings add to the growing body of literature showing altered incentive processing in social anxiety and extend previous findings to include non-social reward and punishment; however, our results were not exactly as expected. As predicted, greater social anxiety corresponded with reduced activity in the ventral striatum during anticipation of loss, suggesting reduced anticipatory reward-related processing when potentially avoiding an aversive stimulus. However, contrary to our hypothesis based on work linking social anxiety with reduced positive experience, we found little relationship between ventral striatum activity and social anxiety during gain anticipation, except when specifically examining the SAD-General subscale [17,21,22,25,41]. Interestingly, depression, which is defined in large part by decreased positive affect, also does not co-vary with reduced ventral striatum activity in response to anticipation of reward [42,43]. When examining gain and loss outcomes using an ROI of the MPFC, we found no associations between brain activity and social anxiety. Strikingly, however, whole brain analysis revealed positive associations between social anxiety and regions such as the precuneus, PCC, and parietal lobe - areas implicated in the default mode network (DMN) - during both the anticipation and receipt of reward. These associations held even after partialing out variance due to trait anxiety.

Activity in the DMN, a collection of brain areas usually more active during rest and less active during task-focused activities [40], is thought to reflect, among other things, self-referential processing, mind-wandering, and episodic memory [44]. That these areas were more active during reward processing among individuals high in social anxiety may indicate that socially anxious individuals find it difficult to direct attention away from the self and toward positive stimuli. This may be especially true in novel situations and when one fears evaluation by others, as similar findings were observed for both anticipation and outcome phases when using the FNE and SAD-New subscales of the SAS-A, but not when using the SAD-General subscale. It is important to note that in these areas, participants generally showed decreased activity during gain compared to neutral cues, as would be expected in DMN areas. Thus, the 'increased' activity seen in more socially anxious individuals is, more accurately, less of a decrease. Social anxiety may correspond with a smaller shift in processing from self-focused, 'default' processing to generalized reward processing. Interestingly, many participants, particularly those in the upper half of social anxiety scores, actually showed greater activity in DMN areas during gain relative to neutral trials.

Precuneus/PCC activity is increased during self-processing and reflection and decreased during goal-directed, non-self-referential activity [45]. The lower reduction in activity in these brain areas seen in the more socially anxious individuals in our sample may indicate a continued need to maintain self-focused vigilance during a state of anticipatory reward, possibly due to assigning greater motivational salience to anticipation of reward compared to the less socially anxious individuals. This pattern of brain activity was also seen in socially anxious individuals during the outcome phase, suggesting self-focused attention may continue even when a socially anxious person's need to perform is over and a reward is being processed. Indeed, research suggests that individuals with social anxiety show not only a fear of negative evaluation but also a fear of positive evaluation [46], which may be due to socially anxious individuals predicting they will not be able to live up to future standards when they perform well. Because participants in our study maintained high hit rates (around 80%), it is possible that the more socially anxious individuals felt added pressure to continue performing well, which may have been mediated by activity in DMN areas.

Our findings somewhat contrast with a study examining both social and non-social reward processing in people with clinical social anxiety disorder [47]. In that study, individuals with social anxiety disorder ($n = 15$) showed no neural differences from healthy controls ($n = 19$) while anticipating and receiving monetary reward during the MID task. However, decreased activity in the accumbens was observed in the socially anxious group when anticipating social reward (in this case, a picture of smiling face). It is possible that our much larger sample size ($n = 84$) afforded the ability to identify brain regions related to social anxiety during anticipation of monetary reward due to a level of statistical power unavailable in the prior study.

Importantly, other constructs related to social anxiety can alter reward processing during incentive delay tasks. For example, shy individuals exhibit relatively quicker reaction times than non-shy individuals to target stimuli when anticipating rewards compared to punishments or neutral incentives, suggesting increased reward sensitivity in shy people [48]. Similar behavioral differences based on social anxiety levels were not found in our study, however. Instead, our more socially anxious participants trended toward slower reaction times for reward incentives. It is possible that shyness differs from social anxiety in some way relevant to reaction times - perhaps shy people lack the same fear of evaluation that may hinder performance in socially anxious individuals. In other work, adolescents who had been classified as behaviorally inhibited in childhood showed increased striatal activity when anticipating incentives compared to those who had not been classified as behaviorally inhibited [49]. These (and our own) findings run counter to our hypothesis that socially anxious people should show decreased reward sensitivity. Importantly, however, Guyer et al. suggest that the increased striatal activity in behaviorally inhibited adolescents is due to heightened concern about making errors - that behaviorally inhibited participants may have been more vigilant during larger incentives due to fear of failure. Corroborating this was the finding that affective ratings for gain cues given after the experiment did not differ between the two groups (that is, behaviorally inhibited individuals did not rate gain cues more positively than non-behaviorally inhibited individuals), suggesting that increased striatal activity did not correspond with increased self-reports of positive experiences.

In the present study, social anxiety showed fewer and less consistent relationships with brain activity during both loss anticipation and loss outcomes. This seems counter-intuitive, given that fear-related disorders are prominently characterized by anxiety about upcoming negative events. Whether this is due to an actual absence of a relationship between social anxiety and punishment processing, due to our lack of a clinically socially anxious group, or due to the high hit rates in our sample is unclear. Of note, when taking an ROI approach, social anxiety corresponded with decreased activity in the ventral striatum during anticipation of loss. Anticipation of punishment generally does not recruit ventral striatum activity [27], as was the case in our sample. This suggests that the more socially anxious individuals in our sample experienced a decrease in ventral striatum activity during loss anticipation compared to neutral anticipation, rather than just less of an increase. However, loss outcomes (in which participants generally successfully avoided punishment) did not show differential MPFC activity related to social anxiety. As always, the observations described here should be considered tentative pending replication. This is perhaps particularly true given the number and complexity of analyses we have performed.

Conclusions

In sum, we found that higher levels of social anxiety were associated with increased activity in default mode network areas during anticipation and receipt of reward. Our findings and those of others suggest that social anxiety may be characterized not by decreased approach-oriented, appetitive motivation so much as by increased self-focused vigilance in the presence of potential rewards. Importantly, the MID task is not an overtly social task - potential gains and losses are of money only. These results suggest that social anxiety, even at subclinical levels, may affect reward processing more generally, not just processing explicitly related to social situations. Yet, it is worth noting that any task performed in an experimental setting is implicitly social - the presence of the experimenter and fMRI technician constitutes a social, or at least not isolated, situation. In other words, although the MID task does not involve social interaction, it does involve an evaluative context. Thus, the altered reward processing seen in socially anxious individuals may be particularly evident in performance or self-evaluative contexts, such as the MID task employed in our study, even in the absence of overt social interaction or cues.

Additional files

Additional file 1: Supplementary analyses for anticipation and outcome phases.

Additional file 2: Table S1. Main effects of gain > neutral and neutral > gain anticipation contrasts using whole brain analysis. **Table S2.** Negative associations with social anxiety in gain large > gain small anticipation contrast using whole brain analysis. **Table S3.** Positive associations with FNE and SAD-New subscales in gain > neutral anticipation contrast using whole brain analysis. **Table S4.** Main effects of loss > neutral and neutral > loss anticipation contrasts using whole brain analysis. **Table S5.** Main effects of gain > neutral and neutral > gain outcome contrasts using whole brain analysis. **Table S6.** Positive associations with social anxiety in gain large > gain small outcome contrast using whole brain analysis. **Table S7.** Positive associations with FNE and SAD-New subscales in gain > neutral outcome contrast using whole brain analysis. **Table S8.** Main effects of loss > neutral and neutral > loss outcome contrasts using whole brain analysis. **Table S9.** Positive associations with FNE and SAD-General subscales in loss > neutral outcome contrast using whole brain analysis. **Table S10.** Positive associations with social anxiety in gain > loss outcome contrast using whole brain analysis.

Abbreviations

ACC: Anterior cingulate cortex; BET: Brain Extraction Tool; BOLD: Blood oxygen level-dependent; DMN: Default mode network; FEAT: fMRI Expert Analysis Tool; FLIRT: FMRIB Linear Image Registration Tool; fMRI: Functional magnetic resonance imaging; FNE: Fear of Negative Evaluation subscale; FSL: FMRIB Software Library; MID: Monetary incentive delay; MNI: Montreal Neurological Institute; MPFC: Medial prefrontal cortex; PCC: Posterior cingulate cortex; RT: Reaction time; SAD-General: Social Avoidance and Distress in General Situations subscale; SAD-New: Social Avoidance and Distress in New Situations subscale; SAS-A: Social Anxiety Scale for Adolescents; SMC: Supplementary motor cortex; STAI: State-Trait Anxiety Inventory.

Competing interests

The authors declare no competing interests.

Authors' contributions

ELM participated in study conception, contributed to data collection, conducted the data analysis, and took the lead on writing the manuscript. JPA helped conceive of the study design and coordination, aided in data collection, and contributed to writing the manuscript. JAC helped conceive of the study design and coordination, provided financial support, assisted in data interpretation, and contributed to writing the manuscript. All authors read and approved the final manuscript.

Acknowledgements

The authors would like to acknowledge Casey Brown for coordinating the study, Lane Beckes and Madelon Hendricx-Riem for assistance with statistical analyses, and Marlen Z. Gonzalez and Bethany A. Teachman for providing insightful comments during manuscript preparation. This work was supported by a grant from the National Institute of Mental Health (R01MH080725) awarded to James A. Coan and grants from the National Institute of Child Health and Human Development and the National Institute of Mental Health (9R01 HD058305-11A1 & R01-MH58066) awarded to Joseph P. Allen.

References

1. Watson D, Clark LA: **Negative affectivity: the disposition to experience aversive emotional states.** *Psychol Bull* 1984, **96:**465–490.
2. Gray EK, Watson D: **Assessing positive and negative affect via self-report.** In *Handbook of Emotion Elicitation and Assessment.* Edited by Coan JA, Allen JJB. New York, NY: Oxford University Press; 2007:171–183.
3. McNaughton N: *The Neuropsychology of Anxiety: An Enquiry into the Function of the Septo-Hippocampal System.* New York, NY: Oxford University Press; 2003.

4. Davidson RJ: **Affective style and affective disorders: perspectives from affective neuroscience.** *Cognition and Emotion* 1998, **12**:307–330.
5. Gray J, McNaughton N: *The Neuropsychology of Anxiety: An Enquiry into the Functions of the Septo-Hippocampal System.* New York, NY: Oxford University Press; 2000.
6. Carver CS, White TL: **Behavioral inhibition, behavioral activation, and affective responses to impending reward and punishment: the BIS/BAS Scales.** *J Pers Soc Psychol* 1994, **67**:319.
7. Ollendick TH, Hirshfeld-Becker DR: **The developmental psychopathology of social anxiety disorder.** *Biol Psychiatry* 2002, **51**:44–58.
8. van Brakel AM, Muris P, Bögels SM, Thomassen C: **A multifactorial model for the etiology of anxiety in non-clinical adolescents: Main and interactive effects of behavioral inhibition, attachment and parental rearing.** *J Child Fam Stud* 2006, **15**:568–578.
9. Schwartz CE, Snidman N, Kagan J: **Adolescent social anxiety as an outcome of inhibited temperament in childhood.** *J Am Acad Child Adolesc Psychiatry* 1999, **38**:1008–1015.
10. Coan JA, Allen JJ: **Frontal EEG asymmetry and the behavioral activation and inhibition systems.** *Psychophysiology* 2003, **40**:106–114.
11. Clark LA, Watson D: **Tripartite model of anxiety and depression: psychometric evidence and taxonomic implications.** *J Abnorm Psychol* 1991, **100**:316–336.
12. Heller W, Nitscke JB: **The puzzle of regional brain activity in depression and anxiety: The importance of subtypes and comorbidity.** *In Cognition and Emotion* 1998, **12**:421–447.
13. Shankman SA, Klein DN: **The relation between depression and anxiety: an evaluation of the tripartite, approach-withdrawal and valence-arousal models.** *Clin Psychol Rev* 2003, **23**:605–637.
14. Weinstock LM, Whisman MA: **Neuroticism as a common feature of the depressive and anxiety disorders: a test of the revised integrative hierarchical model in a national sample.** *J Abnorm Psychol* 2006, **115**:68–74.
15. Clark LA, Watson D, Mineka S: **Temperament, personality, and the mood and anxiety disorders.** *J Abnorm Psychol* 1994, **103**:103–116.
16. Watson D, Wiese D, Vaidya J, Tellegen A: **The two general activation systems of affect: Structural findings, evolutionary considerations, and psychobiological evidence.** *J Pers Soc Psychol* 1999, **76**:820.
17. Chorpita BF: **The tripartite model and dimensions of anxiety and depression: an examination of structure in a large school sample.** *J Abnorm Child Psychol* 2002, **30**:177–190.
18. Henriques JB, Davidson RJ: **Decreased responsiveness to reward in depression.** *Cognition and Emotion* 2000, **14**:711–724.
19. Stewart JL, Coan JA, Towers DN, Allen JJ: **Frontal EEG asymmetry during emotional challenge differentiates individuals with and without lifetime major depressive disorder.** *J Affect Disord* 2011, **129**:167–174.
20. Brown TA, Chorpita BF, Barlow DH: **Structural relationships among dimensions of the DSM-IV anxiety and mood disorders and dimensions of negative affect, positive affect, and autonomic arousal.** *J Abnorm Psychol* 1998, **107**:179.
21. Farmer AS, Kashdan TB: **Social anxiety and emotion regulation in daily life: spillover effects on positive and negative social events.** *Cogn Behav Ther* 2012, **41**:152–162.
22. Kashdan TB, Steger MF: **Expanding the topography of social anxiety. an experience-sampling assessment of positive emotions, positive events, and emotion suppression.** *Psychol Sci* 2006, **17**:120–128.
23. Kimbrel NA, Mitchell JT, Nelson-Gray RO: **An examination of the relationship between behavioral approach system (BAS) sensitivity and social interaction anxiety.** *J Anxiety Disord* 2010, **24**:372–378.
24. Kimbrel NA: **A model of the development and maintenance of generalized social phobia.** *Clin Psychol Rev* 2008, **28**:592–612.
25. Freitas-Ferrari MC, Hallak JE, Trzesniak C, Filho AS, Machado-de-Sousa JP, Chagas MH, Nardi AE, Crippa JA: **Neuroimaging in social anxiety disorder: a systematic review of the literature.** *Prog Neuropsychopharmacol Biol Psychiatry* 2010, **34**:565–580.
26. Knutson B, Westdorp A, Kaiser E, Hommer D: **FMRI visualization of brain activity during a monetary incentive delay task.** *Neuroimage* 2000, **12**:20–27.
27. Knutson B, Adams CM, Fong GW, Hommer D: **Anticipation of increasing monetary reward selectively recruits nucleus accumbens.** *J Neurosci* 2001, **21**:RC159.
28. Knutson B, Fong GW, Adams CM, Varner JL, Hommer D: **Dissociation of reward anticipation and outcome with event-related fMRI.** *Neuroreport* 2001, **12**:3683–3687.
29. Dillon DG, Holmes AJ, Jahn AL, Bogdan R, Wald LL, Pizzagalli DA: **Dissociation of neural regions associated with anticipatory versus consummatory phases of incentive processing.** *Psychophysiology* 2008, **45**:36–49.
30. Allen JP, Chango J, Szwedo D, Schad M, Marston E: **Predictors of susceptibility to peer influence regarding substance use in adolescence.** *Child Dev* 2012, **83**:337–350.
31. Marsh P, McFarland FC, Allen JP, McElhaney KB, Land D: **Attachment, autonomy, and multifinality in adolescent internalizing and risky behavioral symptoms.** *Dev Psychopathol* 2003, **15**:451–467.
32. La Greca AM, Lopez N: **Social anxiety among adolescents: linkages with peer relations and friendships.** *J Abnorm Child Psychol* 1998, **26**:83–94.
33. Inderbitzen-Nolan HM, Walters KS: **Social Anxiety Scale for Adolescents: normative data and further evidence of construct validity.** *J Clin Child Psychol* 2000, **29**:360–371.
34. Spielberger CD: *Manual for the State-Trait Anxiety Inventory (Form Y).* Palo Alto, NM: Consulting Psychologists Press; 1983.
35. Jenkinson M, Bannister P, Brady M, Smith S: **Improved optimization for the robust and accurate linear registration and motion correction of brain images.** *Neuroimage* 2002, **17**:825–841.
36. Spreckelmeyer KN, Krach S, Kohls G, Rademacher L, Irmak A, Konrad K, Kircher T, Grunder G: **Anticipation of monetary and social reward differently activates mesolimbic brain structures in men and women.** *Soc Cogn Affect Neurosci* 2009, **4**:158–165.
37. Norris CJ, Coan JA, Johnstone T: **Functional Magnetic Resonance Imaging and The Study of Emotion.** In *Handbook of Emotion Elicitation and Assessment.* Edited by Coan JA, Allen JJB. New York: Oxford University Press; 2007:440–460.
38. Lieberman MD, Cunningham WA: **Type I and Type II error concerns in fMRI research: re-balancing the scale.** *Soc Cogn Affect Neurosci* 2009, **4**:423–428.
39. Forman SD, Cohen JD, Fitzgerald M, Eddy WF, Mintun MA, Noll DC: **Improved assessment of significant activation in functional magnetic resonance imaging (fMRI): use of a cluster-size threshold.** *Magn Reson Med* 1995, **33**:636–647.
40. Raichle ME, MacLeod AM, Snyder AZ, Powers WJ, Gusnard DA, Shulman GL: **A default mode of brain function.** *Proc Natl Acad Sci U S A* 2001, **98**:676–682.
41. Kashdan TB: **Social anxiety spectrum and diminished positive experiences: theoretical synthesis and meta-analysis.** *Clin Psychol Rev* 2007, **27**:348–365.
42. Knutson B, Bhanji JP, Cooney RE, Atlas LY, Gotlib IH: **Neural responses to monetary incentives in major depression.** *Biol Psychiatry* 2008, **63**:686–692.
43. Pizzagalli DA, Holmes AJ, Dillon DG, Goetz EL, Birk JL, Bogdan R, Dougherty DD, Iosifescu DV, Rauch SL, Fava M: **Reduced caudate and nucleus accumbens response to rewards in unmedicated individuals with major depressive disorder.** *Am J Psychiatry* 2009, **166**:702–710.
44. Buckner RL, Andrews-Hanna JR, Schacter DL: **The brain's default network: anatomy, function, and relevance to disease.** *Ann NY Acad Sci* 2008, **1124**:1–38.
45. Cavanna AE, Trimble MR: **The precuneus: a review of its functional anatomy and behavioural correlates.** *Brain* 2006, **129**:564–583.
46. Weeks JW, Heimberg RG, Rodebaugh TL, Norton PJ: **Exploring the relationship between fear of positive evaluation and social anxiety.** *J Anxiety Disord* 2008, **22**:386–400.
47. Richey JA, Rittenberg A, Hughes L, Damiano CR, Sabatino A, Miller S, Hanna E, Bodfish JW, Dichter GS: **Common and distinct neural features of social and non-social reward processing in autism and social anxiety disorder.** *Soc Cogn Affect Neurosci* 2041, **9**:367–377.
48. Hardin MG, Perez-Edgar K, Guyer AE, Pine DS, Fox NA, Ernst M: **Reward and punishment sensitivity in shy and non-shy adults: relations between social and motivated behavior.** *Pers Individ Dif* 2006, **40**:699–711.
49. Guyer AE, Nelson EE, Perez-Edgar K, Hardin MG, Roberson-Nay R, Monk CS, Bjork JM, Henderson HA, Pine DS, Fox NA, Ernst M: **Striatal functional alteration in adolescents characterized by early childhood behavioral inhibition.** *J Neurosci* 2006, **26**:6399–6405.

13

Correlations between psychological tests and physiological responses during fear conditioning and renewal

Karen G Martínez[1*†], Melissa Castro-Couch[3†], José A Franco-Chaves[1], Brenda Ojeda-Arce[1], Gustavo Segura[4], Mohammed R Milad[5] and Gregory J Quirk[1,2]

Abstract

Background: Anxiety disorders are characterized by specific emotions, thoughts and physiological responses. Little is known, however, about the relationship between psychological/personality indices of anxiety responses to fear stimuli.

Methods: We studied this relationship in healthy subjects by comparing scores on psychological and personality questionnaires with results of an experimental fear conditioning paradigm using a visual conditioned stimulus (CS). We measured skin conductance response (SCR) during habituation, conditioning, and extinction; subsequently testing for recall and renewal of fear 24 hours later.

Results: We found that multiple regression models explained 45% of the variance during conditioning to the CS+, and 24% of the variance during renewal of fear to the CS+. Factors that explained conditioning included lower levels of conscientiousness, increased baseline reactivity (SCL), and response to the shock (UCR). Low levels of extraversion correlated with greater renewal. No model could be found to explain extinction learning or extinction recall to the CS+.

Conclusions: The lack of correlation of fear extinction with personality and neuropsychological indices suggests that extinction may be less determined by trait variables and cognitive state, and may depend more on the subject's current emotional state. The negative correlation between fear renewal and extraversion suggests that this personality characteristic may protect against post-treatment relapse of symptoms of anxiety disorders.

Keywords: Fear, Conditioning, Extinction, Anxiety, Skin conductance, Personality traits

Background

There is increasing evidence that people with anxiety disorders show exaggerated fear responses during experimental fear conditioning, in which a visual cue is paired with a mild shock to elicit increases in startle or skin conductance [1-5]. For example, subjects with post-traumatic stress disorder (PTSD) have shown increased fear conditioning [6], as well as deficient extinction of conditioned fear responses [7], and reduced recall of extinction memories [4]. One way to further understand the clinical relevance of conditioned fear responses is to determine their relation to anxiety phenotypes and personality traits. Anxious thoughts and behaviors can be assessed with questionnaires such as the Beck Anxiety Inventory (BAI) and the State-Trait Anxiety Inventory (STAI) [8]. Anxiety disorders have also been associated with personality characteristics such as neuroticism and extraversion [9], and decreased performance in cognitive processes such as conflict resolution and attention to threat [8].

Recent studies have begun to examine the relationship between some of these anxiety phenotypes and fear responses. Healthy subjects' level of conditioning showed a positive correlation with trait anxiety, surveys of worry/avoidance, low extraversion, and high neuroticism [10-12]. Extinction has shown the opposite relationship with

* Correspondence: Karen.martinez4@upr.edu
†Equal contributors
[1]Department of Psychiatry, University of Puerto Rico School of Medicine, P.O. Box 365067, San Juan, PR 00936, USA
Full list of author information is available at the end of the article

extraversion and neuroticism [12]. In addition, an anxious state is associated with decreased SCR response during fear conditioning and, conversely, elevated SCR response during extinction [13]. These studies focused exclusively on the response to the conditioned stimulus, and did not take into account responses to the unconditioned stimulus or differential learning (CS + minus CS-). Moreover, no prior study has attempted to explain the renewal of fear after extinction, which occurs with changes in context; an emerging model of clinical relapse [14].

To address these issues, we administered a battery of tests to healthy volunteers prior to fear conditioning, extinction, and renewal. To measure thoughts and behaviors associated with anxiety, we used the BAI and STAI. Personality characteristics were assessed with the NEO Five Factor Inventory (NEO-FFI). For cognitive processes, we used two Stroop-type conflict detection tests: 1) The Multi-Source Interference Task (MSIT), which activates conditioning-related areas of anterior cingulate cortex [15], and 2) the emotional Stroop (EST), which activates extinction-related areas of the cingulate and perigenual cortices [16]. We hypothesized that indices of anxiety (high STAI and BAI scores, high neuroticism, and low extraversion) would correlate positively with conditioning measures (i.e., conditioning, renewal), and negatively with extinction. The Stroop conflict tests, which reflect prefrontal engagement, might correlate with conditioning and/or extinction.

Methods

Participants

Healthy Puerto Rican subjects were recruited from the local community via advertisements. Exclusion criteria included a history of neurological conditions, current psychoactive medications, or Axis I diagnosis within the past 6 months. A Structured Clinical Interview for DMS-IV (SCID-I-RV) was used to confirm the absence of an Axis-I diagnosis. Subjects who failed to condition (2 or more trials with SCR > 0.05 μS, n = 2) or were outliers in their SCR values (greater than 2 standard deviations from the mean, n = 1) were also excluded. The final sample consisted of 46 subjects (30 females and 16 males) ranging in age from 21–57 (Mean age females = 28.5 ± 9.6; Mean age males = 25.4 ± 3.5 years). Written informed consent was obtained from all participants in accordance with the requirements of the Institutional Review Board at the University of Puerto Rico, School of Medicine and methods were approved as protocol A5280110.

Neuropsychological tests

All tests were validated for use with Spanish speaking subjects. Testing was performed over two days as outlined in Figure 1.

a. Anxiety symptoms scales
   We used the BAI and STAI to measure anxiety symptoms. The BAI Spanish version used in our study has similar psychometric properties to the original English version [17,18] and the version of the STAI used for our study has been validated for Puerto Ricans [19].
b. NEO Five Factor Inventory (NEO-FFI)
   The NEO-FFI is a 60-item self-report measure of personality traits across five dimensions: neuroticism, extraversion, agreeableness, conscientiousness and

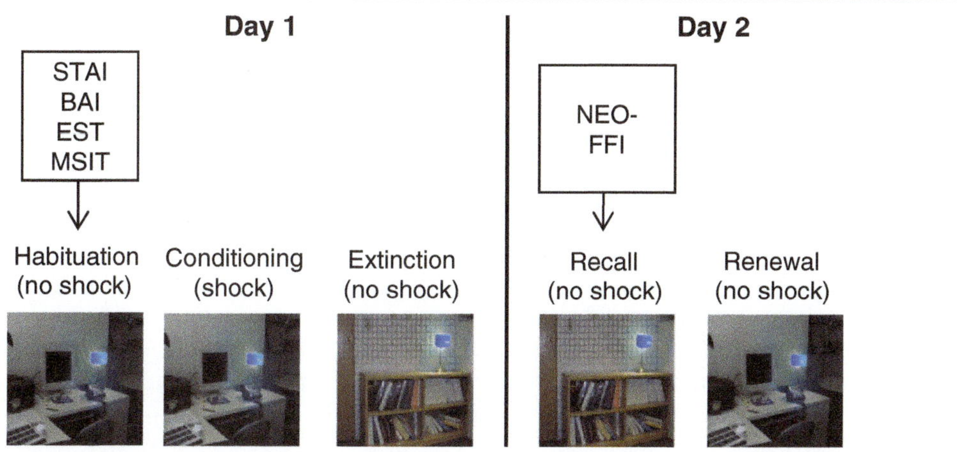

Figure 1 Schematic of experimental protocol. On each day, subjects performed psychological tests, and then underwent fear conditioning and extinction. Pictures of an office and a library represented conditioning and extinction contexts respectively, whereas the blue (or red) light represented the CS that was paired with the shock and later extinguished. STAI = State-Trait Anxiety Inventory, BAI = Beck Anxiety Inventory, EST = Emotional Stroop Task, MSIT = Multi-Source Interference Task, NEO-FFI = NEO Five Factor Personality Inventory.

openness to experience [20]. The Spanish version of the NEO-FFI has been previously validated for Puerto Ricans [21]. Raw scores for each personality dimension were calculated and subsequently transformed into T-scores (M = 50, SD = 10) to adjust for sex differences.

c. Emotional Stroop Task (EST)
We designed a Spanish version of the EST using SuperLab software (Cedrus, Phoenix, Arizona). Participants were instructed to identify the ink color of a series of computer generated words as quickly as possible. Two types of words were used: threat-related and neutral words. The average reaction time (RT) was recorded by a key punch (ms), and a RT difference between threat and neutral words was calculated (RT threat minus RT neutral).

d. Multi-Source Interference Task (MSIT)
The MSIT is a numerical-based Stroop task measuring cognitive interference, designed to specifically activate the dorsal anterior cingulate cortex [15]. Subjects were presented with a set of three numbers (0, 1, 2, or 3), and were instructed to quickly select the one number that differed from the other two. In congruent trials, the position of the target number always matched the position of the key (i.e., 100, 020, 003). During interference trials, the position of the target never matched the position of the key (i.e., 010, 002, 300). Mean response latencies (in msec) for both congruent and incongruent trials were subtracted to yield a difference score (incongruent – congruent).

Fear conditioning and extinction

We used a fear-learning paradigm previously described [22], in which subjects were tested over two consecutive days. On day 1, subjects completed habituation, conditioning, and extinction. The habituation phase consisted of 8 trials in which the conditioned stimuli (red or blue desk lights) were presented in two separate contextual (library and office), without any shock. The contextual stimulus appeared 6 sec prior to the onset of the desk light, which lasted for 12 sec, after which the screen went blank. The average inter-trial interval was 16 sec (range 12–21 sec). Habituation was immediately followed by conditioning, where one of the desk lights (e.g., red CS+) was paired with a mild shock to the second and third fingers of the dominant hand. Conditioning occurred within a specific context (e.g., office) (see Figure 1). The alternative desk light (e.g., blue CS-) was presented without any shock. The color of the stimulus for the CS + (blue vs. red light), as well as the conditioning context (library vs. office), were counter balanced across subjects. The shock lasted 0.5 sec and started immediately after CS + offset. The electric current was generated by a Coulbourn transcutaneous aversive finger stimulator (E13-22) powered by a 9-V dry cell battery. The intensity of the current was pre-set by each participant to be "highly annoying, but not painful". The electrodes remained attached to the subject's fingers during all phases of the experiment, and subjects were instructed prior to each phase that they "may or may not receive a shock". Subjects were given 10 trials of conditioning (5 CS + and 5 CS-). After a few minutes, they received 20 trials of extinction (10 CS + and 10 CS-), in which the CS + and CS- were presented without shocks, in the alternate context (e.g., library).

On Day 2, subjects were brought back to the lab in order to test their retention of the extinction memory. Subjects were shown the context stimulus alone, followed 6 sec later by the CS + without any shock. Extinction memory was tested in two phases: recall and renewal, each consisting of 10 trials (5 CS + and 5 CS-). During the recall phase, the CS + was presented in the extinction context (recall of safety), whereas during the renewal phase, the CS + was presented in the conditioning context (recall of danger). The order of testing (recall vs. renewal) was counterbalanced across subjects.

Physiological measures

The baseline skin conductance level (SCL) consisted of the average skin conductance during the 5 seconds prior to the first habituation trial. The skin conductance response (SCR) to each stimulus (CS + and CS-) was assessed as previously described [6,22,23]. The average skin conductance during the 6 sec context presentation was subtracted from the average skin conductance during the 12 sec CS + context presentation. We applied a minimum conditioning criteria that required subjects to show an SCR to the CS + greater than 0.05 μS in 2 or more conditioning trials [22,24].

Statistical analyses

For each phase, the average SCR to the CS + and CS- were calculated as follows; 1) Habituation: average SCR of the first two trials habituation; 2) Conditioning: maximum SCR during conditioning; 3) Extinction: average SCR of trials 1–2 of extinction minus the average SCR of trials 9–10 of extinction; 4) Percent recall: average SCR in trials 1–2 of recall, divided by the peak SCR during conditioning; 5) Percent renewal: average SCR in trials 1–2 of renewal, divided by the peak SCR during conditioning [22]. Differential responses were calculated in the same way, except that the CS- was subtracted from the CS +.

ANOVAs with repeated measures were used to evaluate differences in SCRs to the CS + and CS-. Two-factor ANOVA's (stimulus vs. trial) were performed for each phase of the experiment, to test for main effects and interactions. The stimulus main effect and stimulus X trial interaction effect were tested using the multivariate criterion of Wilk's lambda (Λ). Paired-samples *t* tests were conducted to follow up the significant interactions. We controlled for familywise error rate across these tests by using Holm's sequential Bonferroni approach (SPSS, version 19.0)

The relationship between psychological tests and physiological measures for each phase was evaluated using simple linear regressions, followed by stepwise multiple linear regression analysis using combinations of tests (SPSS, version 16.0). Simple linear regressions yielded an R^2 representing the amount of variance explained by the test variable, and a beta coefficient (β) representing the correlation coefficient (r) between that test variable and the SCR. We performed a forward stepwise procedure in which variables were added to the model in two steps [25]. The first step included the psychological test variables: BAI, STAI, NEO personality factors, and the neuropsychological measures (MSIT, EST). The second step added additional variables that could have an effect on physiological responses such as sex, age, shock level, baseline SCL, and unconditioned responses to shock. This yielded a unique set of predictor variables for each phase. Multicollinearity between the predictor variables was evaluated by calculating the tolerance criteria [25]. β coefficients were determined for each factor in the model, and R^2 values were adjusted for small sample size [25].

Results

Psychological test results

Our sample of healthy subjects scored within the normal range on all psychological and neuropsychological tests. Anxiety questionnaires showed no evidence of clinically relevant anxiety symptoms (mean BAI score = 3.5, mean state anxiety = 27.22%ile, mean trait anxiety = 30.52%ile) , and personality scores (mean neuroticism T score = 47, mean extraversion T score = 56 and mean conscientiousness T score = 47) were within normal limits [20]. Performance on the MSIT (mean reaction time = 340 msec) was similar to previous studies with healthy subjects [15]. The results of the EST showed no interference effect, on average, as expected from previous studies [26].

Fear conditioning

Day 1: Habituation, conditioning and extinction

During habituation, there were no differences in SCR to the CS + (stimuli paired with shock) and the CS- (stimuli never paired with shock) [$\Lambda = .99$, $F_{(1,45)} = 0.48$, $p = 0.49$]. During conditioning, responses to the CS + were significantly higher than those to the CS- (see Figure 2A).

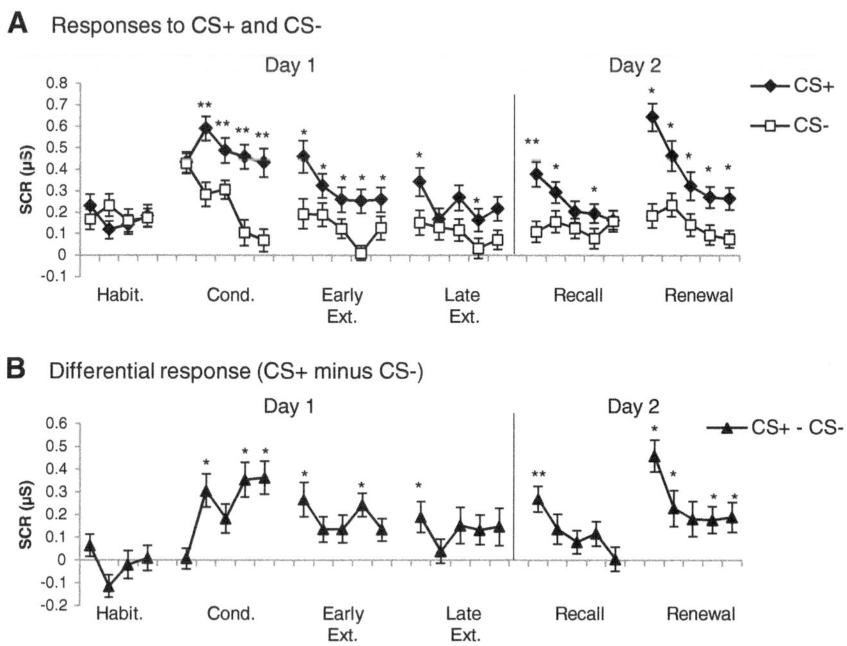

Figure 2 Skin conductance responses (SCR) across all experimental phases. A. Responses to CS + and CS- (single trials shown). On day 2, the order of recall and renewal was counterbalanced between subjects to correct for order effects. **B**. Differential SCR (CS + minus CS-). Differential learning in all phases was compared to last habituation trial. Habit. = Habituation, Cond. = Conditioning, Ext. = Extinction, µS = microsiemens, *p < 0.05; **p < 0.01.

ANOVA during the conditioning phase revealed significant main effects for stimulus [Λ = .50, $F_{(1,45)} = 44.24$, $p < 0.001$] and trials [Λ = .77, $F_{(4, 42)} = 3.20$, $p = 0.022$], as well as a significant stimulus X trial interaction [Λ = .62, $F_{(4,42)} = 6.34$, $p < 0.001$]. Post hoc comparisons revealed that CS + responses were significantly larger than CS-responses during trials 2–5 of conditioning (all $p < 0.01$), demonstrating successful acquisition of conditioned learning.

During the ten trials of extinction, responses to the CS + declined significantly. In extinction (trials 1–10), repeated measures ANOVA revealed significant main effects of stimulus [Λ = .64, $F_{(1,45)} = 25.91$, $p < 0.001$] and trials [Λ = .67, $F_{(9,37)} = 2.01$, $p = 0.065$] and a non-significant stimulus X trial interaction [Λ = .70, $F_{(9,37)} = 1.73$, $p = 0.115$]. Post hoc comparisons revealed that responses to the CS + remained significantly larger than to CS- during all early extinction trials (all $p < 0.02$). During late extinction, significant differences were observed for trials 6 and 9 only (both $p < 0.05$).

Day 2: Recall of extinction and renewal

The following day, subjects were returned to the laboratory to test for recall and renewal, in counterbalanced order. During the recall phase, in which the CS + was presented in the extinction context, ANOVA revealed a significant main effect of stimulus [Λ = .73, $F_{(1,45)} = 16.67$, $p < 0.001$], but not trials [Λ = .682, $F_{(4,42)} = 2.24$, $p = 0.081$], and a significant interaction [Λ = .71, $F_{(4,42)} = 4.27$, $p = 0.05$]. Post-hoc analysis showed that the response to the CS + was significantly higher than to the CS- in trials 1 ($p < 0.001$), 2 ($p = 0.047$) and 4 ($p = 0.036$). Responses to the CS + returned to habituation baseline by the fifth trial.

During the renewal phase, in which the CS + was presented in the conditioning context, the responses to the CS + dramatically increased. ANOVA revealed significant main effects of stimulus [Λ = .58, $F_{(1,45)} = 31.47$, $p < 0.001$] and trials [Λ = .59, $F_{(4,42)} = 7.32$, $p < 0.001$], with a significant stimulus X trial interaction [Λ = .72, $F_{(4,42)} = 4.01$, $p = 0.008$]. Post hoc comparisons revealed that responses to the CS + were significantly larger than to the CS- on all renewal trials (all $p < 0.05$) demonstrating prolonged effects of altering the context.

Differential response

The differential response (CS + minus CS-) reflects the degree of associative learning to the CS + (Figure 2B). Compared with the last trial of habituation, pairwise comparisons revealed significant differential responding during trials 2, 4, and 5 of conditioning (all $p < 0.01$), trials 1, 4, and 6 of extinction (all $p < 0.05$), the first trial of recall ($p = 0.005$), and trials 1, 2, 4, and 5 of renewal (all $p < 0.05$).

Regression analysis

Simple linear regression

We first used simple linear regressions to evaluate the degree to which individual tests could account for variance in SCL or SCR in the different phases, calculating a regression coefficient (R^2). Most psychological measures were not significantly correlated with SCL or SCR responses in any experimental phase (see Table 1). When significant correlations did occur, they accounted for only 8 to 15% of SCR variance. The variance of SCL (15%) was explained by extraversion ($ß = -0.41$, $p = 0.005$). For conditioning memory, conscientiousness could explain 7% of the variance ($ß = -0.30$, $p = 0.043$), whereas for extinction learning, the EST could explain 7% of the variance ($ß = 0.30$, $p = 0.036$). Percent renewal showed similar weak correlations with extraversion ($ß = -0.413$, $p = 0.004$; 17%). No test could account for significant variance in recall or habituation phases.

Multiple regression

We next conducted multiple regression analyses, using a stepwise approach. The possible predictor variables were added to the model in two steps [25]. The first step included the psychological, personality, and neuropsychological test variables. A second step added additional variables that could have an effect on physiological responses such as sex, age, shock level, baseline SCL, and unconditioned responses to shock. This process yielded a unique set of predictor variables for each phase. For the conditioning phase (peak conditioning), a significant model was found which accounted for 45% of the SCR variance across subjects (adjusted $R^2 = 0.446$, $p < 0.001$) (see Figure 3A). Significant variables in the model included one personality trait

Table 1 Results of simple regressions for CS + responses

Tests	SCL	Cond.	Extinction	Recall	Renewal
	R^2	R^2	R^2	R^2	R^2
Trait Anxiety	−0.022	0.009	0.022	−0.008	−0.023
State Anxiety	0.056	0.013	0.004	−0.005	−0.018
Beck Anxiety	−0.020	0.003	0.007	0.001	0.037
Neuroticism	0.021	0.000	0.041	0.000	0.000
Extraversion	**0.145****	0.001	0.016	0.063	**0.170****
	$\beta = -0.405$				$\beta = -0.413$
Conscientiousness	−0.021	**0.071***	0.063	0.019	0.019
		$\beta = -0.304$			
EST Reaction Time	−0.023	0.001	**0.072***	0.035	0.008
			$\beta = 0.304$		
MSIT Reaction Time	−0.010	0.028	0.009	0.037	0.014

Shown are values for R^2 (the amount of SCR variance accounted for each test). For significant correlations with SCR, β is shown. SCL = baseline skin conductance level, Cond. = Conditioning, EST = Emotional Stroop Task, MSIT = Multi-Source Interference Task. *$p < 0.05$, **$p < 0.001$.

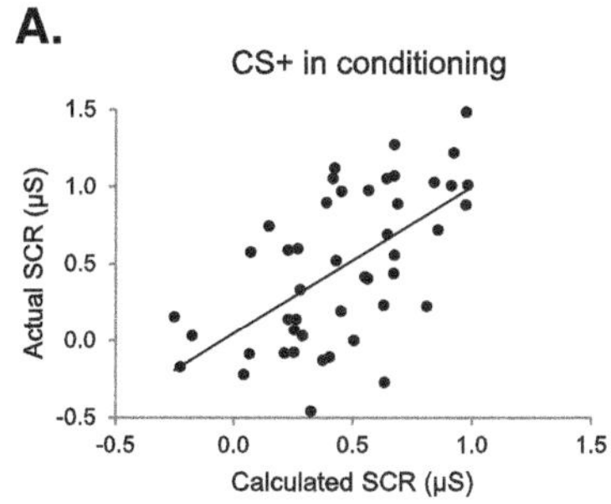

Model for CS+ response during Conditioning	
Factors	Variables chosen for model
Psychological variables entered stepwise: BAI, STAI, NEO, MSIT, EST	Conscientiousness β= -0.292 p=0.011
Physiological and demographic variables entered stepwise: UCR, SCL, sex, age	UCR β= 0.498, p<0.001 SCL β= 0.259, p=0.003
	Adjusted R^2 = 0.446**

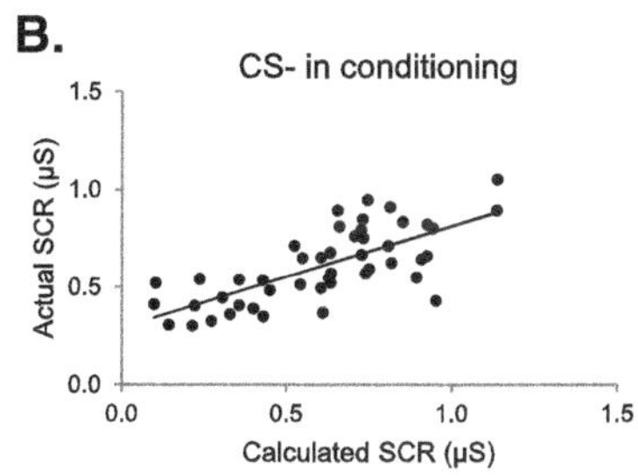

Model for CS- response during Conditioning	
Factors	Variables chosen for model
Psychological variables entered stepwise: BAI, STAI, NEO, MSIT, EST	--------
Physiological and demographic variables entered stepwise: UCR, SCL, sex, age	UCR β= 0.628, p<0.001 SCL β= 0.303, p<0.001
	Adjusted R^2 = 0.499**

Figure 3 Multiple regression models for conditioning. A. Model for CS+. **B**. Model for CS-. Plots compare the correlations between the actual CS responses and those calculated by the multiple regression model. µS = microsiemens, **p < 0.01.

(conscientiousness) and two physiological variables (i.e., UCR, SCL). Lower levels of conditioning were correlated with higher conscientiousness scores and lower UCR and SCL levels. Multicollinearity analysis showed that correlations between the predictor values was not a factor affecting the conditioning model (tolerance scores = 0.931-0.988). For the CS- responses, a significant model was found for peak conditioning consisting only of physiological variables (i.e., UCR, SCL), explaining 50% of the response (Adjusted $R^2 = 0.499$; $p < 0.001$, see Figure 3B).

No models were found that correlated with extinction learning or extinction recall. For the renewal phase, however, a model was found to account for 24% of inter-subject variance in CS + response (Adjusted $R^2 = 0.242$, $p < 0.001$) (see Figure 4). The model consisted of a negative correlation with extraversion and a positive correlation with sex (i.e., being male associated with higher renewal). This model also showed appropriate tolerance criteria (0.945-0.969) minimizing the risk of multicollinearity. There was also a significant (but weaker) model for CS- responses in renewal, using only physiological variables UCR and SCL (Adjusted $R^2 = 0.163$; $p = 0.008$).

Discussion

We have assessed the relationship of several psychological tests related to anxiety phenotypes with physiological indices, both at baseline and during various phases of experimental fear conditioning. While we were unable to find correlations with extinction learning or extinction recall, we were able to explain 24 to 45% of variance in SCR responses during conditioning and renewal, both indicators of the strength of the CS-US association.

The predictive power of our model for conditioning (45%) is consistent with findings from Otto and colleagues, who were able to account for 28% of CS + variance in conditioning, also using multiple regression [10]. This is interesting given that the two models employed different measures. While our model included only conscientiousness and physiological variables associated with reactivity, Otto et al. (2007) found a predictive model that included the Penn State Worry Questionnaire (PSWQ), the Fear Questionnaire (FQ), and the Anxiety Sensitivity Index (ASI). Conscientiousness can be related to PSWQ scores, in that it assesses thoughtfulness and carefulness [20] , and was previously reported to be correlated with conditioning [9]. Thus, together with Otto et al. (2007), we suggest that approximately 28-45% of SCR variance in conditioning may be due to individual characteristics that can be revealed with self-report scales and measures of physiological reactivity. The greater variance explained in our sample was probably due to our taking into account response to the shock and baseline skin conductance.

In contrast to conditioning, we were unable to find significant correlations with extinction learning or extinction recall, using either linear or multiple regression. This differs from Rauch et al. (2005) who reported that recall of extinction was correlated with extraversion

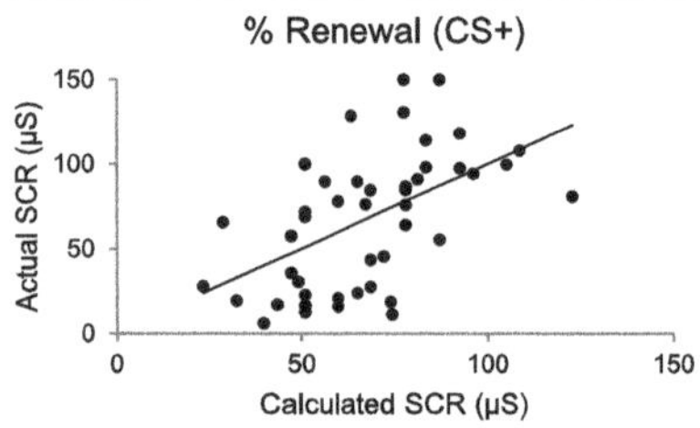

Model for CS+ response during %Renewal	
Factors	Variables chosen for model
Psychological variables entered stepwise: BAI, STAI, NEO, MSIT, EST	Extraversion β= -0.360 p= 0.009
Physiological and demographic variables entered stepwise: UCR, SCL, sex, age	Sex β= 0.330 p= 0.016
	Adjusted R^2 = 0.242**

Figure 4 Multiple regression model for CS + during renewal. Plot shows correlations between the actual SCR responses and those calculated by the multiple regression model for % fear renewal. μS = microsiemens, **$p < 0.001$.

(r = 0.77) and neuroticism (r = −0.61) [12]. The experimental protocols used at the two sites were designed to be identical. Factors that might account for the discrepancy include the larger number of subjects in the current study (46 vs. 14 in Rauch et al.), or an ethnic factor affecting the relationship between personality and extinction (Puerto Rican vs. a largely Caucasian sample in the Boston area). A lack of correlation of extinction with psychological and neuropsychological indices suggests that extinction may be less determined by trait variables, and may depend more on the subject's current emotional state. In support of this idea, Milad et al. (2008) showed that extinction retention deficits in PTSD patients were acquired rather than familial, based on a twin design [27]. Additionally, Vriends et al. (2011) reported decreased extinction in healthy participants who first watched a film intended to induce an anxious emotional state [13]. Our state measure (STAI) showed no correlation with extinction, likely due to the low state anxiety levels of our healthy subjects in the absence of a provocation such as that used in Vriends et al. (2011).

Our most novel finding was the ability to successfully model contextual renewal. Renewal of extinguished fear with a contextual shift is thought to model relapse after treatment with exposure therapy [14]. It has been suggested that the ability to successfully inhibit fear responses when challenged by contextual shifts is the best predictor of clinical response [28]. Extraversion was negatively correlated with renewal, consistent with a protective effect. Individuals with high extraversion scores are more likely to seek stimulation, undertake activities with unknown consequences, and experience positive emotions [20,29]. Extraversion is also positively correlated with the volume of the medial oribitofrontal cortex [30], an area implicated in fear inhibition [31] and reward [32]. Thus, the presence of extraversion may reflect the engagement of structures that modulate fear responses under ambiguous conditions. In addition, sex was also a significant factor in the model (males showed higher renewal). This is an interesting finding given that anxiety disorders are more prevalent in females [8,33]. We are now conducting additional studies on the sex differences we observed in our sample.

We propose several follow-up steps to extend these findings and to address the limitations of our study. In order to state that personality characteristics can predict physiological responses, the predictive power of these models should be tested using predictive model analysis with new subjects. The applicability of these results to subjects with anxiety disorders should also be evaluated. It will be particularly interesting to determine the extent to which conditioning and renewal models are able to predict the severity of anxiety disorders, response to treatment, and/or post-treatment relapse, in longitudinal studies. Factors that could be predictive of renewal, such as low extraversion in our sample, may be used for identifying patients at risk for relapse, who might benefit from preventive measures such as delivering therapy in multiple contexts or providing reminders of the therapeutic context [34].

Conclusion

Using models that included personality characteristics previously associated with the anxiety phenotype as well as physiological responses, we were able to explain up to 45% of variance in experimental fear conditioning and renewal. Understanding the relationships between personality characteristics and fear learning could help in the development of markers to identify people at risk for anxiety disorders and/or risk of relapse after treatment.

Competing interests

The authors declare that they have no competing interests.

Authors' contributions

KGM and MC-C participated in the development of the methodology, implementation of research protocol, statistical analysis and preparation of the manuscript. JAF-C participated in the development of the methodology, implementation of research protocol and statistical analysis. BO-A and GS collected data. MRM and GJQ contributed in the development of the methodology, interpretation of results and preparation of the manuscript. All authors read and approved the final manuscript.

Acknowledgements

We thank George Bush at Harvard Medical School for making the MSIT task available. This work was supported by NIH grant U54 RR026139 from the National Center for Research Resources, and 8U54 MD007587-03 from the

National Institute on Minority Health and Health Disparities to KGM, a post-doctoral master's in clinical research grant R25 RR017589 to KGM, and the UPR Presidents Office to GJQ.

Author details
[1]Department of Psychiatry, University of Puerto Rico School of Medicine, P.O. Box 365067, San Juan, PR 00936, USA. [2]Department of Anatomy & Neurobiology, University of Puerto Rico School of Medicine, San Juan, PR, USA. [3]Clinical Psychology Program, Ponce School of Medicine, Ponce, PR, USA. [4]Clinical Psychology Program, Carlos Albizu University, San Juan, PR, USA. [5]Department of Psychiatry, Massachusetts General Hospital and Harvard Medical School, Charlestown, MA, USA.

References

1. Lissek S, Rabin S, Heller RE, Lukenbaugh D, Geraci M, Pine DS, *et al*: **Overgeneralization of conditioned fear as a pathogenic marker of panic disorder.** *Am J Psychiatry* 2010, **167**:47–55.
2. Michael T, Blechert J, Vriends N, Margraf J, Wilhelm FH: **Fear conditioning in panic disorder: Enhanced resistance to extinction.** *J Abnorm Psychol* 2007, **116**:612–617.
3. Pitman RK, Orr SP, Shalev AY, Metzger LJ, Mellman TA: **Psychophysiological alterations in post-traumatic stress disorder.** *Semin Clin Neuropsychiatry* 1999, **4**:234–241.
4. Milad MR, Pitman RK, Ellis CB, Gold AL, Shin LM, Lasko NB, *et al*: **Neurobiological basis of failure to recall extinction memory in posttraumatic stress disorder.** *Biol Psychiatry* 2009, **66**:1075–1082.
5. Quirk GJ, Martinez KG, Nazario Rodriguez LL: **Translating findings from basic fear research to clinical psychiatry in Puerto Rico.** *P R Health Sci J* 2007, **26**:321–328.
6. Orr SP, Metzger LJ, Lasko NB, Macklin ML, Peri T, Pitman RK: **De novo conditioning in trauma-exposed individuals with and without posttraumatic stress disorder.** *J Abnorm Psychol* 2000, **109**:290–298.
7. Blechert J, Michael T, Vriends N, Margraf J, Wilhelm FH: **Fear conditioning in posttraumatic stress disorder: Evidence for delayed extinction of autonomic, experiential, and behavioural responses.** *Behav Res Ther* 2007, **45**:2019–2033.
8. Craske MG, Rauch SL, Ursano R, Prenoveau J, Pine DS, Zinbarg RE: **What is an anxiety disorder?** *Depress Anxiety* 2009, **26**:1066–1085.
9. Pineles SL, Vogt DS, Orr SP: **Personality and fear responses during conditioning: Beyond extraversion.** *Pers Individ Dif* 2009, **46**:48–53.
10. Otto MW, Leyro TM, Christian K, Deveney CM, Reese H, Pollack MH, *et al*: **Prediction of "fear" acquisition in healthy control participants in a de novo fear-conditioning paradigm.** *Behav Modif* 2007, **31**:32–51.
11. Indovina I, Robbins TW, Nunez-Elizalde AO, Dunn BD, Bishop SJ: **Fear-conditioning mechanisms associated with trait vulnerability to anxiety in humans.** *Neuron* 2011, **69**:563–571.
12. Rauch SL, Milad MR, Orr SP, Quinn BT, Fischl B, Pitman RK: **Orbitofrontal thickness, retention of fear extinction, and extraversion.** *Neuroreport* 2005, **16**:1909–1912.
13. Vriends N, Michael T, Blechert J, Meyer AH, Margraf J, Wilhelm FH: **The influence of state anxiety on the acquisition and extinction of fear.** *J Behav Ther Exp Psychiatry* 2011, **42**:46–53.
14. Bouton ME, Mineka S, Barlow DH: **A modern learning theory perspective on the etiology of panic disorder.** *Psychol Rev* 2001, **108**:4–32.
15. Bush G, Shin LM, Holmes J, Rosen BR, Vogt BA: **The Multi-Source Interference Task: validation study with fMRI in individual subjects.** *Mol Psychiatry* 2003, **8**:60–70.
16. Whalen PJ, Bush G, Shin LM, Rauch SL: **The emotional counting Stroop: a task for assessing emotional interference during brain imaging.** *Nat Protoc* 2006, **1**:293–296.
17. Novy DM, Stanley MA, Averill P, Daza P: **Psychometric comparability of English- and Spanish-language measures of anxiety and related affective symptoms.** *Psychol Assess* 2001, **13**:347–355.
18. Rossello J, Perez D: **Anxiety and social support in a group of young people with insulin-dependent diabetes.** *Bol Asoc Med P R* 2003, **95**:7-10–13-5.
19. Virella B, Arbona C, Novy D: **Psychometric properties and factor structure of the Spanish version of the state-trait anxiety inventory.** *J Pers Assess* 1994, **63**:401–412.
20. Costa PT, McCrae RR: *NEO PI-R Professional Manual.* Florida: Psychological Assessment Resources Inc. 1992.
21. McCrae RR, Terracciano A: **Universal features of personality traits from the observer's perspective: data from 50 cultures.** *J Pers Soc Psychol* 2005, **88**:547–561.
22. Milad MR, Orr SP, Pitman RK, Rauch SL: **Context modulation of memory for fear extinction in humans.** *Psychophysiology* 2005, **42**:456–464.
23. Milad MR, Rauch SL, Pitman RK, Quirk GJ: **Fear extinction in rats: Implications for human brain imaging and anxiety disorders.** *Biol Psychol* 2006, **73**:61–71.
24. Milad MR, Quirk GJ, Pitman RK, Orr SP, Fischl B, Rauch SL: **A role of the human dorsal anterior cingulate cortex in expression of learned fear.** *Biol Psychiatry* 2007, **62**:1191–1194.
25. Neter J, Wasserman W, Kutner M: *Applied Linear Regression Models.* 5th edition. Homewood, IL: RD Irwin; 1983.
26. Bar-Haim Y, Lamy D, Pergamin L, Bakermans-Kranenburg MJ, Van IJzendoorn MH: **Threat-related attentional bias in anxious and nonanxious individuals: a meta-analytic study.** *Psychol Bull* 2007, **133**:1–24.
27. Milad MR, Orr SP, Lasko NB, Chang Y, Rauch SL, Pitman RK: **Presence and acquired origin of reduced recall for fear extinction in PTSD: results of a twin study.** *J Psychiatr Res* 2008, **42**:515–520.
28. Craske MG, Kircanski K, Zelikowsky M, Mystkowski J, Chowdhury N, Baker A: **Optimizing inhibitory learning during exposure therapy.** *Behav Res Ther* 2008, **46**:5–27.
29. Watson D, Clark LA, Chmielewski M: **Structures of personality and their relevance to psychopathology: II. Further articulation of a comprehensive unified trait structure.** *J Pers* 2008, **76**:1545–1586.
30. DeYoung CG, Hirsh JB, Shane MS, Papademetris X, Rajeevan N, Gray JR: **Testing predictions from personality neuroscience. Brain structure and the big five.** *Psychol Sci* 2010, **21**:820–828.
31. Milad MR, Rauch SL: **The role of the orbitofrontal cortex in anxiety disorders.** *Ann N Y Acad Sci* 2007, **1121**:546–561.
32. Rolls ET, Grabenhorst F: **The orbitofrontal cortex and beyond: from affect to decision-making.** *Prog Neurobiol* 2008, **86**:216–244.
33. Canino GJ, Bird HR, Shrout PE, Rubio-Stipec M, Bravo M, Martinez R, *et al*: **The prevalence of specific psychiatric disorders in Puerto Rico.** *Arch Gen Psychiatry* 1987, **44**:727–735.
34. Bouton ME: **Context, ambiguity, and unlearning: sources of relapse after behavioral extinction.** *Biol Psychiatry* 2002, **52**:976–986.

14

Sex differences, gonadal hormones and the fear extinction network: implications for anxiety disorders

Kelimer Lebron-Milad and Mohammed R Milad*

Abstract

Convergent data from rodents and human studies have led to the development of models describing the neural mechanisms of fear extinction. Key components of the now well-characterized fear extinction network include the amygdala, hippocampus, and medial prefrontal cortical regions. These models are fueling novel hypotheses that are currently being tested with much refined experimental tools to examine the interactions within this network. Lagging far behind, however, is the examination of sex differences in this network and how sex hormones influence the functional activity and reactivity of these brain regions in the context of fear inhibition. Indeed, there is a large body of literature suggesting that sex hormones, such as estrogen, do modulate neural plasticity within the fear extinction network, especially in the hippocampus.

After a brief overview of the fear extinction network, we summarize what is currently known about sex differences in fear extinction and the influence of gonadal hormones on the fear extinction network. We then go on to propose possible mechanisms by which sex hormones, such as estrogen, may influence neural plasticity within the fear extinction network. We end with a discussion of how knowledge to be gained from developing this line of research may have significant ramifications towards the etiology, epidemiology and treatment of anxiety disorders.

Keywords: menstrual cycle, sex hormones, estrogen, progesterone, estrus cycle, fear extinction

Background

There are now substantial data indicating that structural, cellular and molecular differences exist between the male and female brains in regions that are important for cognition, memory and affect, such as the hippocampus, amygdala and prefrontal cortex. Some of these differences may have clinical relevance, as marked disparities in disease incidence, manifestation, prognosis and treatment have been observed between the sexes. For example, men have a higher prevalence of conditions that emerge early in development, such as autism, attention deficit hyperactivity disorder and schizophrenia. Women, on the other hand, have a higher prevalence of disorders that emerge in adolescence or adulthood, such as major depression and anxiety disorders. Surprisingly, very little is known about the neural mechanisms that underlie the expression of sex differences in psychiatric disorders. A 2001 report by the Institute of Medicine highlighted the need to conduct scientific studies at the cellular, molecular and whole organism level that take into account sex as a variable to investigate the neural mechanisms that lead to epidemiological differences in psychiatric disorders.

The need to examine sex differences in the network mediating fear learning and its extinction can be surmised from two different perspectives. From a clinical perspective, we need to understand what contributes to the significant epidemiological differences in psychiatric disorders that are characterized by exaggerated fear and anxiety, such as post traumatic stress disorder. From a basic neuroscience perspective, it is essential that we understand how male and female brains differ in processing fundamental neurobiological phenomena such as emotional learning and memory. There is now a clear indication that failure in the function of brain regions that mediate fear learning and fear inhibition may be associated with the psychopathology of anxiety disorders

* Correspondence: milad@nmr.mgh.harvard.edu
Department of Psychiatry, Harvard Medical School & Massachusetts General Hospital, Boston, MA, USA

[1-5]. Sexual dimorphism in the amygdala, hippocampus and medial prefrontal cortices is well documented [6,7]. These brain regions also contain elevated levels of estrogen receptors [8-10]. Thus, the structural and functional differences in these brain regions between the sexes may explain in part, or contribute to, some of the basic and clinical differences observed between men and women. In examining the literature pertinent to learning and memory, fear conditioning, and fear extinction, it is astonishing to note that of all that we have learned about these processes, less than 2% of this research has been focused on the female brain (Figure 1).

The fear extinction network: a brief overview

Review of the fear extinction literature in general is beyond the scope of this article. We direct the reader to some recent reviews on fear extinction that focused on the translational aspects of this line of research [11], the general clinical relevance [12-16] and the molecular machinery of fear extinction [17]. Our review of fear extinction will be brief with the objective of setting the stage for the points we intend to make regarding sex differences in, and estrogen's influence on, the fear extinction network.

Components of the fear extinction network

Early studies of conditioned fear extinction showed that blockade of N-Methyl-D-aspartic acid (NMDA) receptors within the amygdala impair the extinction of fear potentiated startle [18]. A number of studies subsequently showed that lesion or pharmacological manipulations of the basolateral amygdala (BLA) and the intercalated GABAergic neurons within the amygdala interfere with fear extinction learning [19-21]. Electrophysiological data recorded from the BLA during fear extinction indicate the existence of two neural populations: one signals fear and the other signals fear inhibition or extinction [22]. Thus, in addition to its role in fear acquisition [23], the amygdala appears to also play a critical role in fear extinction [24,25].

In addition to the amygdala, the infralimbic (IL) region of the rat ventromedial prefrontal cortex (vmPFC) appears critical for the consolidation and retrieval of the extinction memory after a delay. Lesions [26-28], pharmacological manipulations [24,29,30] and electrophysiological recording [31] studies implicate the IL in extinction memory consolidation and expression. Moreover, electrical stimulation of IL simulates extinction memory [32,33]. Subsequent studies have further supported these findings using different experimental tools, including measuring intrinsic excitability of IL neurons [30,34,35], using metabolic mapping [36], potentiation of thalamic inputs to IL [37], and manipulations of hippocampal inputs to IL [38,39].

Another key structure that plays a role in fear extinction is the hippocampus. While its specific role in fear extinction is currently being investigated, it is likely that the hippocampus learns about the context in which fear learning took place and learns about the context in which extinction learning takes place [40,41]. During extinction recall, the hippocampus can, depending on the context, allow the expression of either the fear memory via activation of the amygdala fear neurons, or safety memory via activation of IL neurons [42]. A number of studies have now shown that the interaction between the hippocampus and IL during fear extinction is key to the success of extinction memory consolidation and expression [41,43-45].

Neuroimaging studies have translated these findings to the human brain using comparable fear conditioning paradigms, some of which use contextual manipulations of fear conditioning and extinction [46-49]. Imaging studies began by implicating the human amygdala in fear

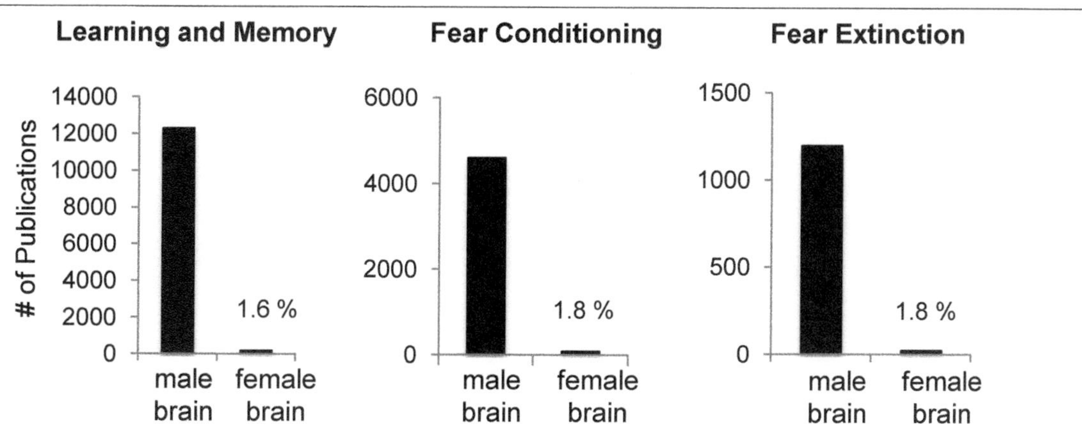

Figure 1 Research studies using males vs females.

conditioning and also during extinction learning [46,50,51]. Recent functional magnetic resonance imaging studies (fMRI) designed specific paradigms to examine extinction recall and found that, like the rat IL, the human vmPFC increased activation to the extinguished cue during extinction recall; the level of activation positively correlates with the extinction recall magnitude [46,47,51]. Thickness of the vmPFC is also correlated with magnitude of extinction recall [52,53]. Like the amygdala and vmPFC, activation of the hippocampus during fear extinction is reported in a number of imaging studies during contextual conditioning [48] and extinction memory recall [47,51]. Deactivation of the hippocampus at the time of the delivery of the unconditioned stimulus (US) has also been reported in humans [54].

The molecular machinery mediating learning not to fear

There now exists a large database regarding the molecular machinery involved in fear extinction within the amygdala, hippocampus and IL in rodents. In BLA, interfering with mitogen activated protein kinase (MAPK), phosphoinositide 3-kinase (PI3-K), immediate early genes cfos and early growth response protein 1 (EGR-1) prevented consolidation of extinction [17,24,41]. Protein synthesis in BLA is also necessary for fear extinction [55]. Extinction training leads to structural changes in BLA. For example, mRNA for the brain-derived neurotrophic factor (BDNF) is up-regulated [56]. Furthermore, rats with lentiviral-induced reduction in BDNF receptors in the BLA can extinguish normally within a session, but were unable to recall extinction the following day, consistent with a role of BLA in consolidation of extinction [56]. In IL, extinction memory requires NMDA receptor activation [57,58], protein kinase A [17], MAPK [59], cannabinoid receptors [60], and protein synthesis [17,29]. In the hippocampus, extinction of context conditioning requires protein synthesis [61] cyclic adenosine monophosphate (c-AMP) [62], BDNF [43] and a number of protein kinases and their regulators [63].

Sex differences during conditioning and its extinction

A number of studies have investigated differences between females and males in learning and memory using a number of behavioral tasks. For example, females acquire eye-blink conditioning at a faster rate relative to males [64]. In inhibitory avoidance tasks, females outperform males in escaping during a one-way avoidance task and a two-way avoidance task [65]. Studies conducted to examine sex differences in the acquisition of cued and contextual fear conditioning showed that male rodents exhibit increased contextual and cued fear conditioning relative to females [66-70], whereas other studies failed to show sex differences in these learning tasks [71].

Relative to fear acquisition, few studies have investigated potential sex differences during extinction learning and recall [72,73]. We showed that sex differences in fear extinction are influenced by the phase of the estrous cycle in female rats and the menstrual cycle in women [74-76]. When not taking cycle phase into consideration, differences in fear extinction recall were not noted in either female rats or in naturally cycling women. When females were divided into low and high endogenous estradiol groups, however, sex differences emerged. During extinction recall, male rats showed comparable levels of extinction retention to female rats with high estradiol; both were significantly higher than females with low estradiol [75]. The same pattern of results was observed in women. That is, men's extinction retention was comparable to that of women with high estradiol; and both groups showed significantly higher levels of extinction retention compared to women with low estradiol [76]. Thus, the lack of sex differences reported in previous studies or the discrepant results between studies may be the result of not taking into consideration the cycle phase of the animals being tested. These data also raise the following question: could sex hormones influence the learning, consolidation and plasticity typically associated with fear extinction in the female brain?

Sex hormones influencing fear extinction in the female rat and in women

The data reviewed above indicate that sex hormones in rodents and humans may contribute to differences in fear learning and fear extinction. In support of this, estrogen treatment in ovariectomized female rats enhanced the acquisition of fear conditioning [70,77] and fear potentiated startle [78]; though elevated estrogen levels have been associated with reduced contextual conditioning in another study [67]. A few studies have shown that estrogen facilitated the extinction of passive avoidance [79] and conditioned taste aversion [80]. To date, there are few published studies that specifically examined the role of sex hormones on fear extinction learning and its subsequent recall. One exception is Chang *et al.*, (2009), who have recently shown that infusion of estrogen into the hippocampus facilitates extinction of context conditioning and enhances hippocampal long term potentiation (LTP) [81].

We have recently conducted a number of experiments examining how endogenous fluctuations and exogenous manipulations of sex hormones, particularly estrogen and progesterone, influence fear extinction in female rats. A diagram of the natural fluctuations of sex hormones during the estrous cycle in rats and the menstrual cycle in women is shown in Figure 2. We observed that naturally cycling females exhibited the least amount of freezing during extinction recall when they underwent extinction learning during the proestrus phase (high estrogen and progesterone) of the estrous cycle [75]. These findings suggest that estrogen and/or progesterone may facilitate the consolidation of extinction learning (Figure 3B). In support of this, systemic pre- or post-extinction administration of estradiol into female rats undergoing extinction learning in the metestrus phase (low estrogen and progesterone) significantly reduced freezing during recall (Figure 4a, b) [75]. Systemic blockade of estrogen receptors alpha (ERα) and estrogen receptor beta (ERβ) in female rats undergoing extinction in the proestrus phase significantly increased freezing [75]. In a later study, we observed that administration of ERβ but not ERα agonists were able to facilitate extinction recall in female rats undergoing extinction training in the metestrus phase of the cycle [74]. These data provide strong evidence that cycling sex hormones, estradiol in particular, in female rats do indeed influence extinction consolidation, possibly via the selective activation of the ERβ receptors.

In women, neuroimaging studies have shown that measures of fear and arousal are associated with changes in hormonal levels throughout the menstrual cycle [67,82,83]. Interestingly, increased vmPFC activation was observed in women in the luteal phase relative to those in the early follicular phase of the menstrual cycle while performing a Go-No-Go Task [84], suggesting that estrogen may facilitate the functional activation of the vmPFC. We have conducted an initial psychophysiological study to assess the influence of the menstrual cycle phase on recall of fear extinction in healthy women, and found that natural fluctuations of gonadal hormones do modulate extinction recall [85]. Women with high estrogen exhibited significantly enhanced extinction recall (that is, less fear) relative to women with low estrogen levels [76] (Figure 3A). In a more recent study, we replicated the effect of facilitated extinction recall in women with high estrogen and found that the increased estrogen levels in these women is associated with increased vmPFC, hippocampal and amygdala activation during extinction recall (Figure 5), further supporting the idea that estrogen may be playing a critical role in extinction memory consolidation [74].

How might estrogen modulate extinction recall?

Estrogen and its receptors

In females, estrogen is primarily produced by the ovaries, while in males testosterone is produce by the testis and then aromatized into estrogen [86]. Estrogen can also be synthesized in brain regions, such as the hippocampus [87]. The most potent circulating estrogen is 17β-estradiol and the most characterized ERs are ERα and ERβ [88]. These receptors belong to the nuclear receptor superfamily and can be localized in the nucleus as well as in the cytoplasm of the cell [88]. ERα and ERβ are coded by different genes but share similar DNA-binding and ligand-binding domains. Estrogen binds to either ERα or ERβ through its estrogen response element DNA binding site. These result in receptor dimerization and subsequence gene transcription [89].

Localization of the estrogen receptors

Both receptors are located throughout the rostral-caudal extent of the brain and spinal cord, including regions of

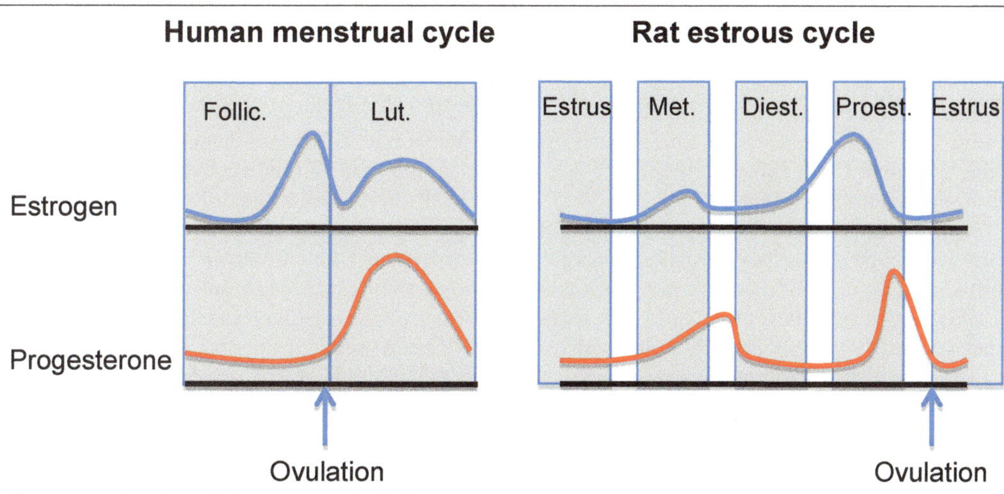

Figure 2 The menstrual cycle and the estrous cycle [164].

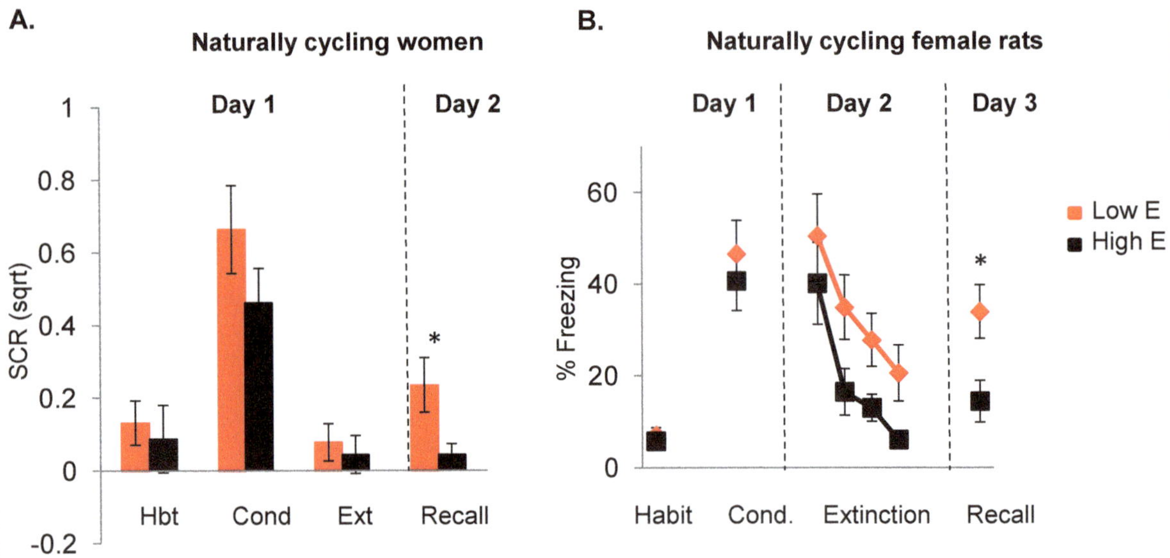

Figure 3 Effects of endogenous estrogen on extinction recall.

the fear circuitry [90,91]. Previous studies have shown that expression of ERα and ERβ overlap in many brain regions, such as the bed nucleus of the stria terminalis, medial and cortical amygdaloid nuclei, periaqueductal grey and locus coeruleus [91]. However, differences in expression have also been shown where one type of receptor is either expressed alone or at higher concentrations relative to the other. For example, ERα is the predominant receptor expressed in the ventromedial nucleus of the hypothalamus while ERβ is most prevalent in the hippocampus [92]. ERα and ERβ are expressed in the amygdala while ERβ is mostly expressed in PFC [93-95]. Activation of these two types of receptors leads to different behavioral consequences. Accumulating evidence now indicates that selective ERβ agonists typically exert potent anxiolytic activity when animals were tested in a number of behavioral paradigms [91,96,97]. In contrast, selective ERα agonists were found to be anxiogenic and correspondingly increased the hormonal stress response [91].

Sex differences in the estrogen receptors

ERα and ERβ have similar distributions in male and female brains, although subcellular distributions of ER to the nucleus, cytoplasm, dendrites and nerve terminals have been reported to be different in male and female human hypothalamus [98]. Although the functional consequences of these differences remain to be determined, this could indicate differential effects of estrogen in the male versus female brains regarding cellular processes, such as neurite extension, synaptic plasticity and mitochondrial energy regulation via mitochondrial ERs. There is also evidence for sex differences in intracellular signaling, expression of co-regulatory proteins, and in the response of the brain ER/aromatase system to injury [88].

Estrogen-induced molecular and cellular changes

The influence of estrogen on molecular and cellular changes in the brain has been examined mostly in the hippocampus [99,100] and in the hypothalamus [88]. Hippocampal estrogen enhances synaptogenesis and long-term potentiation (LTP) [101], increases the formation of dendritic spines [102,103], increases cell proliferation [104], and increases neural excitability [105,106]. Estrogen-induced LTP in the hippocampus is mediated via synaptic transmission of NMDA receptors [107], specifically through the increased expression of the NR2B subunit [108].

Increased estrogen is also associated with increased BDNF expression in the hippocampus [109,110]. It is possible that estrogen-enhanced extinction memory consolidation may be mediated via increasing BDNF expression in the hippocampus or the vmPFC. Indeed, BDNF expression is critical for successful fear extinction in both rodents and humans [111]. Peters *et al.* (2010) showed that hippocampal infusion of BDNF before extinction training enhanced extinction memory in an NMDAr dependent process, suggesting that hippocampal BDNF modulates IL activity during the consolidation of extinction memory [112]. Estrogen and BDNF are known to have similar mechanisms of actions, activate the same cascades, and have the same behavioral effects, especially within the hippocampus. For example, both

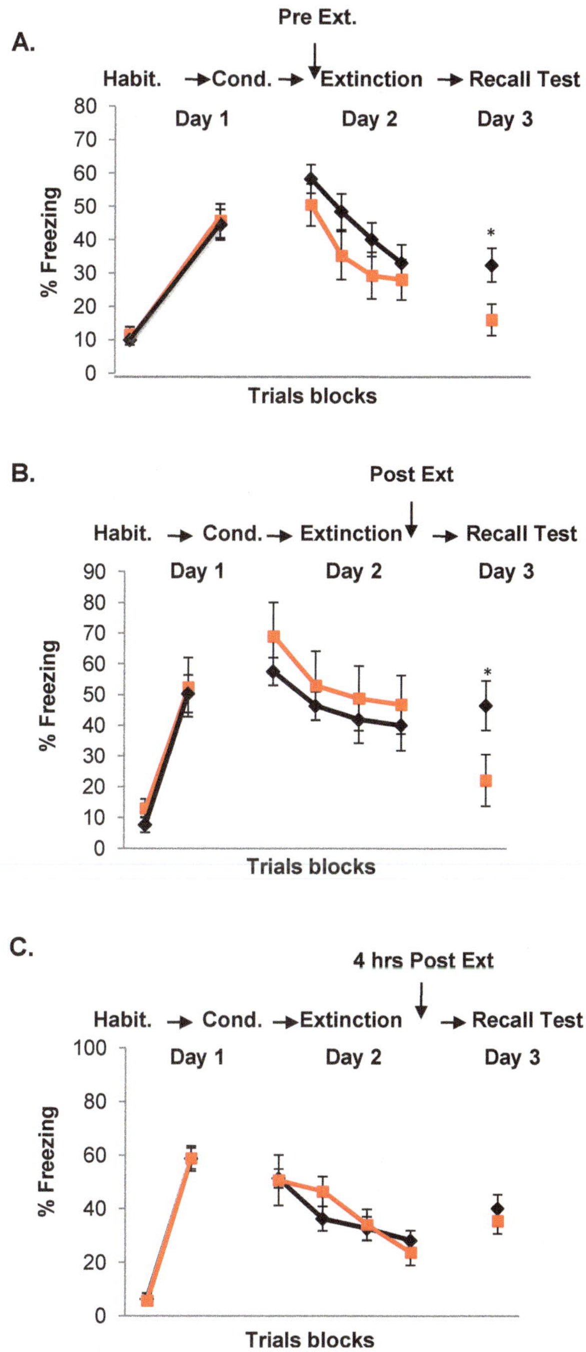

Figure 4 Effects of exogenous estrogen on extinction recall.

estrogen and BDNF enhance hippocampal-dependent learning [109,110]. The direct interaction between estrogen and BDNF during fear extinction has not yet been investigated.

Few studies have examined the influence of estrogen on the function of the vmPFC in the rat. Estrogen has been shown to increase spine density in vmPFC [113], preserve the functional integrity of the IL when

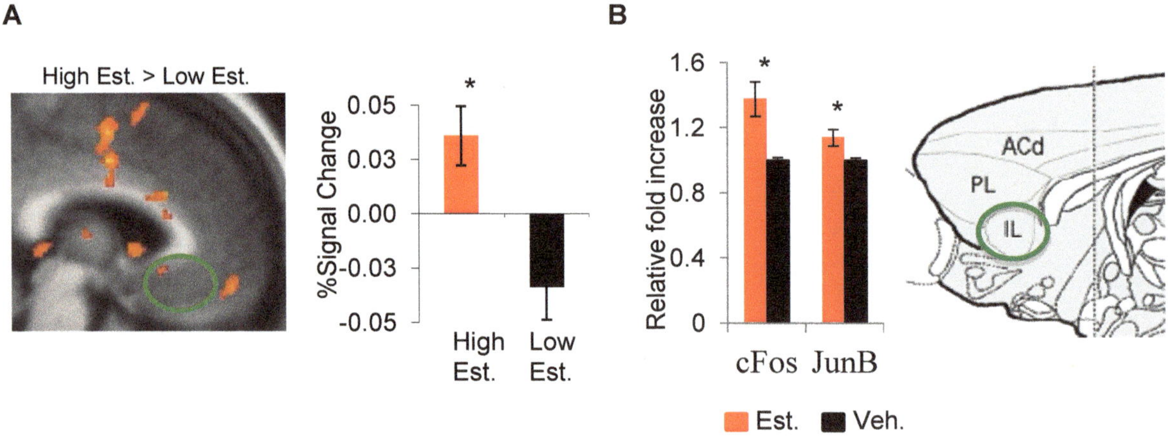

Figure 5 Effects of estrogen in vmPFC activation and gene expression during extinction recall.

subjecting the rats to chronic stress [114], and to enhance working memory [115]. These data indicate that estrogen influences the function of the vmPFC in the rat brain. Markers of neural activity and synaptic plasticity, such as c-Fos, Jun-b and BDNF, have been shown to be modulated by estrogen variance [74,116-118]. Therefore, we propose that estrogen may modulate fear extinction learning and consolidation via its interaction with a number of molecular markers of plasticity, within the fear extinction network.

We recently examined the influence of estradiol administration on c-fos and Jun-b mRNA expression within some components of the fear extinction network. Female rats undergoing fear extinction during the metestrus phase of the cycle (low estrogen) received estradiol immediately post-extinction training and were sacrificed immediately after a brief extinction recall test. The results of this study showed that administration of estradiol after extinction training enhanced c-fos and June-b mRNA expression in IL (Figure 5b) and significantly reduced the expression of both in the amygdala during recall [74]. These data further support the idea that estrogen fluctuations may be a critical modulator of extinction memory consolidation in females. In order to fully understand the role of estrogen in fear extinction, it is necessary to identify the molecular cascades by which estrogen may enhance extinction memory and investigate sex differences in estrogen action within the extinction network.

What about progesterone and testosterone?

Progesterone

Several studies have shown that progesterone administration to ovariectomized female rats facilitates contextual and cued fear conditioning, and enhances cognitive performance in a variety of other behavioral tasks in mice [119]. In healthy young women, administration of progesterone during the early follicular phase (when progesterone and estrogen are at their lowest level) led to increased reactivity in the amygdala while looking at threatening faces [120]. Also, progesterone increased the functional coupling of the amygdala with the mPFC [121], indicating that progesterone influences interactions between the amygdala-PFC circuits. Moreover, progesterone is metabolized into allopregnanolone [122], which acts via $GABA_A$ receptors and appears to have anxiolytic effects when infused into the amygdala or vmPFC before an elevated plus-maze test and shock-probe burying test [122,123]. In other tasks, progesterone facilitates extinction of cocaine self-administration [124]. We have shown that systemic administration of progesterone into female rats (either alone or in conjunction with estrogen) facilitates extinction consolidation [75], suggesting that progesterone appears to also influence the function of brain regions involved in extinction consolidation. Our data gathered in women, however, showed that variance in progesterone levels in two separate cohorts of women did not correlate with extinction recall [74,76]. While progesterone's influence on fear extinction may differ across species, it is important to note that we were not able to fully examine the effects of progesterone independent of estrogen. Thus, it remains possible that progesterone may have an effect on fear extinction consolidation in women directly or perhaps by interacting with estrogen. Additional studies are needed to further examine the role of progesterone in fear extinction in women.

Testosterone

It is established that besides the masculinization/defeminizing role of testosterone during sexual differentiation, this hormone is also critical for the modulation of behavioral and physiological responses to anger [125,126]. Men demonstrating higher dominance express high levels of testosterone. In male primates, dominance is associated with higher testosterone levels and a decrease in stress response, indicating that dominant males find dominance signals less stressful and are more primed to engage in a dominance challenge [127,128]. More interestingly, previous studies have shown that testosterone reduces cortisol response and stress axis reactivity [129,130]. Other studies demonstrated that endogenous as well as exogenous testosterone influence neural reactivity to threatening faces in the amygdala and orbitofrontal cortex (OFC) in males, and in the amygdala in women [128,131]. Exogenous testosterone also increases amygdala reactivity to threatening faces, but reduces functional coupling between the amygdala and OFC in middle-aged women, suggesting that the testosterone may regulate interactions between amygdala and OFC [128]. It is important to note that effects of testosterone may be mediated via direct interactions with androgen receptors or via conversion to other steroids. Testosterone is metabolized to dihydrotestosterone (DHT), which also acts via androgen receptors, and to androstanediol that modulates $GABA_A$ receptor similar to allopregnanolone [132]. Lastly, testosterone is also aromatized into 17b-estradiol, the most potent type of estradiol, and it has been suggested that most of the effects of testosterone are mediated by estrogen [133,134]. Clinical and basic studies are needed to assess the role of testosterone during fear extinction.

Clinical relevance

Increased expression of inappropriate fear is the hallmark of anxiety disorders [135-138]. A large body of evidence from neuroimaging studies indicates that the neural circuits subserving fear conditioning and extinction are impaired across the different anxiety disorders [12]. For example, post-traumatic stress disorder (PTSD) patients exhibit decreased vmPFC and hippocampal activation along with exaggerated amygdala activation during the processing of emotional stimuli in a wide array of paradigms [139-142]. Experimental extinction is also deficient in PTSD patients [10,143-146]. We have recently shown that fear extinction is deficient in PTSD patients and that such deficiency is associated with aberrant activation of the vmPFC, hippocampus and amygdala (in addition to insula and striatal regions) during fear acquisition, extinction learning and extinction recall [1,5,54,74].

Epidemiological data suggest that the prevalence of anxiety disorders is higher in women relative to men. Women are more likely to develop panic disorder (8% vs. 3%), PTSD (12.5% vs. 6%) and generalized anxiety disorder (GAD) (7% vs. 4%) (Pigott, 2003; Breslau *et al.*, 1998;Kinrys and Wygant, 2005). Aside from prevalence, women diagnosed with PTSD have longer symptom duration (48 vs. 12 months) [147], have higher symptom severity and functional impairment [148], and have worse quality of life [149]. Women diagnosed with GAD are more likely to develop comorbid psychiatric disorders and have worse prognoses and impairments [150]. In addition to increased prevalence of panic disorder in women, studies also suggest that panic attacks occur more frequently in women relative to men [151]. These findings point to brain-based differences in the processing of emotional stimuli in women compared to men, and suggest that sex hormones, such as estrogen, play a key role in mediating these differences. Indeed, there are some clinical data suggesting that estrogen therapy improves anxiety symptoms in postnatal depression [152], in recurrent postpartum affective disorder [153], and in menopause [154,155]. Despite these glaring differences, it is puzzling that so few studies have considered sex differences as a critical variable of interest.

Conclusions

The data reviewed herein point to clear sex differences in, and clear influence of, sex hormones, especially estrogen, on fear extinction. The data discussed show that sex hormones may have direct effects on the molecular machinery mediating synaptic plasticity in the hippocampus, and the vmPFC during fear extinction. These data also point to significant clinical implications. Future studies need to develop paradigms to test specific hypotheses based on what we know thus far. For example, does estrogen serve a protective function against elevated fear and anxiety? Could transient periods of low estradiol levels be associated with impaired retention of safety memory? In addition, fear extinction in women using oral contraceptives and in menopausal women with and without hormone replacement therapy should be examined. This is especially important given that the use of oral and intrauterine contraceptives is known to reduce endogenous cycling estradiol levels [156]. Moreover, women appear to be vulnerable to developing mood and anxiety disorders during postpartum [157,158] and menopausal periods [159-163] when endogenous estradiol levels are low. Additional studies investigating the effects of cycling sex hormones and exogenous manipulations of these hormones in animal models of fear inhibition could potentially introduce ways to adapt, improve or produce therapies specifically tailored to women.

Abbreviations

BDNF: brain-derived neurotrophic factor; BLA: basolateral amygdala; cAMP: cyclic adenosine monophosphate; DHT: dihydrotestoterone; EGR-1: early growth response protein 1; ERα: estrogen receptors alpha; ERβ: estrogen receptor beta; fMRI: functional magnetic resonance neuroimaging; GAD: generalize anxiety disorders; IL: infralimbic; ITC: intercalated GABAergic neurons; LTP: long-term potentiation; MAP kinase: mitogen activated protein; NMDAr: N-Methyl-D-aspartic acid receptor; OFC: orbitofrontal cortex; PI 3-kinase: phosphoinositide 3-kinase; PTSD: posttraumatic stress disorders; US: unconditioned stimulus; vmPFC: ventromedial prefrontal cortex

Acknowledgements
We would like to thank Bronwyn Graham, PhD and Alina Tsareva, BS for helpful comments on this manuscript. MRM is supported by NIH grants K01-MH08036 and R01-MH081975 (MGH subcontract), and Department of Defense grant W81XWH-11-2-0079.

Endnotes
There are no endnotes for this manuscript.

Authors' contributions
KLM and MRM contributed equally to this manuscript. Both authors read and approved the final manuscript.

Authors' information
N/A

Competing interests
The authors declare that they have no competing interests.

References

1. Milad MR, Pitman RK, Ellis CB, Gold AB, Shin LM, Lasko NB, Handwerger K, Orr SP, Rauch SL: **Neurobiological basis for failure to recall extinction memory in Posttraumatic Stress Disorder.** *Biol Psychiatry* 2009, **66**:1075-1082.
2. Milad MR, Rauch SL: **The role of the orbitofrontal cortex in anxiety disorders.** *Ann NY Acad Sci* 2007, **1121**:546-561.
3. Milad MR, Quirk GJ, Pitman RK, Orr SP, Fischl B, Rauch SL: **A role for the human dorsal anterior cingulate cortex in fear expression.** *Biol Psychiatry* 2007, **62**:1191-1194.
4. Shin LM, Liberzon I: **The neurocircuitry of fear, stress, and anxiety disorders.** *Neuropsychopharmacology* 2010, **35**:169-191.
5. Rougemont-Bucking A, Linnman C, Zeffiro TA, Zeidan MA, Lebron-Milad K, Rodriguez-Romaguera J, Rauch SL, Pitman RK, Milad MR: **Altered processing of contextual information during fear extinction in PTSD: an fMRI study.** *CNS Neurosci Ther* 2011, **17**:227-236.
6. Goldstein JM, Kennedy DN, Caviness VS Jr: **Images in neuroscience. Brain development, XI: sexual dimorphism.** *Am J Psychiatry* 1999, **156**:352.
7. Goldstein JM, Seidman LJ, Horton NJ, Makris N, Kennedy DN, Caviness VS, Faraone SV, Tsuang MT: **Normal sexual dimorphism of the adult human brain assessed by *in vivo* magnetic resonance imaging.** *Cereb Cortex* 2001, **11**:490-497.
8. Montague D, Weickert CS, Tomaskovic-Crook E, Rothmond DA, Kleinman JE, Rubinow DR: **Oestrogen receptor alpha localisation in the prefrontal cortex of three mammalian species.** *J Neuroendocrinol* 2008, **20**:893-903.
9. Spencer JL, Waters EM, Romeo RD, Wood GE, Milner TA, McEwen BS: **Uncovering the mechanisms of estrogen effects on hippocampal function.** *Front Neuroendocrinol* 2008, **29**:219-237.
10. Walf AA, Frye CA: **A review and update of mechanisms of estrogen in the hippocampus and amygdala for anxiety and depression behavior.** *Neuropsychopharmacology* 2006, **31**:1097-1111.
11. Herry C, Ferraguti F, Singewald N, Letzkus JJ, Ehrlich I, Luthi A: **Neuronal circuits of fear extinction.** *Eur J Neurosci* 2010, **31**:599-612.
12. Graham BM, Milad MR: **The study of fear extinction: implications for anxiety disorders.** *Am J Psychiatry* 2011, **168**:1255-1265.
13. Choi DC, Rothbaum BO, Gerardi M, Ressler KJ: **Pharmacological enhancement of behavioral therapy: focus on posttraumatic stress disorder.** *Curr Top Behav Neurosci* 2010, **2**:279-299.
14. Davis M, Myers KM, Chhatwal J, Ressler KJ: **Pharmacological treatments that facilitate extinction of fear: relevance to psychotherapy.** *NeuroRx* 2006, **3**:82-96.
15. Milad MR, Rauch SL, Pitman RK, Quirk GJ: **Fear extinction in rats: implications for human brain imaging and anxiety disorders.** *Biol Psychol* 2006, **73**:61-71.
16. Rauch SL, Shin LM, Phelps EA: **Neurocircuitry models of posttraumatic stress disorder and extinction: human neuroimaging research–past, present, and future.** *Biol Psychiatry* 2006, **60**:376-382.
17. Quirk GJ, Mueller D: **Neural mechanisms of extinction learning and retrieval.** *Neuropsychopharmacology* 2008, **33**:56-72.
18. Falls WA, Miserendino MJ, Davis M: **Extinction of fear-potentiated startle: blockade by infusion of an NMDA antagonist into the amygdala.** *J Neurosci* 1992, **12**:854-863.
19. Amano T, Unal CT, Pare D: **Synaptic correlates of fear extinction in the amygdala.** *Nat Neurosci* 2010, **13**:489-494.
20. Likhtik E, Popa D, Apergis-Schoute J, Fidacaro GA, Pare D: **Amygdala intercalated neurons are required for expression of fear extinction.** *Nature* 2008, **454**:642-645.
21. Amir A, Amano T, Pare D: **Physiological identification and infralimbic responsiveness of rat intercalated amygdala neurons.** *J Neurophysiol* 2011, **105**:3054-3066.
22. Herry C, Ciocchi S, Senn V, Demmou L, Muller C, Luthi A: **Switching on and off fear by distinct neuronal circuits.** *Nature* 2008, **454**:600-606.
23. Ledoux JE: **Emotion circuits in the brain.** *Annu Rev Neurosci* 2000, **23**:155-184.
24. Myers KM, Davis M: **Mechanisms of fear extinction.** *Mol Psychiatry* 2007, **12**:120-150.
25. Sotres-Bayon F, Quirk GJ: **Prefrontal control of fear: more than just extinction.** *Curr Opin Neurobiol* 2010, **20**:231-235.
26. Lebron K, Milad MR, Quirk GJ: **Delayed recall of fear extinction in rats with lesions of ventral medial prefrontal cortex.** *Learn Mem* 2004, **11**:544-548.
27. Sierra-Mercado D, Padilla-Coreano N, Quirk GJ: **Dissociable roles of prelimbic and infralimbic cortices, ventral hippocampus, and basolateral amygdala in the expression and extinction of conditioned fear.** *Neuropsychopharmacology* 2011, **36**:529-538.
28. Quirk GJ, Russo GK, Barron JL, Lebron K: **The role of ventromedial prefrontal cortex in the recovery of extinguished fear.** *J Neurosci* 2000, **20**:6225-6231.
29. Santini E, Ge H, Ren K, Peña de Ortiz S, Quirk GJ: **Consolidation of fear extinction requires protein synthesis in the medial prefrontal cortex.** *J Neurosci* 2004, **24**:5704-5710.
30. Fontanez-Nuin DE, Santini E, Quirk GJ, Porter JT: **Memory for fear extinction requires mGluR5-mediated activation of infralimbic neurons.** *Cereb Cortex* 2011, **21**:727-735.
31. Milad MR, Quirk GJ: **Neurons in medial prefrontal cortex signal memory for fear extinction.** *Nature* 2002, **420**:70-74.
32. Milad MR, Vidal-Gonzalez I, Quirk GJ: **Electrical stimulation of medial prefrontal cortex reduces conditioned fear in a temporally specific manner.** *Behav Neurosci* 2004, **118**:389-394.
33. Vidal-Gonzalez I, Vidal-Gonzalez B, Rauch SL, Quirk GJ: **Microstimulation reveals opposing influences of prelimbic and infralimbic cortex on the expression of conditioned fear.** *Learn Mem* 2006, **13**:728-733.
34. Santini E, Porter JT: **M-type potassium channels modulate the intrinsic excitability of infralimbic neurons and regulate fear expression and extinction.** *J Neurosci* 2010, **30**:12379-12386.
35. Santini E, Quirk GJ, Porter JT: **Fear conditioning and extinction differentially modify the intrinsic excitability of infralimbic neurons.** *J Neurosci* 2008, **28**:4028-4036.
36. Barrett D, Shumake J, Jones D, Gonzalez-Lima F: **Metabolic mapping of mouse brain activity after extinction of a conditioned emotional response.** *J Neurosci* 2003, **23**:5740-5749.
37. Herry C, Garcia R: **Behavioral and paired-pulse facilitation analyses of long-lasting depression at excitatory synapses in the medial prefrontal cortex in mice.** *Behav Brain Res* 2003, **146**:89-96.
38. Deschaux O, Motanis H, Spennato G, Moreau JL, Garcia R: **Re-emergence of extinguished auditory-cued conditioned fear following a sub-conditioning procedure: effects of hippocampal and prefrontal tetanic stimulations.** *Neurobiol Learn Mem* 2011, **95**:510-518.
39. Deschaux O, Thevenet A, Spennato G, Arnaud C, Moreau JL, Garcia R: **Low-frequency stimulation of the hippocampus following fear extinction impairs both restoration of rapid eye movement sleep and retrieval of extinction memory.** *Neuroscience* 2010, **170**:92-98.

40. Bouton ME, Westbrook RF, Corcoran KA, Maren S: **Contextual and temporal modulation of extinction: behavioral and biological mechanisms.** *Biol Psychiatry* 2006, **60**:352-360.
41. Corcoran KA, Quirk GJ: **Recalling safety: cooperative functions of the ventromedial prefrontal cortex and the hippocampus in extinction.** *CNS Spectr* 2007, **12**:200-206.
42. Corcoran KA, Maren S: **Factors regulating the effects of hippocampal inactivation on renewal of conditional fear after extinction.** *Learn Mem* 2004, **11**:598-603.
43. Peters J, Dieppa-Perea LM, Melendez LM, Quirk GJ: **Induction of fear extinction with hippocampal-infralimbic BDNF.** *Science* 2010, **328**:1288-1290.
44. Corcoran KA, Quirk GJ: **Recalling safety: cooperative functions of the ventromedial prefrontal cortex and the hippocampus in extinction.** *CNS Spectr* 2007, **12**:200-206.
45. Garcia R, Spennato G, Nilsson-Todd L, Moreau JL, Deschaux O: **Hippocampal low-frequency stimulation and chronic mild stress similarly disrupt fear extinction memory in rats.** *Neurobiol Learn Mem* 2008, **89**:560-566.
46. Phelps EA, Delgado MR, Nearing KI, Ledoux JE: **Extinction learning in humans: role of the amygdala and vmPFC.** *Neuron* 2004, **43**:897-905.
47. Kalisch R, Korenfeld E, Stephan KE, Weiskopf N, Seymour B, Dolan RJ: **Context-dependent human extinction memory is mediated by a ventromedial prefrontal and hippocampal network.** *J Neurosci* 2006, **26**:9503-9511.
48. Alvarez RP, Biggs A, Chen G, Pine DS, Grillon C: **Contextual fear conditioning in humans: cortical-hippocampal and amygdala contributions.** *J Neurosci* 2008, **28**:6211-6219.
49. Baas JM, Nugent M, Lissek S, Pine DS, Grillon C: **Fear conditioning in virtual reality contexts: a new tool for the study of anxiety.** *Biol Psychiatry* 2004, **55**:1056-1060.
50. LaBar KS, Gatenby JC, Gore JC, Ledoux JE, Phelps EA: **Human amygdala activation during conditioned fear acquisition and extinction: a mixed-trial fMRI study.** *Neuron* 1998, **20**:937-945.
51. Milad MR, Wright CI, Orr SP, Pitman RK, Quirk GJ, Rauch SL: **Recall of fear extinction in humans activates the ventromedial prefrontal cortex and hippocampus in concert.** *Biol Psychiatry* 2007, **62**:446-454.
52. Milad MR, Quinn BT, Pitman RK, Orr SP, Fischl B, Rauch SL: **Thickness of ventromedial prefrontal cortex in humans is correlated with extinction memory.** *Proc Natl Acad Sci USA* 2005, **102**:10706-10711.
53. Hartley CA, Fischl B, Phelps EA: **Brain structure correlates of individual differences in the acquisition and inhibition of conditioned fear.** *Cereb Cortex* 2011, **21**:1954-1962.
54. Linnman C, Rougemont-Bucking A, Beucke JC, Zeffiro TA, Milad MR: **Unconditioned responses and functional fear networks in human classical conditioning.** *Behav Brain Res* 2011, **221**:237-245.
55. Kim J, Park S, Lee S, Choi S: **Amygdala depotentiation *ex vivo* requires mitogen-activated protein kinases and protein synthesis.** *Neuroreport* 2009, **20**:517-520.
56. Chhatwal JP, Stanek-Rattiner L, Davis M, Ressler KJ: **Amygdala BDNF signaling is required for consolidation but not encoding of extinction.** *Nat Neurosci* 2006, **9**:870-872.
57. Burgos-Robles A, Vidal-Gonzalez I, Santini E, Quirk GJ: **Consolidation of fear extinction requires NMDA receptor-dependent bursting in the ventromedial prefrontal cortex.** *Neuron* 2007, **53**:871-880.
58. Sotres-Bayon F, Diaz-Mataix L, Bush DE, LeDoux JE: **Dissociable roles for the ventromedial prefrontal cortex and amygdala in fear extinction: NR2B contribution.** *Cereb Cortex* 2009, **19**:474-482.
59. Hugues S, Deschaux O, Garcia R: **Postextinction infusion of a mitogen-activated protein kinase inhibitor into the medial prefrontal cortex impairs memory of the extinction of conditioned fear.** *Learn Mem* 2004, **11**:540-543.
60. Lin HC, Mao SC, Su CL, Gean PW: **The role of prefrontal cortex CB1 receptors in the modulation of fear memory.** *Cereb Cortex* 2009, **19**:165-175.
61. Li L, Boddul SV, Patil SS, Zheng JF, An G, Hoger H, Lubec G: **Proteins linked to extinction in contextual fear conditioning in the C57BL/6J mouse.** *Proteomics* 2011, **11**:3706-3724.
62. Wang Z, Phan T, Storm DR: **The type 3 adenylyl cyclase is required for novel object learning and extinction of contextual memory: role of cAMP signaling in primary cilia.** *J Neurosci* 2011, **31**:5557-5561.
63. Radulovic J, Tronson NC: **Molecular specificity of multiple hippocampal processes governing fear extinction.** *Rev Neurosci* 2010, **21**:1-17.
64. Dalla C, Shors TJ: **Sex differences in learning processes of classical and operant conditioning.** *Physiol Behav* 2009, **97**:229-238.
65. Dalla C, Edgecomb C, Whetstone AS, Shors TJ: **Females do not express learned helplessness like males do.** *Neuropsychopharmacology* 2008, **33**:1559-1569.
66. Maren S, De Oca B, Fanselow MS: **Sex differences in hippocampal long-term potentiation (LTP) and Pavlovian fear conditioning in rats: positive correlation between LTP and contextual learning.** *Brain Res* 1994, **661**:25-34.
67. Gupta RR, Sen S, Diepenhorst LL, Rudick CN, Maren S: **Estrogen modulates sexually dimorphic contextual fear conditioning and hippocampal long-term potentiation (LTP) in rats(1).** *Brain Res* 2001, **888**:356-365.
68. Wiltgen BJ, Sanders MJ, Behne NS, Fanselow MS: **Sex differences, context preexposure, and the immediate shock deficit in Pavlovian context conditioning with mice.** *Behav Neurosci* 2001, **115**:26-32.
69. Aguilar R, Gil L, Gray JA, Driscoll P, Flint J, Dawson GR, Gimenez-Llort L, Escorihuela RM, Fernandez-Teruel A, Tobena A: **Fearfulness and sex in F2 Roman rats: males display more fear though both sexes share the same fearfulness traits.** *Physiol Behav* 2003, **78**:723-732.
70. Jasnow AM, Schulkin J, Pfaff DW: **Estrogen facilitates fear conditioning and increases corticotropin-releasing hormone mRNA expression in the central amygdala in female mice.** *Horm Behav* 2006, **49**:197-205.
71. Wiltgen BJ, Sanders MJ, Ferguson C, Homanics GE, Fanselow MS: **Trace fear conditioning is enhanced in mice lacking the delta subunit of the GABAA receptor.** *Learn Mem* 2005, **12**:327-333.
72. Baran SE, Armstrong CE, Niren DC, Hanna JJ, Conrad CD: **Chronic stress and sex differences on the recall of fear conditioning and extinction.** *Neurobiol Learn Mem* 2009, **91**:323-332.
73. Baran SE, Armstrong CE, Niren DC, Conrad CD: **Prefrontal cortex lesions and sex differences in fear extinction and perseveration.** *Learn Mem* 2010, **17**:267-278.
74. Zeidan MA, Igoe SA, Linnman C, Vitalo A, Levine JB, Klibanski A, Goldstein JM, Milad MR: **Estradiol modulates medial prefrontal cortex and amygdala activity during fear extinction in women and female rats.** *Biol Psychiatry* 2011, **70**:920-927.
75. Milad MR, Igoe SA, Lebron-Milad K, Novales JE: **Estrous cycle phase and gonadal hormones influence conditioned fear extinction.** *Neuroscience* 2009, **164**:887-895.
76. Milad MR, Zeidan MA, Contero A, Pitman RK, Klibanski A, Rauch SL, Goldstein JM: **The influence of gonadal hormones on conditioned fear extinction in healthy humans.** *Neuroscience* 2010, **168**:652-658.
77. Morgan MA, Pfaff DW: **Effects of estrogen on activity and fear-related behaviors in mice.** *Horm Behav* 2001, **40**:472-482.
78. Hiroi R, Neumaier JF: **Differential effects of ovarian steroids on anxiety versus fear as measured by open field test and fear-potentiated startle.** *Behav Brain Res* 2006, **166**:93-100.
79. Rivas-Arancibia S, Vazquez-Pereyra F: **Hormonal modulation of extinction responses induced by sexual steroid hormones in rats.** *Life Sci* 1994, **54**: PL363-367.
80. Yuan DL, Chambers KC: **Estradiol accelerates extinction of a conditioned taste aversion in female and male rats.** *Horm Behav* 1999, **36**:1-16.
81. Chang YJ, Yang CH, Liang YC, Yeh CM, Huang CC, Hsu KS: **Estrogen modulates sexually dimorphic contextual fear extinction in rats through estrogen receptor beta.** *Hippocampus* 2009, **19**:1142-1150.
82. Cahill L: **Sex- and hemisphere-related influences on the neurobiology of emotionally influenced memory.** *Prog Neuropsychopharmacol Biol Psychiatry* 2003, **27**:1235-1241.
83. Goldstein JM, Jerram M, Poldrack R, Ahern T, Kennedy DN, Seidman LJ, Makris N: **Hormonal cycle modulates arousal circuitry in women using functional magnetic resonance imaging.** *J Neurosci* 2005, **25**:9309-9316.
84. Protopopescu X, Pan H, Altemus M, Tuescher O, Polanecsky M, McEwen B, Silbersweig D, Stern E: **Orbitofrontal cortex activity related to emotional processing changes across the menstrual cycle.** *Proc Natl Acad Sci USA* 2005, **102**:16060-16065.
85. Milad MR, Goldstein JM, Orr SP, Wedig MM, Klibanski A, Pitman RK, Rauch SL: **Fear conditioning and extinction: influence of sex and menstrual cycle in healthy humans.** *Behav Neurosci* 2006, **120**:1196-1203.
86. Celotti F, Melcangi RC, Negri-Cesi P, Poletti A: **Testosterone metabolism in brain cells and membranes.** *J Steroid Biochem Mol Biol* 1991, **40**:673-678.

87. Fester L, Prange-Kiel J, Jarry H, Rune GM: **Estrogen synthesis in the hippocampus.** *Cell Tissue Res* 2011, **345**:285-294.
88. Gillies GE, McArthur S: **Estrogen actions in the brain and the basis for differential action in men and women: a case for sex-specific medicines.** *Pharmacol Rev* 2010, **62**:155-198.
89. Tsai MJ, O'Malley BW: **Molecular mechanisms of action of steroid/thyroid receptor superfamily members.** *Annu Rev Biochem* 1994, **63**:451-486.
90. Weiser MJ, Foradori CD, Handa RJ: **Estrogen receptor beta activation prevents glucocorticoid receptor-dependent effects of the central nucleus of the amygdala on behavior and neuroendocrine function.** *Brain Res* 2010, **1336**:78-88.
91. Weiser MJ, Foradori CD, Handa RJ: **Estrogen receptor beta in the brain: from form to function.** *Brain Res Rev* 2008, **57**:309-320.
92. Mitra SW, Hoskin E, Yudkovitz J, Pear L, Wilkinson HA, Hayashi S, Pfaff DW, Ogawa S, Rohrer SP, Schaeffer JM, McEwen BS, Alves SE: **Immunolocalization of estrogen receptor beta in the mouse brain: comparison with estrogen receptor alpha.** *Endocrinology* 2003, **144**:2055-2067.
93. Kritzer MF: **Regional, laminar, and cellular distribution of immunoreactivity for ER alpha and ER beta in the cerebral cortex of hormonally intact, adult male and female rats.** *Cereb Cortex* 2002, **12**:116-128.
94. Zhang JQ, Cai WQ, Su BY, Zhou de S: **Immunocytochemical localization of estrogen receptor beta in the rat brain.** *Shi Yan Sheng Wu Xue Bao* 2002, **35**:15-20.
95. Osterlund M, Kuiper GG, Gustafsson JA, Hurd YL: **Differential distribution and regulation of estrogen receptor-alpha and -beta mRNA within the female rat brain.** *Brain Res Mol Brain Res* 1998, **54**:175-180.
96. Krezel W, Dupont S, Krust A, Chambon P, Chapman PF: **Increased anxiety and synaptic plasticity in estrogen receptor beta -deficient mice.** *Proc Natl Acad Sci USA* 2001, **98**:12278-12282.
97. Imwalle DB, Gustafsson JA, Rissman EF: **Lack of functional estrogen receptor beta influences anxiety behavior and serotonin content in female mice.** *Physiol Behav* 2005, **84**:157-163.
98. Kruijver FP, Balesar R, Espila AM, Unmehopa UA, Swaab DF: **Estrogen receptor-alpha distribution in the human hypothalamus in relation to sex and endocrine status.** *J Comp Neurol* 2002, **454**:115-139.
99. Scharfman HE, Hintz TM, Gomez J, Stormes KA, Barouk S, Malthankar-Phatak GH, McCloskey DP, Luine VN, Maclusky NJ: **Changes in hippocampal function of ovariectomized rats after sequential low doses of estradiol to simulate the preovulatory estrogen surge.** *Eur J Neurosci* 2007, **26**:2595-2612.
100. Smith CC, Vedder LC, McMahon LL: **Estradiol and the relationship between dendritic spines, NR2B containing NMDA receptors, and the magnitude of long-term potentiation at hippocampal CA3-CA1 synapses.** *Psychoneuroendocrinology* 2009, **34(Suppl 1)**:S130-S142.
101. McEwen B: **Estrogen actions throughout the brain.** *Recent Prog Horm Res* 2002, **57**:357-384.
102. Murphy DD, Cole NB, Greenberger V, Segal M: **Estradiol increases dendritic spine density by reducing GABA neurotransmission in hippocampal neurons.** *J Neurosci* 1998, **18**:2550-2559.
103. Good M, Day M, Muir JL: **Cyclical changes in endogenous levels of oestrogen modulate the induction of LTD and LTP in the hippocampal CA1 region.** *Eur J Neurosci* 1999, **11**:4476-4480.
104. Tanapat P, Hastings NB, Gould E: **Ovarian steroids influence cell proliferation in the dentate gyrus of the adult female rat in a dose- and time-dependent manner.** *J Comp Neurol* 2005, **481**:252-265.
105. Foy MR, Xu J, Xie X, Brinton RD, Thompson RF, Berger TW: **17beta-estradiol enhances NMDA receptor-mediated EPSPs and long-term potentiation.** *J Neurophysiol* 1999, **81**:925-929.
106. Terasawa E, Timiras PS: **Electrical activity during the estrous cycle of the rat: cyclic changes in limbic structures.** *Endocrinology* 1968, **83**:207-216.
107. Smith CC, McMahon LL: **Estradiol-induced increase in the magnitude of long-term potentiation is prevented by blocking NR2B-containing receptors.** *J Neurosci* 2006, **26**:8517-8522.
108. Smith CC, McMahon LL: **Estrogen-induced increase in the magnitude of long-term potentiation occurs only when the ratio of NMDA transmission to AMPA transmission is increased.** *J Neurosci* 2005, **25**:7780-7791.
109. Scharfman HE, Maclusky NJ: **Similarities between actions of estrogen and BDNF in the hippocampus: coincidence or clue?** *Trends Neurosci* 2005, **28**:79-85.
110. Scharfman HE, MacLusky NJ: **Estrogen and brain-derived neurotrophic factor (BDNF) in hippocampus: complexity of steroid hormone-growth factor interactions in the adult CNS.** *Front Neuroendocrinol* 2006, **27**:415-435.
111. Soliman F, Glatt CE, Bath KG, Levita L, Jones RM, Pattwell SS, Jing D, Tottenham N, Amso D, Somerville L, Voss HU, Glover G, Ballon DJ, Liston C, Teslovich T, Van Kempen T, Lee FS, Casey BJ: **A genetic variant BDNF polymorphism alters extinction learning in both mouse and human.** *Science* 2010, **327**:863-866.
112. Peters J, Dieppa-Perea LM, Melendez LM, Quirk GJ: **Induction of fear extinction with hippocampal-infralimbic BDNF.** *Science* 2010, **328**:1288-1290.
113. Shansky RM, Hamo C, Hof PR, Lou W, McEwen BS, Morrison JH: **Estrogen promotes stress sensitivity in a prefrontal cortex-amygdala pathway.** *Cereb Cortex* 2010, **20**:2560-2567.
114. Gerrits M, Westenbroek C, Koch T, Grootkarzijn A, Ter Horst GJ: **Increased limbic phosphorylated extracellular-regulated kinase 1 and 2 expression after chronic stress is reduced by cyclic 17beta-estradiol administration.** *Neuroscience* 2006, **142**:1293-1302.
115. Sinopoli KJ, Floresco SB, Galea LA: **Systemic and local administration of estradiol into the prefrontal cortex or hippocampus differentially alters working memory.** *Neurobiol Learn Mem* 2006, **86**:293-304.
116. Lokuge S, Frey BN, Foster JA, Soares CN, Steiner M: **The rapid effects of estrogen: a mini-review.** *Behav Pharmacol* 2010, **21**:465-472.
117. Smith CC, Vedder LC, McMahon LL: **Estradiol and the relationship between dendritic spines, NR2B containing NMDA receptors, and the magnitude of long-term potentiation at hippocampal CA3-CA1 synapses.** *Psychoneuroendocrinology* 2009, **34(Suppl 1)**:S130-142.
118. Fan L, Hanbury R, Pandey SC, Cohen RS: **Dose and time effects of estrogen on expression of neuron-specific protein and cyclic AMP response element-binding protein and brain region volume in the medial amygdala of ovariectomized rats.** *Neuroendocrinology* 2008, **88**:111-126.
119. Frye CA, Walf AA: **Progesterone enhances learning and memory of aged wildtype and progestin receptor knockout mice.** *Neurosci Lett* 2010, **472**:38-42.
120. Derntl B, Windischberger C, Robinson S, Lamplmayr E, Kryspin-Exner I, Gur RC, Moser E, Habel U: **Facial emotion recognition and amygdala activation are associated with menstrual cycle phase.** *Psychoneuroendocrinology* 2008, **33**:1031-1040.
121. van Wingen GA, Ossewaarde L, Backstrom T, Hermans EJ, Fernandez G: **Gonadal hormone regulation of the emotion circuitry in humans.** *Neuroscience* 2011, **191**:38-45.
122. Engin E, Treit D: **The anxiolytic-like effects of allopregnanolone vary as a function of intracerebral microinfusion site: the amygdala, medial prefrontal cortex, or hippocampus.** *Behav Pharmacol* 2007, **18**:461-470.
123. Akwa Y, Purdy RH, Koob GF, Britton KT: **The amygdala mediates the anxiolytic-like effect of the neurosteroid allopregnanolone in rat.** *Behav Brain Res* 1999, **106**:119-125.
124. Jackson LR, Robinson TE, Becker JB: **Sex differences and hormonal influences on acquisition of cocaine self-administration in rats.** *Neuropsychopharmacology* 2006, **31**:129-138.
125. Peterson CK, Harmon-Jones E: **Anger and testosterone: evidence that situationally-induced anger relates to situationally-induced testosterone.** *Emotion* 2011.
126. Mazur A: **The role of testosterone in male dominance contests that turn violent.** *Soc Biol* 2006, **53**:24-29.
127. Sapolsky RM: **The influence of social hierarchy on primate health.** *Science* 2005, **308**:648-652.
128. Stanton SJ, Wirth MM, Waugh CE, Schultheiss OC: **Endogenous testosterone levels are associated with amygdala and ventromedial prefrontal cortex responses to anger faces in men but not women.** *Biol Psychol* 2009, **81**:118-122.
129. Rubinow DR, Roca CA, Schmidt PJ, Danaceau MA, Putnam K, Cizza G, Chrousos G, Nieman L: **Testosterone suppression of CRH-stimulated cortisol in men.** *Neuropsychopharmacology* 2005, **30**:1906-1912.

130. Hermans EJ, Putman P, Baas JM, Gecks NM, Kenemans JL, van Honk J: **Exogenous testosterone attenuates the integrated central stress response in healthy young women.** *Psychoneuroendocrinology* 2007, **32**:1052-1061.
131. van Wingen G, Mattern C, Verkes RJ, Buitelaar J, Fernandez G: **Testosterone reduces amygdala-orbitofrontal cortex coupling.** *Psychoneuroendocrinology* 2010, **35**:105-113.
132. Frye CA, Koonce CJ, Edinger KL, Osborne DM, Walf AA: **Androgens with activity at estrogen receptor beta have anxiolytic and cognitive-enhancing effects in male rats and mice.** *Horm Behav* 2008, **54**:726-734.
133. Sharpe RM: **The roles of oestrogen in the male.** *Trends Endocrinol Metab* 1998, **9**:371-377.
134. Jones ME, Boon WC, Proietto J, Simpson ER: **Of mice and men: the evolving phenotype of aromatase deficiency.** *Trends Endocrinol Metab* 2006, **17**:55-64.
135. Pitman RK, Shin LM, Rauch SL: **Investigating the pathogenesis of posttraumatic stress disorder with neuroimaging.** *J Clin Psychiatry* 2001, **62(Suppl 17)**:47-54.
136. Rothbaum BO, Schwartz AC: **Exposure therapy for posttraumatic stress disorder.** *Am J Psychother* 2002, **56**:59-75.
137. Rothbaum BO, Davis M: **Applying learning principles to the treatment of post-trauma reactions.** *Ann NY Acad Sci* 2003, **1008**:112-121.
138. Rauch SL, Shin LM, Whalen PJ, Pitman RK: **Neuroimaging and the neuroanatomy of PTSD.** *CNS Spectr* 1998, **3**:30-41.
139. Bremner JD: **Alterations in brain structure and function associated with post-traumatic stress disorder.** *Semin Clin Neuropsychiatry* 1999, **4**:249-255.
140. Gilbertson MW, Shenton ME, Ciszewski A, Kasai K, Lasko NB, Orr SP, Pitman RK: **Smaller hippocampal volume predicts pathologic vulnerability to psychological trauma.** *Nat Neurosci* 2002, **5**:1242-1247.
141. Shin LM, Orr SP, Carson MA, Rauch SL, Macklin ML, Lasko NB, Peters PM, Metzger LJ, Dougherty DD, Cannistraro PA, Alpert NM, Fischman AJ, Pitman RK: **Regional cerebral blood flow in the amygdala and medial prefrontal cortex during traumatic imagery in male and female Vietnam veterans with PTSD.** *Arch Gen Psychiatry* 2004, **61**:168-176.
142. Shin LM, Shin PS, Heckers S, Krangel TS, Macklin ML, Orr SP, Lasko N, Segal E, Makris N, Richert K, Levering J, Schacter DL, Alpert NM, Fischman AJ, Pitman RK, Rauch SL: **Hippocampal function in posttraumatic stress disorder.** *Hippocampus* 2004, **14**:292-300.
143. Orr SP, Roth WT: **Psychophysiological assessment: clinical applications for PTSD.** *J Affect Disord* 2000, **61**:225-240.
144. Jovanovic T, Norrholm SD, Blanding NQ, Davis M, Duncan E, Bradley B, Ressler KJ: **Impaired fear inhibition is a biomarker of PTSD but not depression.** *Depress Anxiety* 2010, **27**:244-251.
145. Orr SP, Metzger LJ, Lasko NB, Macklin ML, Peri T, Pitman RK: ***De novo* conditioning in trauma-exposed individuals with and without posttraumatic stress disorder.** *J Abnorm Psychol* 2000, **109**:290-298.
146. Milad MR, Orr SP, Lasko NB, Chang Y, Rauch SL, Pitman RK: **Presence and acquired origin of reduced recall for fear extinction in PTSD: results of a twin study.** *J Psychiatr Res* 2008, **42**:515-520.
147. Breslau N, Davis GC, Andreski P, Peterson EL, Schultz LR: **Sex differences in posttraumatic stress disorder.** *Arch Gen Psychiatry* 1997, **54**:1044-1048.
148. Seedat S, Stein DJ, Carey PD: **Post-traumatic stress disorder in women: epidemiological and treatment issues.** *CNS Drugs* 2005, **19**:411-427.
149. Holbrook TL, Hoyt DB, Stein MB, Sieber WJ: **Gender differences in long-term posttraumatic stress disorder outcomes after major trauma: women are at higher risk of adverse outcomes than men.** *J Trauma* 2002, **53**:882-888.
150. Bakish D: **The patient with comorbid depression and anxiety: the unmet need.** *J Clin Psychiatry* 1999, **60(Suppl 6)**:20-24.
151. Reed V, Wittchen HU: **DSM-IV panic attacks and panic disorder in a community sample of adolescents and young adults: how specific are panic attacks?** *J Psychiatr Res* 1998, **32**:335-345.
152. Gregoire AJ, Kumar R, Everitt B, Henderson AF, Studd JW: **Transdermal oestrogen for treatment of severe postnatal depression.** *Lancet* 1996, **347**:930-933.
153. Sichel DA, Cohen LS, Robertson LM, Ruttenberg A, Rosenbaum JF: **Prophylactic estrogen in recurrent postpartum affective disorder.** *Biol Psychiatry* 1995, **38**:814-818.
154. Arpels JC: **The female brain hypoestrogenic continuum from the premenstrual syndrome to menopause. A hypothesis and review of supporting data.** *J Reprod Med* 1996, **41**:633-639.
155. Best NR, Rees MP, Barlow DH, Cowen PJ: **Effect of estradiol implant on noradrenergic function and mood in menopausal subjects.** *Psychoneuroendocrinology* 1992, **17**:87-93.
156. Taneepanichskul S, Patrachai S: **Effects of long-term treatment with depot medroxy progesterone acetate for contraception on estrogenic activity.** *J Med Assoc Thai* 1998, **81**:944-946.
157. Altshuler LL, Hendrick V, Cohen LS: **Course of mood and anxiety disorders during pregnancy and the postpartum period.** *J Clin Psychiatry* 1998, **59(Suppl 2)**:29-33.
158. Altshuler LL, Hendrick V, Cohen LS: **Course of mood and anxiety disorders during pregnancy and the postpartum period.** *J Clin Psychiatry* 1998, **59(Suppl 2)**:29-33.
159. Schnatz PF, Whitehurst SK, O'Sullivan DM: **Sexual dysfunction, depression, and anxiety among patients of an inner-city menopause clinic.** *J Womens Health (Larchmt)* 2010, **19**:1843-1849.
160. Schnatz PF, Whitehurst SK, O'Sullivan DM: **Sexual dysfunction, depression, and anxiety among patients of an inner-city menopause clinic.** *J Womens Health (Larchmt)* 2010, **19**:1843-1849.
161. Schmidt PJ, Rubinow DR: **Sex hormones and mood in the perimenopause.** *Ann N Y Acad Sci* 2009, **1179**:70-85.
162. Schweckendiek J, Klucken T, Merz CJ, Tabbert K, Walter B, Ambach W, Vaitl D, Stark R: **Weaving the (neuronal) web: fear learning in spider phobia.** *Neuroimage* 2011, **54**:681-688.
163. Harsh V, Meltzer-Brody S, Rubinow DR, Schmidt PJ: **Reproductive aging, sex steroids, and mood disorders.** *Harv Rev Psychiatry* 2009, **17**:87-102.
164. Becker JB, Arnold AP, Berkley KJ, Blaustein JD, Eckel LA, Hampson E, Herman JP, Marts S, Sadee W, Steiner M, Taylor J, Young E: **Strategies and methods for research on sex differences in brain and behavior.** *Endocrinology* 2005, **146**:1650-1673.

15

Diminished rostral anterior cingulate cortex activation during trauma-unrelated emotional interference in PTSD

Reid Offringa[1,2], Kathryn Handwerger Brohawn[1,2], Lindsay K Staples[1,2], Stacey J Dubois[1,2], Katherine C Hughes[2], Danielle L Pfaff[1], Michael B VanElzakker[1,2], F Caroline Davis[1,2] and Lisa M Shin[1,2*]

Abstract

Background: Previous research suggests that individuals with posttraumatic stress disorder (PTSD) preferentially attend to trauma-related emotional stimuli and have difficulty completing unrelated concurrent tasks. Compared to trauma-exposed control groups, individuals with PTSD also exhibit lower rostral anterior cingulate cortex (rACC) activation during tasks involving interference from trauma-related stimuli. However, it is not clear whether relatively diminished rACC activation in PTSD also occurs during interference tasks involving trauma-*unrelated* emotional stimuli. The present study employed functional magnetic resonance imaging (fMRI) and an interference task that involves emotional facial expressions and elicits rACC activation in healthy participants.

Findings: While performing a trauma-unrelated emotional interference task, participants with PTSD (n=17) showed less rACC activation than trauma-exposed non-PTSD (TENP; n=18) participants. In the PTSD group, rACC activation was negatively correlated with the severity of re-experiencing symptoms. The two groups did not significantly differ on behavioral measures (i.e., response times and error rates).

Conclusions: These findings suggest that relatively diminished rACC activation in PTSD can be observed in interference tasks involving trauma-unrelated emotional stimuli, indicating a more general functional brain abnormality in this disorder. Future neuroimaging studies need not employ trauma-related stimuli in order to detect rACC abnormalities in PTSD.

Keywords: fMRI, Stroop, Posttraumatic stress disorder, Anterior cingulate, Interference, Trauma

Background

Posttraumatic stress disorder (PTSD) is a debilitating psychiatric disorder that occurs in 9-20% of individuals following a traumatic event [1]. Those with PTSD have difficulty suppressing trauma-related thoughts and suffer from persistent re-experiencing symptoms [2,3]. Such symptoms have been studied in the laboratory with interference tasks in which participants are asked to ignore trauma-related information (e.g., words) while performing an unrelated cognitive task (such as naming the color or number of the words). Indeed, individuals with PTSD have difficulty performing such tasks and show impaired behavioral performance (e.g. [3-5]) and relatively diminished activation in the rostral anterior cingulate cortex (rACC) [6,7]. The rACC is a brain structure that is thought to resolve emotional conflict [8] and/or "decrease the 'weighting' of affective information in the service of optimizing cognitive performance" [9]. Relatively diminished rACC function in PTSD may reflect a failure to (1) appropriately "weight" distracting emotional information and (2) inhibit the amygdala (e.g. [10]). In fact, activation of the rACC has been found to negatively correlate with PTSD symptom severity (e.g. [11,12]).

Previous neuroimaging studies that found reduced rACC activation in PTSD during interference tasks have used trauma-related words as stimuli [6,7]. If the same rACC abnormality could be demonstrated using trauma-

* Correspondence: Lisa.Shin@tufts.edu
[1]Department of Psychology, Tufts University, Medford, MA, USA
[2]Department of Psychiatry, Massachusetts General Hospital, Charlestown, MA, USA

unrelated emotional stimuli, it would suggest the presence of a more global emotional and attentional dysfunction in PTSD, as opposed to a deficit specific to trauma-related stimuli. Two recent studies examined rACC activation in participants with PTSD during trauma-unrelated emotional interference [13,14] but yielded conflicting results.

In the current experiment, we used functional magnetic resonance imaging (fMRI) to study rACC activation in individuals with PTSD and trauma-exposed non-PTSD (TENP) participants during the performance of an interference task using trauma-unrelated emotional stimuli (i.e., faces and words) [8,15]. We hypothesized that the PTSD group would exhibit diminished rACC activation relative to the TENP group when comparing high-interference to low-interference conditions. Given previous findings (e.g., [11-13]), we also hypothesized that, for the PTSD group only, rACC activation would inversely correlate with PTSD symptom severity.

Methods

We recruited 42 right-handed participants who had been exposed to criterion A traumatic events (e.g., assault, motor vehicle accidents, abuse, and witnessing serious injury/death). Of these, 21 had current PTSD and 21 never developed PTSD. Within the PTSD group, two participants were removed due to excessive movement during the scan, one participant stopped the scan before the task began, and one participant failed to respond to an adequate number (75%) of trials. Within the TENP group, two participants were excluded due to a button box malfunction, and one participant was excluded due to excessive errors (greater than 25%). A total of 17 PTSD (14 female) and 18 TENP (13 female) participants were included in the final analyses.

PTSD diagnoses were determined using the Clinician Administered PTSD Scale (CAPS) [16]. All other diagnoses were made using the Structured Clinical Interview for the DSM-IV Axis I Disorders (SCID) [2]. Participants were free of the following: contraindications to MRI (e.g., metallic implants), complicating major medical conditions such as neurological disorders, pregnancy, current use of psychotropic medications, and a history of drug/alcohol abuse in the last six months. None of the TENP participants met criteria for any psychiatric disorders. Some participants with PTSD were also diagnosed with current major depressive disorder (MDD; n=5), specific phobia (n=1), and panic disorder (n=3). Psychometric and clinical data are presented in Table 1. All participants provided written informed consent. This study was in compliance with the Helsinki Declaration and approved by the institutional review board at Partners Healthcare System, Boston, Massachusetts.

Table 1 Demographic and psychometric data

Variable	PTSD Mean (SD)	TENP Mean (SD)	Significance
Age	29.88 (7.8)	27.06 (6.0)	p=0.235
Education	14.94 (2.4)	16.11 (2.1)	p=0.129
BMI	25.44 (4.6)	23.43 (3.4)	p=0.150
Current CAPS*	60.31 (15.1)	1.89 (3.1)	p<0.001
BDI*	13.12 (10.6)	1.27 (1.4)	p<0.001
BAI*	15.00 (9.5)	2.11 (3.6)	p<0.001

An asterisk (*) denotes a significant difference between groups. *BMI*, Body mass index; *CAPS*, Clinician administered PTSD scale; *BDI*, Beck depression inventory [17]; *BAI*, Beck anxiety inventory [18]; *SD*, Standard deviation.

Stimuli and procedures

Stimuli consisted of black and white photographs of 10 faces (5 male), each displaying one happy and one fearful expression [19], with either the word "happy" or "afraid" superimposed on each face (Figure 1). In the Congruent condition (low-interference), the superimposed word matched the facial expression. In the Incongruent condition (high-interference), the superimposed word did not match the facial expression. In the Baseline condition, a string of Xs was superimposed on the facial expression. Presentation timing was jittered using Optseq [20]. Faces were presented for 1300 milliseconds (ms), with a 700 ms inter-stimulus interval, in a pseudorandom order such that the same identity was never presented in succession. Fearful and happy faces were presented an equal number of times for a total of 180 stimuli per run. Interleaved within the facial stimuli were 28 white fixation crosses (null trials), which were presented for either 1300 ms or 3300 ms.

Participants completed four runs (6 minutes and 40 seconds each), but fMRI (and behavioral) analyses included only the first two runs to avoid decrements in

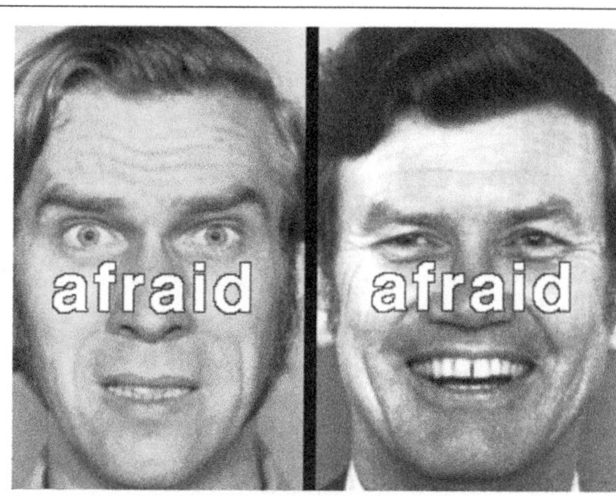

Figure 1 The face on the left is an example of a Congruent trial, in which the word matched the facial expression. The face on the right is an example of an Incongruent trial, in which the word did not match the facial expression.

Table 2 Response time (RT) and error rate (ER) results

	PTSD (n=17)				TENP (n=18)				Mixed-Model ANOVA[a]					
	Congruent		Incongruent		Congruent		Incongruent		Group		Condition		Group x Condition	
	M	SD	M	SD	M	SD	M	SD	F	*p*	F	*p*	F	*p*
RT (ms)	762	76	805	86	804	106	847	111	1.69	.20	102.7	<.001	.016	.89
ER (%)	.76	.74	2.87	2.36	.91	1.12	2.26	2.66	.201	.65	21.20	<.001	1.01	.32

Note that [a]df = 1, 33 for all effects. *ms*, Milliseconds. *RT*, Response time; *ER*, Percent error.

anterior cingulate activation that are known to occur with extended task performance [21]. Face stimuli were displayed using MacStim Carbon 3.2.1 and projected via a Sharp Notevision6 (XG-NV6XU) LCD projector (Osaka, Japan). Participants used a button box to indicate whether faces were happy or afraid. Button assignments for "happy" and "afraid" were counterbalanced across subjects.

Image acquisition

Participants were scanned using a Symphony/Sonata 1.5T whole body high-speed imaging device, equipped for echo planar imaging (Siemens Medical Systems, Iselin, NJ) with a 3-axis gradient head coil. First, we collected an automated scout image and shimmed [22]. Next, we collected two high-resolution three-dimensional magnetization prepared rapid acquisition gradient echo (MPRAGE) sequences (TR/TE/Flip angle=2730 ms/3.39 ms/7°) with 1.33 mm slice thickness. We acquired fMRI blood-oxygen-level dependent (BOLD) signal images [23] using gradient echo T2*-weighted sequences (TR/TE/Flip angle=2000 ms/40 ms/90°) in 22 coronal slices, (thickness=7 mm, 1 mm gap), with interleaved excitation order and foot-to-head phase encoding. To allow longitudinal magnetization to reach equilibrium, four images were acquired and discarded before the start of each functional scan.

Data analysis

Behavioral analyses

Response times were averaged across correct trials within each condition. Separate 2 (Group: PTSD, TENP) × 2 (Condition: Incongruent, Congruent) analyses of variance (ANOVA) were used to analyze response time and error rate data. With regard to error rates, we examined both errors of commission (incorrect response) and errors of omission (failure to respond) in separate ANOVAs.

FMRI analyses

We performed all fMRI statistical analyses using SPM 2.0 software (Wellcome Department of Cognitive Neurology, London, UK). Functional images were slice-time and motion corrected (realigned to the first volume in the time series), co-registered to structural images, spatially normalized into a standard stereotactic space (Montreal Neurological Institute [MNI] template), and smoothed with a Gaussian filter set at 7mm full width at half maximum.

Voxelwise Incongruent vs. Congruent (IvC) contrast images were created for each participant. These contrast images were then submitted to a second-level random effects model to assess differences between groups (PTSD vs. TENP). Trials involving either errors of commission or omission were excluded from all contrasts.

Statistical parametric maps were inspected for activations in rACC and dorsal anterior cingulate cortex (dACC) that exceeded a significance threshold of $p<0.001$ (one-tailed), uncorrected. We included the dACC as a secondary region of interest because previous studies have shown relatively greater dACC activation in PTSD versus non-PTSD groups (e.g., [6,14,24,25]). Consistent with previous research, the rACC was defined as the region superior/anterior to the corpus callosum and inferior to the cingulate sulcus, with a y coordinate greater than +30 [26]. The dACC was defined as the region superior to the corpus callosum and inferior to the cingulate sulcus, with a y coordinate between 0 and +30 [25-27]. Activations observed outside of these predefined regions of interest (ROIs) were subjected to the more conservative threshold of $p<0.00001$, uncorrected. Data from clusters exceeding these thresholds were extracted using MarsBaR (MRC Cognition and Brain Sciences Unit, Cambridge, United Kingdom).

Voxelwise whole brain correlations

To assess the relationship between current CAPS scores and IvC signal change in the PTSD group, we conducted

Table 3 Incongruent vs. Congruent (IvC) contrast within PTSD and TENP groups

Activation in PTSD group			Activation in TENP group		
Region	*MNI (x,y,z)*	*z Score*	*Region*	*MNI (x,y,z)*	*z Score*
rACC	6, 32, 36	2.97 (ns)	rACC	16, 36, 34	4.48
dACC	12, 4, 42	3.40		−4, 34, 42	3.27
				16, 46, 2	3.23
				−10, 42, 32	3.10
			dACC	−12, 4, 44	3.96
				−14, 20, 32	3.33

There were no suprathreshold regions of activation for the inverse (CvI) contrast.

Table 4 Between-group comparison of the IvC contrast

Activation greater in PTSD group			Activation greater in TENP group		
Region	*MNI (x,y,z)*	*z Score*	*Region*	*MNI (x,y,z)*	*z Score*
-	-	-	rACC	18, 32, 32	3.57

the following voxelwise whole brain correlational analyses. First, we computed the IvC contrast within each participant in the PTSD group and correlated those contrast images with total CAPS scores. Because IvC activation could be related differently to different types of PTSD symptoms, we also ran correlations with CAPS-B (re-experiencing), CAPS-C (avoidance/numbing) and CAPS-D (hyper-arousal) subscale scores. We then inspected our regions of interest for significant clusters using the same p-value thresholds as described above.

Findings

Significant main effects of Condition confirmed that response times and error rates were greater in the Incongruent vs. Congruent condition (Table 2). However, groups did not significantly differ on response time or error rate measures (*ps* > 0.32). Only the TENP group exhibited significant rACC activation in the IvC contrast (Table 3). When directly compared to the PTSD group, the TENP group exhibited significantly greater rACC activation (MNI x,y,z coordinates = 18, 32, 32) (Table 4). We extracted data from all significant voxels greater than z=3.09 (p<0.001) in this region for each condition compared to the null trials (i.e., fixation crosses). From these extractions, the TENP group exhibited activation during the Incongruent trials and deactivation during the Congruent trials. Comparatively, the participants of the PTSD group did not show such modulation of activation in the rACC (Figure 2). We also correlated the extracted data from the rACC (18, 32, 32) with symptom severity scores. Within the PTSD group, rACC activation was significantly negatively correlated with CAPS-B subscale scores (r [15]= −0.55, p=0.03) and had a trend-level negative correlation with total CAPS (r [15]= −0.44, p=0.08), but was not significantly correlated with other CAPS subscale scores, BAI scores, or BDI scores (all *ps* > 0.13). Within the TENP group, rACC activation did not significantly correlate with total CAPS scores, CAPS subscale scores, BAI scores, or BDI scores (all *ps* > 0.31).

Voxelwise correlation analyses revealed no significant negative correlation between total CAPS score and rACC activation (IvC) in the PTSD group; however, we did find a significant negative correlation between total CAPS scores and activation of medial frontal gyrus (MFG), just adjacent to the rACC (MNI x,y,z coordinates = −18, 48, 14; z=3.66; Figure 3A), and activation in a more dorsal region of the anterior cingulate cortex (dACC) (MNI x,y,z coordinates = −8, 24, 28; z=3.74; Figure 3B). We also ran voxelwise correlations between IvC and CAPS-B, C and D subscale scores in the PTSD group. The results were similar to those of the correlations with total CAPS scores with one important exception: only CAPS-B (re-experiencing) subscale scores were significantly negatively correlated with activation in the rACC proper (MNI x,y,z coordinates = 16, 36, 30; z=3.28 and 4, 40, 0; z=3.28; Figure 3C and D).

Discussion and conclusion

In support of our primary hypothesis, the PTSD group exhibited lower rACC activation to trauma-*unrelated*

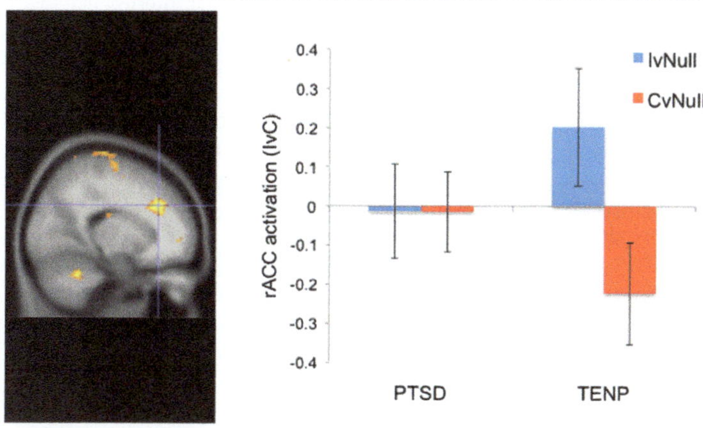

Figure 2 The image on the left shows greater rACC (18, 32, 32) activation in the Incongruent versus Congruent (IvC) contrast in the trauma-exposed non-PTSD (TENP) group compared to the PTSD group. The bar graph on the right breaks down this activation. IvNull shows fMRI signal in the Incongruent condition relative to the Null (focus cross) baseline. CvNull shows fMRI signal in the Congruent condition relative to the Null (focus cross) baseline. Error bars reflect standard error of the mean.

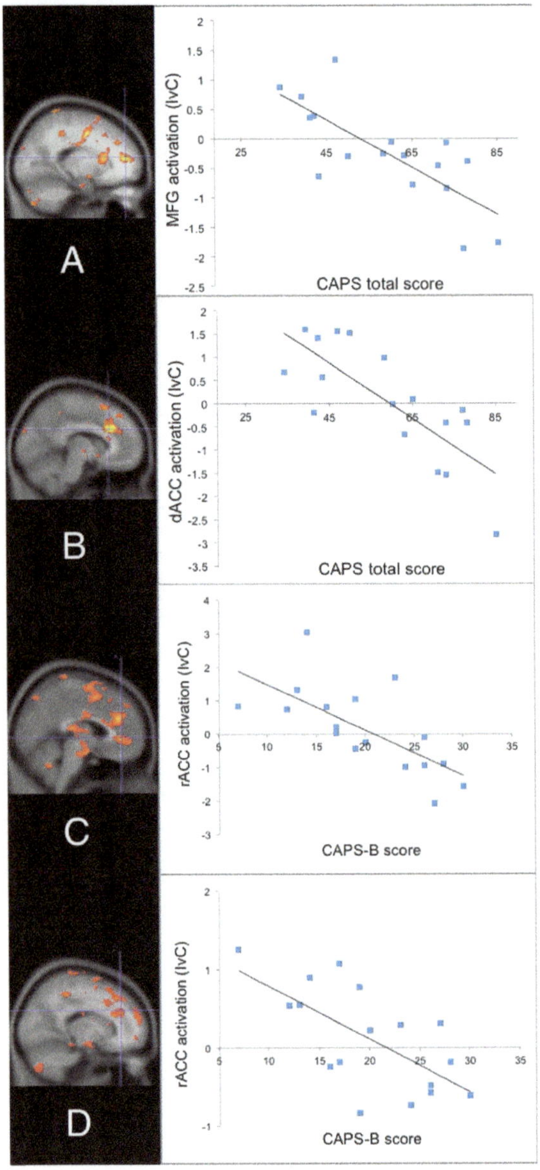

Figure 3 In the PTSD group for the lvC contrast, total CAPS symptom severity scores negatively correlated with activation in the (A) medial frontal gyrus (MFG) (−18, 48, 14) and (B) dorsal anterior cingulate cortex (dACC) (−8, 24, 28). In addition, CAPS-B scores (re-experiencing symptom severity) negatively correlated with rACC activation at (**C**) 4,40,0 and (**D**) 16,36,30.

interference, as compared to the TENP group. These results are consistent with those of Kim and colleagues [13] and suggest that diminished rACC function may reflect a more general abnormality in processing emotional material in PTSD.

We did not find any significant between-group differences on response times or error rates. It is possible that rACC dysfunction in PTSD is not behaviorally apparent until stimuli are more salient (trauma-related). Indeed, a recent meta-analysis has suggested that trauma-unrelated emotional word stimuli do not elicit greater behavioral interference in PTSD participants, as compared to controls [28]. However, previous studies that used trauma-related stimuli also failed to find significant behavioral impairment despite showing diminished rACC activation in PTSD [6,7]. It should be noted, however, that the latter study measured only accuracy (not response times) and the former study did report greater group differences in behavioral interference than the current study. Thus, it remains possible that behavioral evidence of rACC dysfunction is stronger when the stimuli are more salient. Regardless, the lack of behavioral differences in the present study suggests that our neuroimaging results cannot be attributed to group differences in behavioral performance.

Consistent with previous research, we found a trend toward a negative correlation between total symptom severity and activation in the rACC proper [11-13]. We also found significant negative correlations between total symptom severity and activation of structures adjacent to the rACC: the MFG and the dACC. Previous studies have revealed negative correlations between symptom severity and MFG activation (e.g., [29,30]). The observed dACC cluster lies 6mm away from the rACC boundary as defined herein. Given the smoothing kernel (7 mm), this cluster could reflect function of the rACC. Importantly, we also found that only re-experiencing symptom severity (CAPS-B) was significantly negatively correlated with activation in rACC proper. That the degree of diminished rACC activation during emotional interference may reflect the severity of re-experiencing symptoms per se makes sense given that emotional interference tasks were originally intended to tap into the cognitive processes underlying re-experiencing symptoms of PTSD [3].

If the rACC deficit in PTSD is more general (i.e., not specific to trauma-related material), then rACC activation to emotional interference should correlate negatively with PTSD symptom severity regardless of whether the emotional stimuli are trauma-related. Consistent with this hypothesis, Kim et al. [13] found that rACC activation to trauma-unrelated emotional stimuli is negatively correlated with PTSD symptom severity. In addition, we found a similar negative correlation in the current study between rACC activation and CAPS-B re-experiencing symptoms. Unfortunately, correlations between brain activation and symptom severity were not reported in other previous neuroimaging studies of emotional interference in PTSD [6,7,14].

In summary, our findings suggest that relatively diminished rACC function in PTSD may reflect a more generalized abnormality that can be observed even when emotional stimuli are unrelated to trauma. This finding also has implications for the planning of future neuroimaging studies that examine rACC function in groups with diverse trauma histories. Individually tailoring stimuli to match each participant's traumatic event may not be necessary as emotional interference tasks need not contain trauma-related stimuli in order to reveal rACC abnormalities in PTSD.

Abbreviations
ANOVA: Analysis of variance; BOLD: Blood oxygenation level dependent; CAPS: Clinician administered PTSD scale; dACC: Dorsal anterior cingulate cortex; DSM-IV: Diagnostic and statistical manual of mental disorders, fourth edition; fMRI: Functional magnetic resonance imaging; IvC: Incongruent versus Congruent contrast; MDD: Major depressive disorder; MFG: Medial frontal gyrus; MRI: Magnetic resonance imaging; PTSD: Posttraumatic stress disorder; rACC: Rostral anterior cingulate cortex; ROIs: Regions of interest; SCID: Structured clinical interview for the DSM-IV; TENP: Trauma-exposed non-PTSD.

Competing interests
The authors declare that they have no competing interests.

Authors' contributions
RO collected and analyzed the data and drafted the manuscript. KHB collected and analyzed the data and edited the manuscript. LKS, SJD, KCH, DLP, MBV, and FCD assisted with data analysis and edited the manuscript. LMS designed and piloted the task, collected and analyzed the data, and edited the manuscript. All authors read and approved the final manuscript.

Acknowledgements
The authors would like to thank Mary O'Hara and Larry White of the Martinos Center for their technical assistance. This study was supported by funding from Tufts University.

References
1. Breslau N, Kessler RC, Chilcoat HD, Schultz LR, Davis GC, Andreski P: **Trauma and posttraumatic stress disorder in the community: the 1996 Detroit area survey of trauma.** *Arch Gen Psychiatry* 2004, **55**(7):626–632.
2. First MB, Spitzer RL, Gibbon M, Williams J: *Structured Clinical Interview for DSM-IV Axis I Disorders - Patient Edition (SCID-I/P Version 2.0).* New York: New York State Psychiatric Institute, Biometrics Research Department; 1995.
3. McNally RJ: **Experimental approaches to cognitive abnormality in posttraumatic stress disorder.** *Clin Psychol Rev* 1998, **18**(8):971–982.
4. Foa EB, Feske U, Murdock TB, Kozak MJ, McCarthy PR: **Processing of threat-related information in rape victims.** *J Abnorm Psychol* 1991, **100**(2):156–162.
5. Bryant RA, Harvey AG: **Processing threatening information in posttraumatic stress disorder.** *J Abnorm Psychol* 1995, **104**(3):537–541.
6. Shin LM, Whalen PJ, Pitman RK, Bush G, Macklin ML, Lasko NB, Orr SP, McInerney SC, Rauch SL: **An fMRI study of anterior cingulate function in posttraumatic stress disorder.** *Biol Psychiatry* 2001, **50**(12):932–942.
7. Bremner JD, Vermetten E, Vythilingam M, Afzal N, Schmahl C, Elzinga B, Charney DS: **Neural correlates of the classic color and emotional stroop in women with abuse-related posttraumatic stress disorder.** *Biol Psychiatry* 2004, **55**(6):612–620.
8. Etkin A, Egner T, Peraza DM, Kandel ER, Hirsch J: **Resolving emotional conflict: a role for the rostral anterior cingulate cortex in modulating activity in the amygdala.** *Neuron* 2006, **51**(6):871–882.
9. Whalen PJ, Bush G, McNally RJ, Wilhelm S, McInerney SC, Jenike MA, Rauch SL: **The emotional counting stroop paradigm: a functional magnetic resonance imaging probe of the anterior cingulate affective division.** *Biol Psychiatry* 1998, **44**(12):1219–1228.
10. Rauch SL, Shin LM, Phelps EA: **Neurocircuitry models of posttraumatic stress disorder and extinction: human neuroimaging research–past, present, and future.** *Biol Psychiatry* 2006, **60**(4):376–382.
11. Hopper JW, Frewen PA, van der Kolk BA, Lanius RA: **Neural correlates of reexperiencing, avoidance, and dissociation in PTSD: symptom dimensions and emotion dysregulation in responses to script-driven trauma imagery.** *J Trauma Stress* 2007, **20**(5):713–725.
12. Shin LM, Wright CI, Cannistraro PA, Wedig MM, McMullin K, Martis B, Macklin ML, Lasko NB, Cavanagh SR, Krangel TS, Orr SP, Pitman RK, Whalen PJ, Rauch SL: **A functional magnetic resonance imaging study of amygdala and medial prefrontal cortex responses to overtly presented fearful faces in posttraumatic stress disorder.** *Arch Gen Psychiatry* 2005, **62**(3):273–281.
13. Kim MJ, Chey J, Chung A, Bae S, Khang H, Ham B, Yoon SJ, Jeong DU, Lyoo IK: **Diminished rostral anterior cingulate activity in response to threat-related events in posttraumatic stress disorder.** *J Psychiatr Res* 2008, **42**(4):268–277.
14. Hayes JP, Labar KS, Petty CM, McCarthy G, Morey RA: **Alterations in the neural circuitry for emotion and attention associated with posttraumatic stress symptomatology.** *Psychiatr Res Neuroimaging* 2009, **172**(1):7–15.
15. Haas BW, Omura K, Constable RT, Canli T: **Interference produced by emotional conflict associated with anterior cingulate activation.** *Cogn Affect Behav Neurosci* 2006, **6**(2):152–156.
16. Blake DD, Weathers FW, Nagy LM, Kaloupek DG, Gusman FD, Charney DS, Keane TM: **The development of a clinician-administered PTSD scale.** *J Trauma Stress* 1995, **8**(1):75–90.
17. Beck AT, Steer RA: *Manual for the revised Beck Depression Inventory.* San Antonio, TX: The Psychological Corporation; 1987.
18. Beck AT, Steer RA: *Beck Anxiety Inventory Manual.* San Antonio, Tex: Psychological Corp; 1990.
19. Ekman P, Friesen WV: *Pictures of Facial Affect.* Palo Alto, CA: Consulting Psychologists Press; 1976.
20. *The Optseq Program.* http://surfer.nmr.mgh.harvard.edu/optseq/.
21. Bush G, Whalen PJ, Rosen BR, Jenike MA, McInerney SC, Rauch SL: **The counting stroop: an interference task specialized for functional neuroimaging–validation study with functional MRI.** *Hum Brain Mapp* 1998, **6**(4):270–282.
22. Reese TG, Davis TL, Weisskoff RM: **Automated shimming at 1.5 T using echo-planar image frequency maps.** *J Magn Reson Imaging* 1995, **5**(6):739–745.
23. Kwong KK, Belliveau JW, Chesler DA, Goldberg IE, Weisskoff RM, Poncelet BP, Kennedy DN, Hoppel BE, Cohen MS, Turner R: **Dynamic magnetic resonance imaging of human brain activity during primary sensory stimulation.** *Proc Natl Acad Sci U S A* 1992, **89**(12):5675–5679.
24. Shin LM, Bush G, Whalen PJ, Handwerger K, Cannistraro PA, Wright CI, Martis B, Macklin ML, Lasko NB, Orr SP, Pitman RK, Rauch SL: **Dorsal anterior cingulate function in posttraumatic stress disorder.** *J Trauma Stress* 2007, **20**(5):701–712.
25. Shin LM, Bush G, Milad MR, Lasko NB, Brohawn KH, Hughes KC, Macklin ML, Gold AL, Karpf RD, Orr SP, Rauch SL, Pitman RK: **Exaggerated activation of dorsal anterior cingulate cortex during cognitive interference: a monozygotic twin study of posttraumatic stress disorder.** *Am J Psychiatry* 2011, **168**(9):979–985.
26. Bush G, Luu P, Posner M: **Cognitive and emotional influences in anterior cingulate cortex.** *Trends Cogn Sci* 2000, **4**(6):215–222.
27. Bush G, Vogt BA, Holmes J, Dale AM, Greve D, Jenike MA, Rosen BR: **Dorsal anterior cingulate cortex: a role in reward-based decision making.** *Proc Natl Acad Sci U S A* 2002, **99**(1):523–528.
28. Cisler JM, Wolitzky-Taylor KB, Adams TG Jr, Babson KA, Badour CL, Willems JL: **The emotional Stroop task and posttraumatic stress disorder: a meta-analysis.** *Clin Psychol Rev* 2011, **31**(5):817–828.
29. Britton JC, Phan KL, Taylor SF, Fig LM, Liberzon I: **Corticolimbic blood flow in posttraumatic stress disorder during script-driven imagery.** *Biol Psychiatry* 2005, **57**(8):832–840.
30. Shin LM, Orr SP, Carson MA, Rauch SL, Macklin ML, Lasko NB, Peters PM, Metzger LJ, Dougherty DD, Cannistraro PS, Alpert NM, Fischman AJ, Pitman RK: **Regional cerebral blood flow in the amygdala and medial prefrontal cortex during traumatic imagery in male and female Vietnam veterans with PTSD.** *Arch Gen Psychiatry* 2004, **61**(2):168–176.

Effects of genetic deletion of the Kv4.2 voltage-gated potassium channel on murine anxiety-, fear- and stress-related behaviors

Carly Kiselycznyk[1*], Dax A Hoffman[2] and Andrew Holmes[1]

Abstract

Background: Potassium channels have been proposed to play a role in mechanisms of neural plasticity, and the Kv4.2 subunit has been implicated in the regulation of action-potential back-propagation to the dendrites. Alterations in mechanisms of plasticity have been further proposed to underlie various psychiatric disorders, but the role of Kv4.2 in anxiety or depression is not well understood.

Methods: In this paper, we analyzed the phenotype Kv4.2 knockout mice based on their neurological function, on a battery of behaviors including those related to anxiety and depression, and on plasticity-related learning tasks.

Results: We found a novelty-induced hyperactive phenotype in knockout mice, and these mice also displayed increased reactivity to novel stimulus such as an auditory tone. No clear anxiety- or depression-related phenotype was observed, nor any alterations in learning/plasticity-based paradigms.

Conclusions: We did not find clear evidence for an involvement of Kv4.2 in neuropsychiatric or plasticity-related phenotypes, but there was support for a role in Kv4.2 in dampening excitatory responses to novel stimuli.

Background

The excitability and functional plasticity of specific brain circuits in cortical, limbic, and midbrain regions is thought to mediate behavioral responses to environmental threats, and to enable adaptation to stressors. At the cellular level, voltage- and calcium-activated potassium (K+) channels provide an important means of modulating neuronal activity and synaptic plasticity. Their function is further refined via the presence of multiple Kv primary and auxiliary subunits that differ in their voltage-dependence, post-translational regulation, sub-cellular localization and regional pattern of expression in the brain to accomplish distinct physiological functions.

A-type K+ channels composed of Kv4 subunits transmit a rapidly activating and inactivating current [1]. Kv4.2 mRNA is expressed in the periphery and in various brain regions involved in mediating stress-related behaviors, including the medial prefrontal cortex (mPFC), hippocampus and hypothalamus [2]. In CA1 hippocampal neurons, Kv4.2 protein is primarily localized on dendrites [3] where they exert their strongest functional effects [4]. Gene deletion of Kv4.2 (*Kcnd2*) in mice eliminates most of the A-type K+ current in hippocampal and cortical neurons [5-7], and increases back-propagation of the action potential from the axon to the somatodendritic region [6]. These and other effects of Kv4.2 knockout (KO) may be countered to some extent by compensatory increases in the expression of other Kv subunits [8], and increased inhibitory transmission in the hippocampus [9]. Notwithstanding, loss of Kv4.2 function produces a net increase in neuronal, and particularly dendritic, hyperexcitability in the mPFC and hippocampus, and possibly other brain regions in which this subunit is expressed.

Synaptic plasticity is also altered by Kv4.2 deletion, as evidenced by the enhanced CA1 hippocampal long-term potentiation (LTP) and increased threshold for long-term depression (LTD) seen in Kv4.2 (KO) mice [6,10]. Further demonstrating an important contribution to hippocampal plasticity, Kv4.2 channels are internalized during LTP induction, and Kv4.2 overexpression or deletion alters synaptic expression of N-Methyl-D-

* Correspondence: kiselycznykc@mail.nih.gov
[1]Laboratory of Behavioral and Genomic Neuroscience, National Institute on Alcohol Abuse and Alcoholism, NIH, Bethesda, MD, USA
Full list of author information is available at the end of the article

aspartate (NMDA) receptor subunits (GluN2A, GluN2B) to respectively constrain or promote hippocampal LTP [11,12]. Conversely, NMDAR throughput decreases hippocampal Kv4.2 through degradation [13,14] whereas concurrently causing an increase in Kv4.2 translation [15]. The reciprocal relationship between Kv4.2 and NMDA receptor subunits is particularly intriguing in the context of prior studies showing that gene KO of GluN2A [16] or GluN2B [17] disrupts anxiety-related behaviors and adaptations to stress.

Behaviorally, Kv4.2 KO mice are viable and appear grossly normal [18]. However, Kv4.2 KO mice show augmented nociceptive responses to thermal and mechanical stimulation [8] and increased sensitivity to the pro-convulsive effects of kainate, with no apparent increase in spontaneous seizures [19]. Furthermore, in a recent study assessing Kv4.2 KO mice on a 129S6/SvEv-Tac (129S6) background on a range of behavioral assays, Lockridge *et al.* found that the KO mice had reduced grip strength on a wire-hang test and increased locomotor activity in a brightly illuminated open field, but not in a dimly illuminated one [20]. Although the KO mice displayed an increased tendency to enter into the aversive central area of the open field, consistent with an anxiolytic-like phenotype, the mutants were no different from the wild-type (WT) controls in the increased plus-maze test for anxiety-such as behavior. This study also found that Kv4.2 KO mice showed increased immobility in the forced-swim test (FST) (but not the tail-suspension test) for 'depression-related' behavior, and were insensitive to the anti-immobility effects of the antidepressant fluoxetine, but not imipramine or desipramine, in the FST. In addition, *ex vivo* slice physiological recordings indicated that a form of 5-hydroxytryptamine (5-HT)2A receptor-mediated excitatory synaptic transmission in mPFC pyramidal neurons was attenuated in Kv4.2 KO mice after a single forced swim exposure, but only after repeated exposures in WT controls. Based on these findings, Lockridge *et al.* concluded that Kv4.2 deletion produces abnormal behavioral responses to stress, and suggested that this might be related to excessive 5-HT release.

The aim of the present study was to confirm and extend the characterization of Kv4.2 KO mice in stress- and other 'emotion'-related phenotypes. KO mice and WT littermate controls were compared for a battery of sensory and neurological tests (including hot-plate nociception, acoustic startle and prepulse inhibition of startle, and home-cage locomotion), exploratory and anxiety-related behaviors (novel open field, light/dark exploration, elevated plus-maze tests), pavlovian fear conditioning and extinction, and 'depression-related' behavioral responses (single and repeated inescapable forced-swim exposure). Phenotyping was conducted after the mutants were backcrossed onto a C57BL/6J background strain. This is important because genetic background can strongly influence the phenotype of mutant mice [21,22], and the aforementioned studies by Lockridge and colleagues tested the KO mice on a different genetic background (129S6).

Methods

Experimental procedures were performed in accordance with the NIH Guide for Care and Use of Laboratory Animals and were approved by the local Animal Care and Use Committee.

Animals

Kv4.2 KO mice were generated in a 129S6 genetic background as described previously [19]. For the current experiments, mice were backcrossed to the C57BL/6J strain for nine generations. To control for potential effects of maternal genotype [22], KO mice and WT controls were littermates bred from heterozygous parents. Males and females were used. Mice were housed in same-sex groupings in a temperature- and humidity-controlled vivarium under a 12-hour light/dark cycle (lights on at 06.00 hours) and testing conducted during the light phase after 1 hour of acclimation to the test room. Three separate, naïve cohorts were tested. One cohort of mice was screened on a battery of neurological measures, including prepulse inhibition and home-cage activity, and basal home-cage corticosterone levels. A second cohort was tested on a battery of assays for anxiety-, fear- and stress-related phenotypes, with putatively more stressful tests conducted later in the sequence and at least 6 days between each test: novel open field, light/dark exploration, elevated plus maze, pavlovian fear conditioning and extinction, and forced-swim test/swim-induced corticosterone response. A third cohort was tested for behavioral responses to repeated inescapable forced swims. The experimenter remained blinded to genotype during testing. The number of mice tested in each assay is given in the corresponding figure legends.

Initial phenotypic screen

Neurological test battery

Functional observational battery Gross physical and neurological abnormalities were examined using a simple functional observation battery, as described previously [16,23,24]. Basic physical health was evaluated by examining for missing whiskers, bald patches, piloerection, exophthalmus, straub tail, kinked tail, kyphosis, lordosis, core body temperature, reactivity to handling, and body weight. Simple sensory reflexes were measured via orienting responses to an approaching hand and to physical touch via palpebral closure on touch of the eye, twitch of pinna on touch, and an orienting response to tail pinch. Mice were observed for splayed limbs, and forepaw and hind limb clutch when suspended upside-down by the tail, and wild running, freezing, trembling, sniffing, licking, rearing, jumping, seizures, defecation, urination, head bobbing, circling, abnormal gait, retropulsion, and prancing forelimbs when placed in a novel, bare, standard holding cage (130 × 135 × 350 mm) for 1 minute.

Nociception Pain perception was tested using the hot-plate test. a flat plate (Columbus Instruments, Columbus, OH, USA) was heated to 55°C, and the mouse placed upon it. The latency to first hind-paw lick was manually timed, with a maximum response latency of 30 seconds. and genotypes statistically compared via Student's t-test.

Acoustic startle and prepulse inhibition of startle Acoustic startle and prepulse inhibition of startle (PPI) was tested as described previously [25]. The mouse was placed in a clear Plexiglas holding cylinder (San Diego Instruments SR-LAB System; San Diego, CA, USA) for an acclimation period of 5 minutes. A 65-dB broadband background noise was presented during acclimation and throughout the test session. Five pulse-alone trials (120 dB broadband sound pulse for 40 ms) began and ended the session, and were not included in the analysis. Testing consisted of presentation of 120 dB startle trials and prepulse + startle trials (noise prepulse sound for 20 ms, followed 100 ms later by the 40 ms 120-dB broadband sound pulse). There were three different prepulse intensities (3, 6 and 12 dB above background), each presented 10 times with a variable interval (range 12-30 seconds) between each presentation. There were vie pulse-alone trials before and after each prepulse + startle trial. Basal activity in the startle chambers was measured during the no-stimulus trials. Startle amplitude was measured starting from the onset of the startle stimulus via whole-body vibrations (sampled every 1 ms over 65 ms), transduced into analog signals by a piezoelectric unit attached to the platform on which the cylinders rested. This was used to derive an average startle amplitude over the 65 ms recording period. PPI at each prepulse intensity was calculated as:

$$100 - \frac{\text{startle response for prepulse + startle trials}}{\text{startle response for startle} - \text{alone trials}} \times 100$$

The effects of genotype and PPI intensity were analyzed using two-way analysis of variance (ANOVA), with repeated measures for PPI intensity.

Home-cage activity The mouse was individually housed in a standard holding cage as before, and left undisturbed for a 48-hour acclimation period under normal vivarium conditions. Activity was measured over 24 hours using a photocell-based activity monitor (Opto M3; Columbus Instruments, Columbus, OH, USA) and expressed as the 12-hour average activity during the light and dark phase, as described previously [26]. The effects of genotype and circadian phase were analyzed using two-way ANOVA, with repeated measures for cycle.

Battery of anxiety-, fear-, and stress-related behaviors

Anxiety-related behaviors

Novel open field The novel open-field test [27] was conducted as described previously [28] in a 400 × 400 × 350 mm square arena (60 lux) constructed of white Plexiglas. Testing was conducted under 65 dB white noise to minimize external noise disturbances (Sound Screen, Marpac Corporation, Rocky Point, NC, USA). The mouse was placed in the perimeter and allowed to explore the apparatus for 30 minutes. Total distance traveled and time spent in the center square (200 × 200 mm) was measured by a video-tracking system (Ethovision; Noldus Information Technology Inc., Leesburg, VA, USA).

Light-dark exploration test The light-dark exploration test [24] was conducted as described previously [29]. The mouse began the test in an opaque black Plexiglas shelter (390 × 130 × 160 mm) with a 130 × 80 mm opening at floor level that opened onto a large white Plexiglas square arena (390 × 390 × 350 mm) illuminated to approximately 90 lux. Percentage time spent in the lighted compartment, frequency of entering the lighted compartment, and total distance traveled in the entire apparatus over a 15 min session were measured by a video-tracking system (Ethovision Noldus Information Technology Inc). Mice that did not enter the lighted compartment were recorded as having a latency to exit time of 900 seconds. Genotypes were compared using Student's t-test.

Elevated plus-maze The elevated plus-maze test [30] was conducted as described previously [31]. The apparatus consisted of two open arms (300 × 50 mm; 90 lux) and two closed arms (300 × 50 × 150 mm; 20 lux), extending from a 50 × 50 mm central area and elevated 200 mm from the ground (San Diego Instruments, San Diego, CA, USA). The walls were made from black acrylonitrile butadiene styrene (ABS) plastic and the floor from white ABS plastic. A 50 mm high raised lip around the perimeter of the open arms prevented the mice from falling off the maze. Testing was conducted under 65 dB white noise (Sound Screen, Marpac Corporation, Rocky Point, NC, USA) to minimize external noise disturbance. The mouse was placed in the center of the maze facing an open arm, and allowed to explore the apparatus for 6 minutes. Time spent in the open arms and number of entries into the open and closed arms were measured by a video-tracking system (Ethovision Noldus Information

Technology Inc). Genotypes were compared using Student's t-test.

Fear-related behaviors

Pavlovian fear conditioning and extinction Pavlovian fear conditioning and extinction was assessed as described previously [32,33]. The mouse was placed in context A: a 270 × 270 × 110 mm chamber with transparent walls and a metal rod floor. To provide a distinctive olfactory environment, the chamber was cleaned between subjects with a 79% ethanol/20% water/1% vanilla extract solution. After acclimation period of 180 seconds, the mouse received three pairings (interval of 60-120 seconds after each pairing) of an auditory tone (30 seconds, 80 dB, white noise) and footshock (2 seconds, 0.6 mA scrambled footshock), in which the shock was presented during the last 2 seconds of the tone. The presentation of stimuli was controlled by a freeze monitoring system (Med Associates Inc, Georgia, VT, USA).

Twenty-four hours later, expression of fear to the tone and subsequent within-session extinction was tested. Mice were placed in context B: a novel context (Plexiglas cylinder with black/white-checkered walls and a solid floor, cleaned with a 1% acetic acid/99% water solution) housed in a novel room. After an initial acclimation period of 180 seconds, the mouse received 500 presentations of the tone alone (each tone for 30 seconds, with a no-stimulus interval of 5 seconds). Twenty-four hours later, extinction retrieval was probed with three tone presentations in context A. Four hours later, mice were presented with three tones in context B to assess fear renewal.

Freezing (no visible movement except that required for respiration) in response to the tone was manually scored every 5 seconds and converted to a percentage:

(number of freezing observations/total number of observations × 100).

Freezing during extinction trials were averaged into 100 five-trial blocks for analysis, and the first and last trial blocks compared. The effect of genotype and trial/trial block during conditioning and extinction were analyzed using two-factor ANOVA, with repeated measures for trial/trial block, followed by Bonferroni *post hoc* tests. The effect of genotype on extinction retrieval and fear renewal were analyzed using Student's t-test.

Responses to swim stressors

Forced-swim test behavior and corticosterone response The forced-swim test [34] was conducted as described previously [35]. The mouse was gently lowered into a 200 mm-diameter cylinder filled with water 24 ± 1.0°C for test lasting 6 minutes. Immobility (cessation of limb movements except for minor movement necessary to keep the mouse afloat) was manually scored every 5 seconds during minute 3 to 6. Genotypes were compared using Student's t-test.

Mice were returned to the home cage for 30 minutes after forced swim, and then killed via cervical dislocation and decapitated. The trunk blood was collected, left to coagulate at room temperature for 1-2 hours, and then separated by centrifugation at 4°C for 30 seconds at 13,000 rpm (20000 x g). Serum was collected and analyzed for corticosterone (bound and free) using a commercial radioimmunoassay (MP Biomedicals, Orangeburg, NY) as described previously [36]. Genotypes were compared using Student's t-test.

Repeated inescapable forced swim The repeated inescapable forced-swim (riFS) test was conducted as described previously [17]. The mouse was gently lowered into a cylinder filled with water at 24 ± 1.0°C. The cylinder was of a larger diameter (300 mm) than that used for the forced-swim test used above (200 mm) and had a 40 × 40 mm escape hole located 40 mm above the waterline and out of reach for the mouse. A platform (plastic wiffle ball) was magnetically held 100 mm below the water, also out of reach. After 1 minute, the platform was remotely released (by turning off the magnet) and quickly (within < 2 seconds) floated vertically upwards along a pole to sit on top of the water, directly under the escape hole. If the mouse attempted to climb onto or hold the platform, it sank below the water. The test terminated 20 seconds after the platform was presented, regardless of the number of attempts by the mouse to use it to reach the escape hole. There was one trial per day (10.00 to 12.00 hours) for 10 consecutive days. Immobility was manually scored every 5 seconds during the 1 minute before platform presentation. The effect of genotype and trial were analyzed using two-way ANOVA, with repeated measures for trial.

Statistical analysis

Knockout and wildtype mice were compared using Student's t-test with the exception of the prepulse inhibition of startle, home cage activity, fear conditioning and extinction, and riFS testing, which was analyzed using a 2-factor analysis of variance (ANOVA) with Bonferroni posttest. The threshold for statistical significance was $P < .05$. GraphPad Prism 5 statistical software (La Jolla, CA) was used for all statistical analysis.

Results

Normal gross behavior and neurological functions

The different genotypes did not differ on most measures of physical health, gross behavior, or neurological functions (Table 1), with the exception of increased rearing seen in KO mice relative to WT controls when placed in an empty cage for 1 min ($t_{(16)} = 2.21$, $P < 0.05$) (Figure 1A). Hot-plate nociception was not different between genotypes (Figure 1B). KO mice also showed

Table 1 Empty-cage behaviors, physical health, sensory reflexes, and neurological functions

Empty-cage behaviors[a]	WT[b]	KO[c]
Freezing	0	0
Trembling	0	0
Sniffing	100	100
Licking	0	0
Rearing	80	100
Jumping	0	0
Seizure	0	0
Defecation	60	25
Urination	0	0
Head bobbing	0	0
Circling	0	0
Abnormal gait	0	0
Retropulsion	0	0
Physical health		
Missing whiskers	0	0
Bald patches	0	0
Exopthalmus	0	0
Straub tail	0	0
Kinked tail	0	0
Kyphosis	0	0
Lordosis	0	0
Body weight, g[e]	23.6 ± 0.8	23.9 ± 1.3
Core body temp, °C[e]	36.2 ± 0.3	36.8 ± 0.1
Sensory reflexes		
Approach response	100	100
Touch response	100	100
Palpebral response	100	100
Pinna reflex	100	100
Tail pinch response	100	100
Motor, neurological		
Splayed limbs	100	100
Forepaw clutch	0	0
Hind-paw clutch	0	0

[a]Data denote the percentage of animals showing a response unless specified otherwise,
[b]Wild-type.
[c]Knockout.
[e]Mean ± SD.

no alterations in acoustic startle compared with WT controls (Figure 1C). There was a significant effect of prepulse intensity ($F_{(2,32)}$ = 35.65, $P < 0.01$) but not of genotype, and no intensity × genotype interaction for PPI (Figure 1D). There was a significant effect of circadian phase for home-cage activity ($F_{(1,15)}$ = 23.94, $P <$ 0.01), with both genotypes showing more activity during the dark phase than the light phase (Figure 1E) (after one mouse per genotype with outlying scores (> 2 SD) were excluded). There was no effect of genotype or phase × genotype interaction for home-cage activity.

Increased exploratory locomotion and test-specific decreased anxiety-like behavior

In the novel open-field test, time-course analysis revealed a significant effect of genotype ($F_{(1,18)}$ = 13.70, $P < 0.01$) and time bin ($F_{(5,90)}$ = 14.13, $P < 0.01$), but no interaction for distance traveled (Figure 2A). KO mice traveled significantly farther than WT controls over the whole session ($t_{(18)}$ = 3.70, $P < 0.01$) (Figure 2B). Genotypes did not differ in the time spent in the center of the open field (Figure 2C).

In the light/dark exploration test, genotypes did not differ in percentage time (Figure 2D) or entries into (Figure 2E) the lighted compartment during the first or last (data not shown) 5 minutes. Genotypes also did not differ in distance traveled in both compartments during the first (data not shown) or last 5 minutes of the session (Figure 2F).

In the elevated plus maze, KO mice spent significantly more time in the open arms ($t_{(17)}$ = 2.30, $P < 0.05$) (Figure 2G), and made significantly more entries into the open arms ($t_{(17)}$ = 2.52, $P < 0.05$) (Figure 2H), compared with WT controls. Genotypes did not differ in the number of entries into the closed arms (Figure 2I). One WT mouse with outlying (> 2 SD) was excluded from each of the three elevated plus maze measures (time in open arms, open-arm entries, closed-arm entries).

Increased freezing to unconditioned auditory tones

During conditioning, there was significant interaction between the conditioned stimulus (CS) trial and genotype ($F_{(1,21)}$ = 6.28, $P < 0.05$) for freezing to the CS tone. *Post hoc* tests revealed higher freezing to the first (that is, before any foot shock) and second CS trial but not to the third CS trial in KO mice (Figure 3A).

During extinction training, there was a significant effect of trial block ($F_{(9,189)}$ = 15.25, $P < 0.01$), and significant reduction in freezing to the last five tones compared with the first five ($F_{(1,21)}$ = 61.35, $P < 0.01$). However, there was no effect of genotype or trial block × genotype interaction for freezing (Figure 3B).

Genotypes did not differ in freezing to the CS during either the extinction-retrieval (Figure 3C) or context-renewal tests (Figure 3D). Freezing during the baseline pre-CS periods was negligible, and was not different between genotypes for extinction training (WT = 9.5 ± 2.4, KO = 6.4 ± 1.4) or retrieval (WT = 4.2 ± 1.2, KO = 1.2 ± 1.2).

Exaggerated swim-induced corticosterone and normal 'depression-related' responses to single and repeated forced swim

During a single forced-swim exposure, genotypes did not differ in percentage of time spent immobile (Figure 4A). However, serum corticosterone levels after this

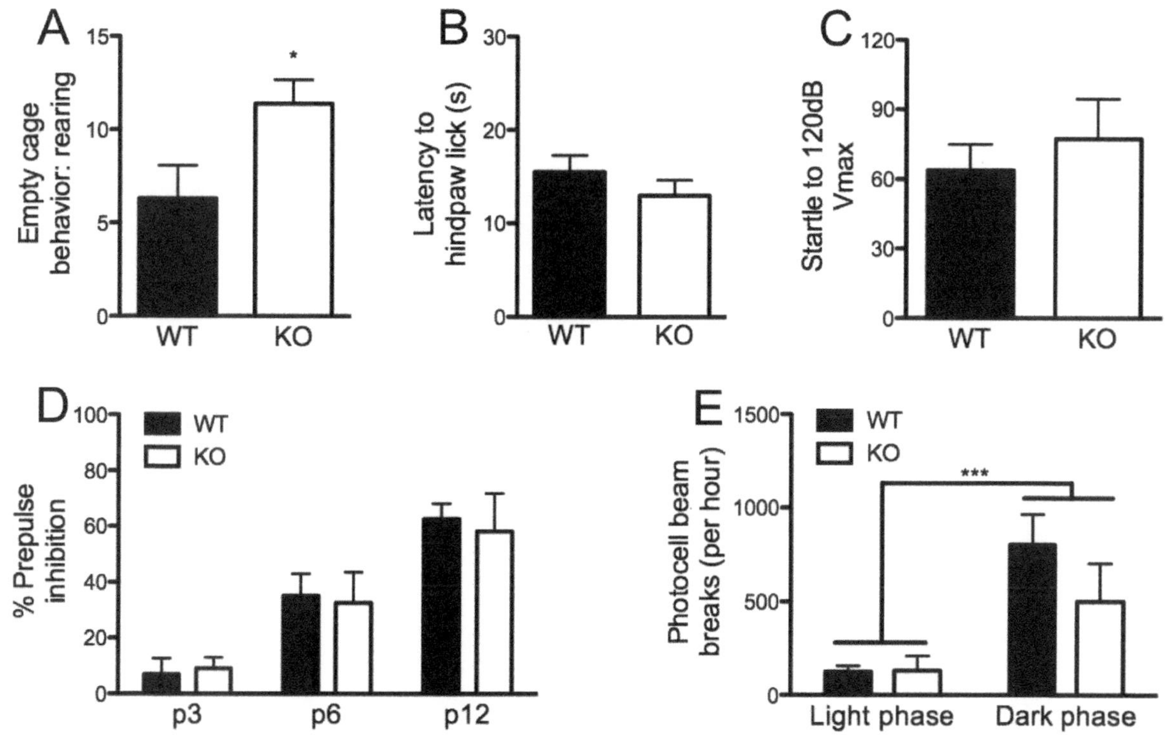

Figure 1 Increased exploratory rearing in Kv4.2 knockout (KO) mice. (A) KO mice showed more rearing behavior than wild-type (WT) controls in a novel empty-cage environment. **(B)** Genotypes did not differ in nociception as measured by the hot-plate tes, or in **(C)** the acoustic startle response **(D)** or prepulse inhibition of startle. **(E)** Light and dark phase home-cage activity was similar between genotypes. Data are mean ± SEM; n = 8-10/genotype. $^*P < 0.05$; $^{**}P < 0.01$.

swim exposure were significantly higher in KO mice than WT controls ($t_{(19)} = 3.27$, $P < 0.01$) (Figure 4B). Based on this genotype difference, a separate cohort of stress-naïve mice was killed immediately on removal from the cage for corticosterone analysis. Corticosterone levels did not differ between genotypes under these non-stressed conditions (WT = 40.4 ± 4.3 mg/mL, KO = 109.5 ± 41.8 mg/mL). Three WT and one KO sample were removed because of errors in the blood-collection assay.

On the riFS test, there was a significant effect of trial ($F_{(9,270)}$_ = 27.85, $P < 0.01$) but not of genotype, and no trial × genotype interaction for percentage immobility (Figure 4D).

Discussion

The aim of the current study was to examine the effects of deleting the A-type voltage-gated K+ channel Kv4.2 on multiple stress- and other 'emotion'-related phenotypes. We found a complex set of significant phenotypic alterations in Kv4.2 mice. These included increased exploratory activity in novel environments, test-specific decreases in anxiety-like behavior, increased fear response to auditory stimuli, and an exaggerated corticosterone response to stress.

Consistent with previous studies [19], an initial observational battery showed no gross alterations in various measures of health or sensory function in the Kv4.2 knockout; however, this analysis did reveal increased rearing in the KO mice, suggestive of heightened levels of exploratory behavior. Similarly, exploratory locomotion in a novel open field was robustly increased in the KO mice, at least over a 30 minute session (longer sessions were not examined). These genotype effects did not seem to reflect generalized locomotor hyperactivity in the mutants, as evidenced by normal levels of activity in the familiar and low-stress environment of the home cage. Rather, these data suggest that Kv4.2 deletion produced an augmented behavioral reaction to novel and/ or stressful environments.

This behavioral phenotype may be related to the neural abnormalities that have been reported in Kv4.2 KO mice. For example, these mice have been found to exhibit neuronal and dendritic hyperexcitability due to increased axonal back-propagation [6]. Interestingly in this context, we have previously identified a similar

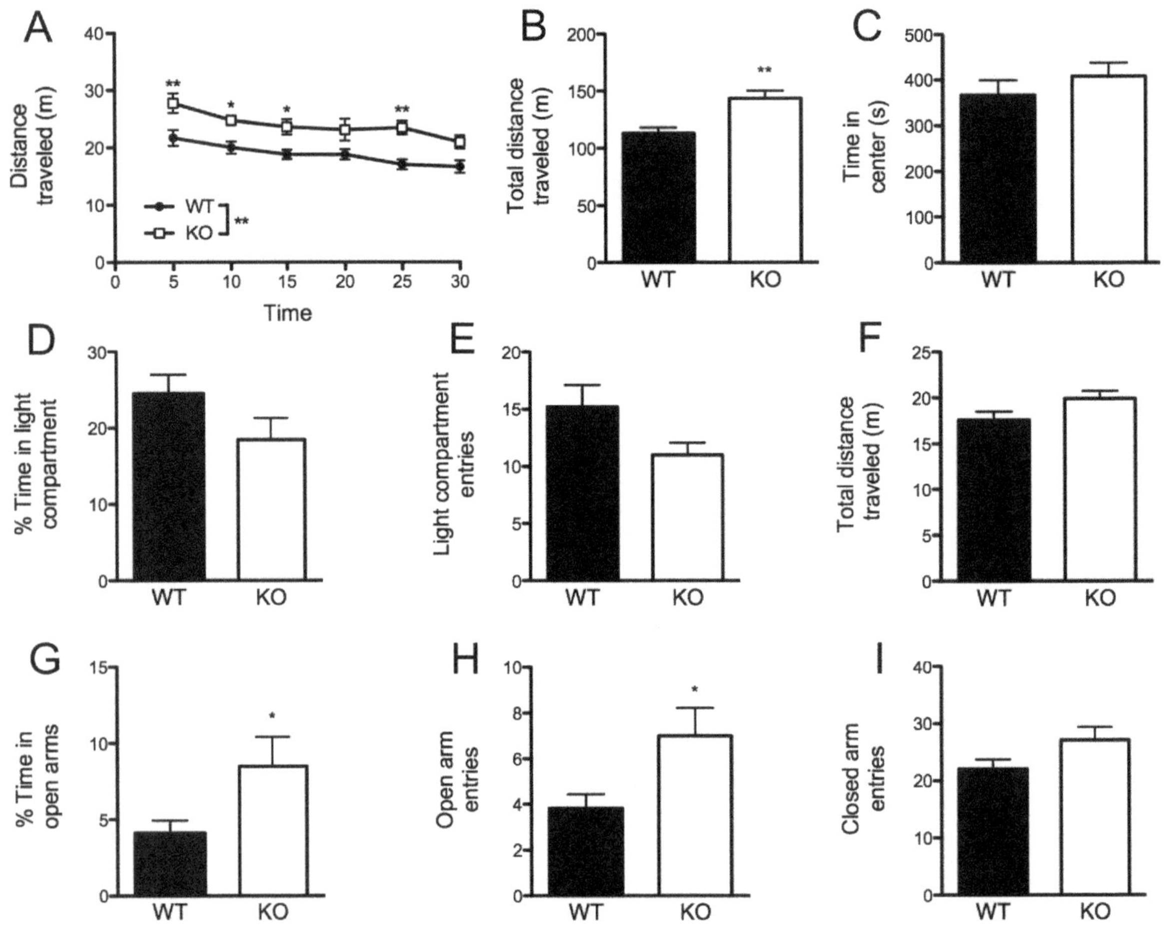

Figure 2 Increased open-field locomotor activity and test-specific decreases in anxiety-like behavior in Kv4.2 knockout (KO) mice. KO mice traveled farther than wild-type (WT) controls in a novel open-field test, as shown via **(A)** a time-course analysis) and **(B)** over the full session. **(C)** Time spent in the center of the open field did not differ between genotypes. In the light/dark exploration test, genotypes did not differ in **(D)** percentage time spent in the lighted compartment, **(E)** entries into the lighted compartment or **(F)** distance traveled throughout the apparatus. In the elevated plus maze, KO mice spent a greater percentage of the session **(G)** in the open arms and made more entries into **(H)** the open arms, but not into **(I)** the closed arms, compared with wild-type (WT) controls. Data are mean ± SEM; n = 8-12/genotype. *$P < 0.05$; **$P < 0.01$.

profile in the same behavioral assays after deletions of other genes involved in regulating neuronal excitability, such as components of the glutamate signaling system [16,37,38]. This overlap indicates that genetic loss of molecules involved in regulating neuronal excitability and synaptic plasticity produces some convergent phenotypic effects on novelty-driven behavioral reactivity. Although hyperlocomotion in a novel environment is often taken as a measure relevant to schizophrenia [39,40], the Kv4.2 KO mice in the present study did not show changes in another schizophrenia-relevant measure, prepulse inhibition of startle, unlike our findings in previous studies of glutamate deletions. Therefore, without additional experiments to interrogate this issue further, it would be premature discuss the Kv4.2 KO phenotype in terms of potential relevance to that disease.

Novelty-induced hyperactivity can confound interpretation of behavior in tests for anxiety-like behavior due to non-specific increases in activity [41]. However, we found that Kv4.2 KO mice were no different from WT controls in the light/dark exploration test and showed increased open-arm exploration in the elevated plus maze, which was not associated with increased general locomotor activity in this test (as measured by the number of closed-arm entries). This suggests a test-specific anxiolytic-like phenotype in the KO mice, albeit with the caveat that the classic conflict-based assays for

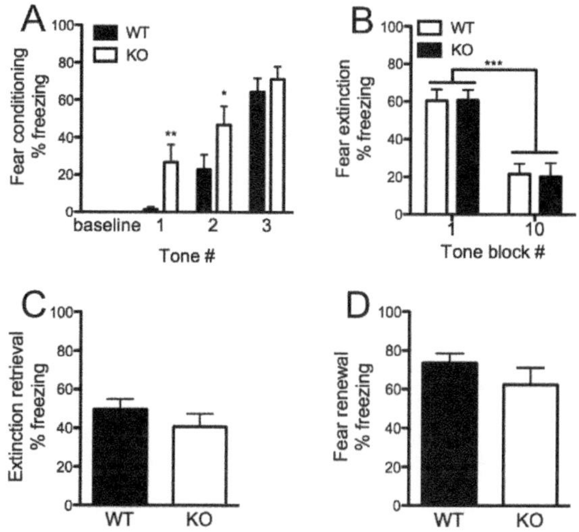

Figure 3 Increased freezing to unconditioned tones in Kv4.2 knockout (KO) mice. (A) During conditioning KO mice froze more than wild-type (WT) controls during the first (before conditioning) and second conditioned stimulus (CS) presentation trials. **(B)** Genotypes showed equivalent initial freezing and similar reductions in freezing from the first to the last five CS trial block during extinction training. Genotypes did not differ in freezing during **(C)** extinction retrieval or **(D)** fear renewal. Data are mean ± SEM; n = 8-12/genotype. *$P < 0.05$; **$P < 0.01$.

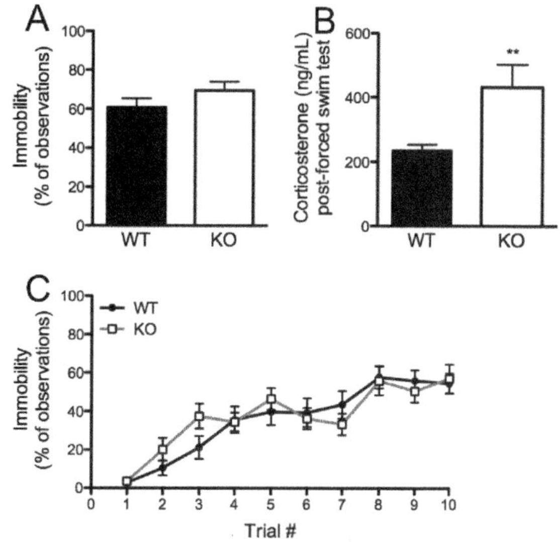

Figure 4 Exaggerated swim-induced corticosterone and normal responses to swim stressors in Kv4.2 knockout (KO) mice. (A) Genotypes did not differ in percentage immobility during a single 6-minute forced-swim exposure (n = 9-13/genotype). **(B)** KO mice had significantly raised serum corticosterone levels after the single forced-swim exposure (n = 9-13/genotype). **(C)** Genotypes had a similar increase in percentage immobility increased over 10 × 1-min inescapable forced swim exposures (n = 14-18/genotype). Data are mean ± SEM. **$P < 0.01$.

anxiety-like behavior cannot unequivocally parse an anxiety-like decrease in avoidance from a novelty-driven increase in approach [41]. Notwithstanding, the test-specific nature of this phenotype is notable, and echoes earlier studies showing that the elevated plus maze can be particularly sensitive to certain gene mutations, possibly because it is inherently more stressful than ostensibly similar tests such as the light/dark exploration [42]. This would generally fit with a profile of exaggerated behavioral responses of Kv4.2 KO mice, particularly under conditions of strong environmental 'provocation.'

Consistent with this interpretation, the KO mice showed increased unconditioned freezing to an auditory stimulus, and an augmented corticosterone response to a single exposure to the forced-swim test. By contrast, the behavioral response (immobility) to forced swim, a very stressful and 'provocative' situation, was normal in the KO mice. Increases in immobility produced by repeated, brief, forced-swim exposures were also similar between KO mice and WT controls. Thus, increased behavioral reactivity in the mutants does not generalize to altered immobility during various forms of forced-swim exposure. One explanation is enhanced tonic inhibitory transmission [9] served to mitigate the penetrance of the phenotype under forced-swim conditions.

The absence of changes in forced-swim tests in the current study differs from the previous finding by Lockridge *et al.* that these mice showed increased immobility in the forced-swim test [20]. Indeed, whereas the earlier report found, as we did, novel open field hyperactivity, some other differences were seen in the earlier study, including no change in elevated plus maze anxiety-like behavior. Other than methodological variations, the principal salient factor potentially explaining these apparent discrepancies is genetic background. Kv4.2 KO mice were bred on a C57BL/6J background for the current study and a 129S6 background for the previous study. Genetic background can have a profound influence on the penetrance and expression of emotion-related phenotypes in mutant mice, because of epistatic interactions between a mutation and modifier genes [21,22]. It seems likely that such interactions shaped the phenotypic profile of the Kv4.2 KO mice, and it would be interesting to explore this further by identifying the responsible modifiers.

Another important avenue for future studies will involve assessment of Kv4.2 KO mice for learning and memory. The mutants have enhanced hippocampal synaptic plasticity [6,10], which is associated with altered synaptic expression of synaptic proteins that are strongly implicated in learning by mutant studies [23,43-45], such as the NMDA receptor GluN2A and GluN2B subunits [11-13]. In the current study we found that the KO mice displayed normal amygdala-mediated fear learning and mPFC-mediated fear extinction. Given the localization of synaptic alterations to the hippocampus, it will be valuable to supplement these findings by assessing Kv4.2 KO mice for hippocampal-dependent forms of learning.

Conclusions

In summary, we found that constitutive deletion of the A-type voltage-gated K+ channel Kv4.2 produced a behavioral phenotype principally characterized by increased behavioral reactivity to exposure to some but not all novel environmental situations. This largely confirms earlier evaluation of these mice, although some discrepancies were found, possibly due to the influence of genetic background. These behavioral abnormalities extend the finding that deletion of Kv4.2 leads to exaggerated neuronal excitability in cortical and hippocampal regions involved in emotion regulation. These data shed further light on the role of Kv4.2 in regulating neural and behavioral functions.

List of abbreviations

5-HT: 5-hydroxytryptamine; ABS: acrylonitrile butadiene styrene; CS: conditioned stimulus; KO: knockout; LTD: long-term depression; LTP: long-term potentiation; mPFC: medial prefrontal cortex; NMDA: N-Methyl-D-aspartate; PPI: prepulse inhibition of startle; WT: wild-type.

Acknowledgements

We thank Begum Choudhary and Heather Cameron for technical assistance. Funding was provided by the National Institute of Mental Health and the National Institute of Alcohol Abuse and Alcoholism Intramural Research Program.

Author details

[1]Laboratory of Behavioral and Genomic Neuroscience, National Institute on Alcohol Abuse and Alcoholism, NIH, Bethesda, MD, USA. [2]Molecular Neurophysiology and Biophysics Unit, Laboratory of Cellular and Synaptic Neurophysiology, Eunice Kennedy Shriver National Institute of Child Health and Human Development, NIH, Bethesda, MD, USA.

Authors' contributions

CK carried out the behavioral testing and drafted the manuscript, DH generated the Kv4.2 mice and aided in manuscript revision, and AH conceived of the study and helped draft the manuscript. All authors read and approved the final manuscript.

Competing interests

The authors declare that they have no competing interests.

References

1. Shah MM, Hammond RS, Hoffman DA: **Dendritic ion channel trafficking and plasticity.** *Trends Neurosci* 2010, **33(7)**:307-16.
2. Serodio P, Rudy B: **Differential expression of Kv4 K+ channel subunits mediating subthreshold transient K+ (A-type) currents in rat brain.** *J Neurophysiol* 1998, **79(2)**:1081-91.
3. Sheng M, *et al*: **Subcellular segregation of two A-type K+ channel proteins in rat central neurons.** *Neuron* 1992, **9(2)**:271-84.
4. Hoffman DA, *et al*: **K+ channel regulation of signal propagation in dendrites of hippocampal pyramidal neurons.** *Nature* 1997, **387(6636)**:869-75.
5. Kim J, Wei DS, Hoffman DA: **Kv4 potassium channel subunits control action potential repolarization and frequency-dependent broadening in rat hippocampal CA1 pyramidal neurones.** *J Physiol* 2005, **569(Pt 1)**:41-57.
6. Chen X, *et al*: **Deletion of Kv4.2 gene eliminates dendritic A-type K+ current and enhances induction of long-term potentiation in hippocampal CA1 pyramidal neurons.** *J Neurosci* 2006, **26(47)**:12143-51.
7. Nerbonne JM, *et al*: **Electrical remodelling maintains firing properties in cortical pyramidal neurons lacking KCND2-encoded A-type K+ currents.** *J Physiol* 2008, **586(6)**:1565-79.
8. Hu HJ, *et al*: **The kv4.2 potassium channel subunit is required for pain plasticity.** *Neuron* 2006, **50(1)**:89-100.
9. Andrasfalvy BK, *et al*: **Altered synaptic and non-synaptic properties of CA1 pyramidal neurons in Kv4.2 knockout mice.** *J Physiol* 2008, **586(16)**:3881-92.
10. Zhao C, *et al*: **Dendritic mechanisms controlling the threshold and timing requirement of synaptic plasticity.** *Hippocampus* 2010.
11. Kim J, *et al*: **Regulation of dendritic excitability by activity-dependent trafficking of the A-type K+ channel subunit Kv4.2 in hippocampal neurons.** *Neuron* 2007, **54(6)**:933-47.
12. Jung SC, Hoffman DA: **Biphasic somatic A-type K channel downregulation mediates intrinsic plasticity in hippocampal CA1 pyramidal neurons.** *PLoS One* 2009, **4(8)**:e6549.
13. Lei Z, *et al*: **Downregulation of Kv4.2 channels mediated by NR2B-containing NMDA receptors in cultured hippocampal neurons.** *Neuroscience* 2010, **165(2)**:350-62.
14. Lei Z, Deng P, Xu ZC: **Regulation of Kv4.2 channels by glutamate in cultured hippocampal neurons.** *J Neurochem* 2008, **106(1)**:182-92.
15. Lee HY, *et al*: **Bidirectional regulation of dendritic voltage-gated potassium channels by the fragile x mental retardation protein.** *Neuron* 2011, **72(4)**:630-42.
16. Boyce-Rustay JM, Holmes A: **Genetic inactivation of the NMDA receptor NR2A subunit has anxiolytic- and antidepressant-like effects in mice.** *Neuropsychopharmacology* 2006, **31(11)**:2405-14.
17. Kiselycznyk CL, *et al*: **Genetic, pharmacological and lesion analyses reveal a selective role for corticohippocampal GLUN2B in a novel repeated swim stress paradigm.** *Neuroscience* 2011.
18. Guo W, *et al*: **Targeted deletion of Kv4.2 eliminates I(to, f) and results in electrical and molecular remodeling, with no evidence of ventricular hypertrophy or myocardial dysfunction.** *Circ Res* 2005, **97(12)**:1342-50.
19. Barnwell LF, *et al*: **Kv4.2 knockout mice demonstrate increased susceptibility to convulsant stimulation.** *Epilepsia* 2009, **50(7)**:1741-51.
20. Lockridge A, Su J, Yuan LL: **Abnormal 5-HT modulation of stress behaviors in the Kv4.2 knockout mouse.** *Neuroscience* 2010, **170(4)**:1086-97.
21. Holmes A, Hariri AR: **The serotonin transporter gene-linked polymorphism and negative emotionality: placing single gene effects in the context of genetic background and environment.** *Genes Brain Behav* 2003, **2(6)**:332-5.
22. Crusio WE, *et al*: **Standards for the publication of mouse mutant studies.** *Genes Brain Behav* 2009, **8(1)**:1-4.
23. Brigman JL, *et al*: **Loss of GluN2B-containing NMDA receptors in CA1 hippocampus and cortex impairs long-term depression, reduces dendritic spine density, and disrupts learning.** *J Neurosci* 2010, **30(13)**:4590-600.
24. Crawley JN, Paylor R: **A proposed test battery and constellations of specific behavioral paradigms to investigate the behavioral phenotypes of transgenic and knockout mice.** *Horm Behav* 1997, **31(3)**:197-211.
25. Millstein RA, *et al*: **Effects of repeated maternal separation on prepulse inhibition of startle across inbred mouse strains.** *Genes Brain Behav* 2006, **5(4)**:346-54.
26. Feyder M, *et al*: **Association of mouse Dlg4 (PSD-95) gene deletion and human DLG4 gene variation with phenotypes relevant to autism spectrum disorders and Williams' syndrome.** *Am J Psychiatry* 2010, **167(12)**:1508-17.
27. Hall C, Ballachey EL: **A study of the rat's behavior in a field. A contribution to method in comparative psychology.** University of California Publications in Psychology; 1932:**6**:1-12.

28. Karlsson RM, *et al*: **Assessment of glutamate transporter GLAST (EAAT1)-deficient mice for phenotypes relevant to the negative and executive/cognitive symptoms of schizophrenia.** *Neuropsychopharmacology* 2009, **34(6)**:1578-89.
29. Mozhui K, *et al*: **Strain differences in stress responsivity are associated with divergent amygdala gene expression and glutamate-mediated neuronal excitability.** *J Neurosci* 2010, **30(15)**:5357-67.
30. Handley SL, Mithani S: **Effects of alpha-adrenoceptor agonists and antagonists in a maze-exploration model of 'fear'-motivated behaviour.** *Naunyn Schmiedebergs Arch Pharmacol* 1984, **327(1)**:1-5.
31. Fegley DB, *et al*: **Increased fear- and stress-related anxiety-like behavior in mice lacking tuberoinfundibular peptide of 39 residues.** *Genes Brain Behav* 2008, **7(8)**:933-42.
32. Davis AR, *et al*: **Yohimbine impairs extinction of cocaine-conditioned place preference in an alpha2-adrenergic receptor independent process.** *Learn Mem* 2008, **15(9)**:667-76.
33. Yang RJ, *et al*: **Variation in Mouse Basolateral Amygdala Volume is Associated With Differences in Stress Reactivity and Fear Learning.** *Neuropsychopharmacology* 2008.
34. Porsolt RD, Bertin A, Jalfre M: **"Behavioural despair" in rats and mice: strain differences and the effects of imipramine.** *Eur J Pharmacol* 1978, **51(3)**:291-4.
35. Brigman JL, *et al*: **Pharmacological or genetic inactivation of the serotonin transporter improves reversal learning in mice.** *Cereb Cortex* 2010, **20(8)**:1955-63.
36. Boyce-Rustay JM, Cameron HA, Holmes A: **Chronic swim stress alters sensitivity to acute behavioral effects of ethanol in mice.** *Physiol Behav* 2007, **91(1)**:77-86.
37. Karlsson RM, Heilig M, Holmes A: **Loss of Glial Glutamate and Aspartate Transporter (Excitatory Amino Acid Transporter 1) Causes Locomotor Hyperactivity and Exaggerated Responses to Psychotomimetics: Rescue by Haloperidol and Metabotropic Glutamate 2/3 Agonist.** *Biol Psychiatry* 2008.
38. Wiedholz LM, *et al*: **Mice lacking the AMPA GluR1 receptor exhibit striatal hyperdopaminergia and 'schizophrenia-related' behaviors.** *Mol Psychiatry* 2008, **13(6)**:631-40.
39. Arguello PA, Gogos JA: **Modeling madness in mice: one piece at a time.** *Neuron* 2006, **52(1)**:179-96.
40. Powell CM, Miyakawa T: **Schizophrenia-relevant behavioral testing in rodent models: a uniquely human disorder?** *Biol Psychiatry* 2006, **59(12)**:1198-207.
41. Cryan JF, Holmes A: **The ascent of mouse: advances in modelling human depression and anxiety.** *Nat Rev Drug Discov* 2005, **4(9)**:775-90.
42. Holmes A, *et al*: **Galanin GAL-R1 receptor null mutant mice display increased anxiety like behavior specific to the elevated plus maze.** *Neuropsychopharmacology* 2003, **28(6)**:1031-44.
43. Brigman JL, *et al*: **Impaired discrimination learning in mice lacking the NMDA receptor NR2A subunit.** *Learn Mem* 2008, **15(2)**:50-4.
44. Bannerman DM, *et al*: **NMDA Receptor Subunit NR2A Is Required for Rapidly Acquired Spatial Working Memory But Not Incremental Spatial Reference Memory.** *J Neurosci* 2008, **28(14)**:3623-30.
45. von Engelhardt J, *et al*: **Contribution of hippocampal and extra-hippocampal NR2B-containing NMDA receptors to performance on spatial learning tasks.** *Neuron* 2008, **60(5)**:846-60.

17

Reconceptualizing major depressive disorder as an infectious disease

Turhan Canli[1,2,3,4]

Abstract

In this article, I argue for a reconceptualization of major depressive disorder (major depression) as an infectious disease. I suggest that major depression may result from a parasitic, bacterial, or viral infection and present examples that illustrate possible pathways by which these microorganisms could contribute to the etiology of major depression. I also argue that the reconceptualization of the human body as an ecosystem for these microorganisms and the human genome as a host for non-human exogenous sequences may greatly amplify the opportunity to discover genetic links to the illness. Deliberately speculative, this article is intended to stimulate novel research approaches and expand the circle of researchers taking aim at this vexing illness.

Keywords: Genomics, Virus, Bacterial, Parasite, Depression

Background

Despite decades of substantial research efforts, major depressive disorder (MDD) remains among the most common mental disorders, with a 16.6% lifetime prevalence rate [1]. Pharmacological treatment approaches have not changed during this period, targeting primarily receptor-ligand interactions [2]. These types of antidepressants may bring relief to patients with severe symptoms but are not clinically more effective than placebos in mild to moderate cases [3]. Indeed, recurrence rates of 50% for first-episode patients and of 80% for second-episode patients [4] suggest that the core of the illness goes untreated.

Given this track record, I argue that it is time for an entirely different approach. Instead of conceptualizing MDD as an emotional disorder, I suggest to reconceptualize it as some form of an infectious disease. I propose that future research should conduct a concerted search for parasites, bacteria, or viruses that may play a causal role in the etiology of MDD. I present three arguments why this may be a fruitful endeavor. I have outlined the idea in much greater detail elsewhere [5], but will highlight some key points here.

Correspondence: turhan.canli@stonybrook.edu
[1]Department of Psychology, Stony Brook University, Stony Brook, NY 11794, USA
[2]Department of Radiology, Stony Brook University, Stony Brook, NY 11794, USA
Full list of author information is available at the end of the article

Main text

My first argument is that patients with MDD exhibit sickness behavior. Patients experience loss of energy; they commonly have difficulty getting out of bed and lose interest in the world around them. Although our Western conceptualization puts affective symptoms front-and-center, non-Western patients who meet DSM criteria for major depression report primarily somatic symptoms [6-11], reflecting in part cultural differences in the stigmatization of mental illness.

Yet, studies of inflammatory biomarkers in major depression strongly suggest an illness-related origin. For example, a meta-analysis of 24 studies confirmed prior reports of elevated TNFα and IL-6 in patients with major depression [12]. A second meta-analysis of 29 studies further extended the list of significantly elevated inflammatory markers to also include the soluble interleukin-2 receptor [13].

Several postmortem studies report the presence of inflammatory markers in the brains of depressed or mood-disordered patients. For example, compared to controls, female suicide victims showed elevated levels of IL-4 and male suicide victims showed elevated levels of IL-13 in Brodmann Area (BA) 11 [14], a brain region previously associated with suicidal ideation [15,16]. Compared to age-matched controls, patients diagnosed with major depression showed elevated levels of transmembrane TNFα (tmTNFα) in BA46 [17], a region associated with emotion regulation [18-20]. Patients with major depression, relative to controls, showed differential expression of a large set of both anti- and pro-inflammatory markers (including IL1α, 2, 3, 5, 8, 9, 10, 12A, 13, 15, 18, and IFNγ) in BA10 [21], a region associated with reward processing [22].

These inflammatory markers may represent activation of the immune system in response to some kind of pathogen, which could be a parasite, bacterium, or virus, and which could play a causal role in the etiology of depression. There is currently no direct evidence that major depression is caused by such microorganisms, but nature has offered some examples to illustrate that such a process is conceivable.

Thus, my second argument is that nature has already provided examples by which parasites, bacteria, or viruses can affect emotional behavior. The best-known example of a parasite that affects emotional behavior and that is relevant to human health is *Toxoplasma gondii. T. gondii* lives in the feline intestinal tract, where it lays its eggs, which are dispersed into the environment upon excretion. When a rat comes in contact with these eggs and becomes infected, it becomes attracted to the scent of cat urine [23,24]. This manipulation of the rat's behavior involves the deposit of parasitic cysts across the rodent brain including the amygdala [25]. The mechanism for loss of fear to the scent of cat urine appears to involve a reduction in circulating corticosterone and dendritic retraction in the basolateral amygdala [26]. The mechanism for the rat's attraction to the odor may involve activation of sexual arousal pathways [27].

The specificity of the behavioral change in the rat's behavior appears to reflect functional changes that are limited to catecholaminergic neurons [28]. Infected animals have elevated levels of dopamine [29], but *T. gondii* can only synthesize tyrosine hydroxylase (which converts tyrosine to L-DOPA), and would therefore need to rely on catecholaminergic neurons to provide the needed DOPA decarboxylase to convert the L-DOPA to dopamine.

Human exposure to *T. gondii* is pervasive, with one-third of the world's population [30] and one-fifth of the U.S. population [31] believed to be infected. Infection is associated with elevated inflammatory cytokines IL-6, IL-12, TNF, and IFN-γ [32,33], similarly as observed in depressed patients. A study of 20 European countries reported a positive correlation between *T. gondii* prevalence rates and national suicide rates [34]. Among patients with diagnosed major depression or bipolar disorder, those with a history of suicide attempt had higher *T. gondii* antibody titers [35]. Yet, large-scale studies of major depression and *T. gondii* or systematic searches to discover other potential parasitic infections have not yet been conducted.

Bacteria could be another causal factor for major depression. Studies of bacterial colonies residing in the gastrointestinal tract have begun to examine links to emotional behavior. In the first study of this kind, germ-free (GF), specific pathogen-free (SPF), and gnotobiotic mice were compared in their response to restraint stress [36]. GF mice exhibited higher levels of plasma ACTH and corticosterone and had lower levels of brain-derived neurotrophic factor in the cortex and hippocampus, compared to SPF mice. The elevated stress response of GF mice was normalized with administration of the bacterium *Bifidobacterium infantis.* Another rodent study showed that administration of *B. infantis* in rats reduced the levels of IFN-γ, TNF-α, and IL-6 following mitogen stimulation and altered tryptophan, 5-HIAA, and DOPAC levels in the frontal cortex and amygdala [37]. Administration of the *Lactobacillus rhamnosus* strain in mice was shown to alter GABAergic expression in the brain: elevating $GABA_{B1b}$ mRNA in the cingulate and prelimbic cortices, while reducing it in hippocampus and amygdala, among other regions [38].

The 'leaky gut' hypothesis proposes a mechanism by which gastrointestinal bacteria may contribute to major depression [39,40]. According to this hypothesis, cytokines or other stressors may render the intestinal tract permeable to lipopolysaccharides (LPS) from gram-negative bacteria to activate the immune system. Indeed, the model is supported by data showing elevated serum concentrations of IgM and IgA against LPS of the gram-negative enterobacteria in depressed patients [39,40]. These studies were conducted with relatively small numbers of patients and suggested that this mechanism may apply to some subgroups of patients but not others. It would be useful to expand the search using large patient cohorts and a wide range of different antibodies. Future work should then examine potential neural mechanisms.

Viruses represent the third pathogenic route in the etiology of major depression. A meta-analysis of 28 studies explicitly examined the link between infectious agents and depression [41]. Among viruses that had significant associations with the illness were the Borna disease virus (BDV), herpes simplex virus-1, varicella zoster virus, and Epstein-Barr virus. Among these, BDV has been studied most extensively and was 3.25 times more likely to be found in depressed patients than in normal controls [41]. One postmortem study reported BDV infection in 2 out of 30 depressed patients in the frontal and temporal cortex, olfactory bulb, and hippocampus [42], although a larger study failed to detect any infection [43]. A small open-label study of BDV-infected depressed patients reported a reduction in both depressive symptoms and BDV infection upon treatment with the antiviral drug amantadine [44].

The mechanism between BDV infection and depression could involve glutaminergic transmission, because amantadine is an antagonist of the N-methyl-D-aspartate (NMDA) receptor, one of the receptors targeted by glutamate. The related NMDA antagonist memantine has been evaluated in a randomized, double-blind study of patients diagnosed with bipolar depression, where it was applied to augment treatment with the presynaptic glutamate release inhibitor lamotrigine, and found to accelerate treatment response [45]. Another NMDA receptor antagonist, ketamine, also has antidepressant effects [46], which appear to be mediated by changes in mTOR signaling [47]. However, the literature on BDV infection and depression remains controversial, with several studies failing to replicate any association between the two [48-51].

My third argument is that reconceptualizing major depression as being causally linked to parasites, bacteria, or viruses is useful when thinking about the genetics of this illness. Evidence from twin studies notwithstanding, the search for specific genes linked to major depression has come up empty [52,53]. Perhaps, we have been looking at the wrong organism. Genetic studies to date have focused the search on human genes within our genome. Yet, 8% of the human genome is based on exogenous sequences from retroviruses [54]. These retroviral insertions may sometimes benefit the human host and therefore be protected from mutational degeneration [55]. Indeed, the BDV discussed earlier inserted some of its sequences into vertebrate genomes approximately 40 million years ago [56], and presence of these sequences correlates with disease resistance to BDV. Parasites could also add exogenous sequences to the human genome through the process of horizontal gene transfer [57]. It is possible that polymorphisms within such exogenous sequences, or interactions between these exogenous sequences and other variables such as human gene polymorphisms or stressful life experiences, could render some individuals vulnerable to major depression.

Furthermore, if we view the human body as an ecosystem that is a host to numerous microorganisms which may be passed across generations, the opportunity for genetic discoveries is vastly amplified. For example, an estimated thousand species of bacteria reside in the human gastrointestinal tract [58], and these could be passed during birth or through common environmental exposure between parents and offspring [59]. Humans also carry vast numbers of viruses, which can be unknown and go undetected until subjected to a concerted search using new approaches such as deep sequencing [60].

Conclusions

In light of the above considerations, an important point of reflection concerns the relation between the immune response and MDD and the specificity of any putative mechanism. The literature implicating the immune system in MDD [61] can be read as suggesting that the immune response itself is the causal mechanism in depression. Indeed, conditions such as hypoxia known to produce sterile inflammation ([62], i.e., activation of the immune system sans a pathogen) may increase the risk of depression [61] in conditions such as obstructive sleep apnea [63] or chronic obstructive pulmonary disease [64]. Yet, most cases of MDD are not attributable to sterile inflammation. Thus, I suggest that some unknown pathogen(s) could play a causal role, and that the immune response is secondary to the infection; interventions that only target the immune response may bring symptom relief but would not address the root cause of the illness.

If a pathogen played a causal role in MDD, the next question would concern the specificity of the mechanism. One perspective would favor a very general, non-specific mechanism. For example, chronic fatigue syndrome (CFS)—which is characterized by sickness behavior that may include depressive symptoms—has been hypothesized to be caused by vagus nerve infection, regardless of the type of pathogen [65]. My view is that, for MDD, the type of pathogen may matter a great deal, and that it plays a very specific causal role: the examples I presented above suggest plausible mechanisms by which pathogens may alter neurotransmission. However, there may not be a single pathogen that causes all cases of MDD. Instead, there may be a class of pathogens, similar to those discussed above, which share common modes of action. This class of pathogens would specifically target the nervous system in a manner that causally contributes to MDD. I use the term 'contribute' to indicate that these pathogens may act in concert with other variables. For example, an individual may carry a latent infection and be asymptomatic for depressive symptoms. This individual would be characterized by susceptibility to MDD which may only emerge after the pathogen was activated by other factors such as stressful life events; this activation could then also trigger a concomitant immune response. It is possible that such a pathogen-driven mechanism is not limited to MDD but may contribute to other psychopathologies. For example, posttraumatic stress disorder could be one such extension of the same mechanism: not every individual develops the disorder in response to a traumatic experience (suggesting individual differences in susceptibility), and the illness is accompanied by immune system activation [66,67].

In closing, I think it would be worthwhile to conduct large-scale studies of carefully characterized depressed patients and healthy controls, using gold-standard clinical and infectious disease-related study protocols, as have already been developed for bacteria [68,69] and viruses [70-76]. Such efforts, if successful, would represent the 'end of the beginning', as any such discovery would represent the first step toward developing a vaccination for major depression.

Abbreviations
BA: Brodmann Area; BDV: Borna disease virus; GABA: gamma-aminobutyric acid; IFN-γ: interferon gamma; IgA: immunoglobulin A; IgM: immunoglobulin M; IL: interleukin; L-DOPA: L −3,4-dihydroxyphenylalanine; LPS: lipopolysaccharides; MDD: major depressive disorder; NMDA: N-methyl-D-aspartate; TNFα: tumor necrosis factor alpha; tmTNFα: transmembrane tumor necrosis factor alpha.

Competing interests
The author declares that he has no competing interests.

Author details
[1]Department of Psychology, Stony Brook University, Stony Brook, NY 11794, USA.
[2]Department of Radiology, Stony Brook University, Stony Brook, NY 11794, USA.
[3]Program in Genetics, Stony Brook University, Stony Brook, NY 11794, USA.
[4]Program in Neuroscience, Stony Brook University, Stony Brook, NY 11794, USA.

References

1. Kessler RC, Petukhova M, Sampson NA, Zaslavsky AM, Wittchen H-U: **Twelve-month and lifetime prevalence and lifetime morbid risk of anxiety and mood disorders in the United States.** *Int J Methods Psychiatr Res* 2012, **21**:169–184.
2. Agid Y, Buzsaki G, Diamond DM, Frackowiak R, Giedd J, Girault JA, Grace A, Lambert JJ, Manji H, Mayberg H, Popoli M, Prochiantz A, Richter-Levin G, Somogyi P, Spedding M, Svenningsson P, Weinberger D: **How can drug discovery for psychiatric disorders be improved?** *Nat Rev Drug Discov* 2007, **6**:189–201.
3. Kirsch I, Deacon BJ, Huedo-Medina TB, Scoboria A, Moore TJ, Johnson BT: **Initial severity and antidepressant benefits: a meta-analysis of data submitted to the food and drug administration.** *PLoS Med* 2008, **5**:e45.
4. Burcusa SL, Iacono WG: **Risk for recurrence in depression.** *Clin Psychol Rev* 2007, **27**:959–985.
5. Canli T: **Is depression an infectious disease?** In *The Oxford Handbook of Molecular Psychology.* Edited by Canli T. New York: Oxford University Press; 2014. Online Publication Date: Sep 2014. doi:10.1093/oxfordhb/9780199753888.013.28. [http://www.oxfordhandbooks.com/view/10.1093/oxfordhb/9780199753888.001.0001/oxfordhb-9780199753888-e-28]
6. Seifsafari S, Firoozabadi A, Ghanizadeh A, Salehi A: **A symptom profile analysis of depression in a sample of Iranian patients.** *Iran J Med Sci* 2013, **38**:22–29.
7. Wilkowska-Chmielewska J, Szelenberger W, Wojnar M: **Age-dependent symptomatology of depression in hospitalized patients and its implications for DSM-5.** *J Affect Disord* 2013, **150**:142–145.
8. Raguram R, Weiss MG, Channabasavanna SM, Devins GM: **Stigma, depression, and somatization in South India.** *Am J Psychiatry* 1996, **153**:1043–1049.
9. Rao D, Young M, Raguram R: **Culture, somatization, and psychological distress: symptom presentation in South Indian patients from a public psychiatric hospital.** *Psychopathology* 2007, **40**:349–355.
10. Heredia Montesinos A, Rapp MA, Temur-Erman S, Heinz A, Hegerl U, Schouler-Ocak M: **The influence of stigma on depression, overall psychological distress, and somatization among female Turkish migrants.** *Eur Psychiatry* 2012, **27**(Suppl 2):S22–S26.
11. Bagayogo IP, Interian A, Escobar JI: **Transcultural aspects of somatic symptoms in the context of depressive disorders.** *Adv Psychosom Med* 2013, **33**:64–74.
12. Dowlati Y, Herrmann N, Swardfager W, Liu H, Sham L, Reim EK, Lanctot KL: **A meta-analysis of cytokines in major depression.** *Biol Psychiatry* 2010, **67**:446–457.
13. Liu Y, Ho RC, Mak A: **Interleukin (IL)-6, tumour necrosis factor alpha (TNF-alpha) and soluble interleukin-2 receptors (sIL-2R) are elevated in patients with major depressive disorder: a meta-analysis and meta-regression.** *J Affect Disord* 2012, **139**:230–239.
14. Tonelli LH, Stiller J, Rujescu D, Giegling I, Schneider B, Maurer K, Schnabel A, Moller HJ, Chen HH, Postolache TT: **Elevated cytokine expression in the orbitofrontal cortex of victims of suicide.** *Acta Psychiatr Scand* 2008, **117**:198–206.
15. Mann JJ: **Neurobiology of suicidal behaviour.** *Nat Rev Neurosci* 2003, **4**:819–828.
16. Oquendo MA, Placidi GP, Malone KM, Campbell C, Keilp J, Brodsky B, Kegeles LS, Cooper TB, Parsey RV, van Heertum RL, Mann JJ: **Positron emission tomography of regional brain metabolic responses to a serotonergic challenge and lethality of suicide attempts in major depression.** *Arch Gen Psychiatry* 2003, **60**:14–22.
17. Dean B, Tawadros N, Scarr E, Gibbons AS: **Regionally-specific changes in levels of tumour necrosis factor in the dorsolateral prefrontal cortex obtained postmortem from subjects with major depressive disorder.** *J Affect Disord* 2010, **120**:245–248.
18. Silvers JA, Weber J, Wager TD, Ochsner KN: **Bad and worse: neural systems underlying reappraisal of high- and low-intensity negative emotions.** *Soc Cogn Affect Neurosci* first published online March 5, 2014 doi:10.1093/scan/nsu043.
19. Belden AC, Luby JL, Pagliaccio D, Barch DM: **Neural activation associated with the cognitive emotion regulation of sadness in healthy children.** *Dev Cogn Neurosci* 2014, **9**:136–147.
20. Kohn N, Eickhoff SB, Scheller M, Laird AR, Fox PT, Habel U: **Neural network of cognitive emotion regulation–an ALE meta-analysis and MACM analysis.** *Neuroimage* 2014, **87**:345–355.
21. Shelton RC, Claiborne J, Sidoryk-Wegrzynowicz M, Reddy R, Aschner M, Lewis DA, Mirnics K: **Altered expression of genes involved in inflammation and apoptosis in frontal cortex in major depression.** *Mol Psychiatry* 2011, **16**:751–762.
22. Rogers RD, Owen AM, Middleton HC, Williams EJ, Pickard JD, Sahakian BJ, Robbins TW: **Choosing between small, likely rewards and large, unlikely rewards activates inferior and orbital prefrontal cortex.** *J Neurosci* 1999, **19**:9029–9038.
23. Berdoy M, Webster JP, Macdonald DW: **Fatal attraction in rats infected with Toxoplasma gondii.** *Proc Biol Sci Royal Soc* 2000, **267**:1591–1594.
24. Vyas A, Kim SK, Giacomini N, Boothroyd JC, Sapolsky RM: **Behavioral changes induced by Toxoplasma infection of rodents are highly specific to aversion of cat odors.** *Proc Natl Acad Sci U S A* 2007, **104**:6442–6447.
25. Berenreiterova M, Flegr J, Kubena AA, Nemec P: **The distribution of Toxoplasma gondii cysts in the brain of a mouse with latent toxoplasmosis: implications for the behavioral manipulation hypothesis.** *PLoS One* 2011, **6**:e28925.
26. Mitra R, Sapolsky RM, Vyas A: **Toxoplasma gondii infection induces dendritic retraction in basolateral amygdala accompanied by reduced corticosterone secretion.** *Dis Model Mech* 2013, **6**:516–520.
27. House PK, Vyas A, Sapolsky R: **Predator cat odors activate sexual arousal pathways in brains of Toxoplasma gondii infected rats.** *PLoS One* 2011, **6**:e23277.
28. McConkey GA, Martin HL, Bristow GC, Webster JP: **Toxoplasma gondii infection and behaviour - location, location, location?** *J Exp Biol* 2013, **216**:113–119.
29. Stibbs HH: **Changes in brain concentrations of catecholamines and indoleamines in Toxoplasma gondii infected mice.** *Ann Trop Med Parasitol* 1985, **79**:153–157.
30. Montoya JG, Liesenfeld O: **Toxoplasmosis.** *Lancet* 2004, **363**:1965–1976.
31. Centers for Disease Control and Prevention (CDC): **Parasites - toxoplasmosis (toxoplasma infection).** [http://www.cdc.gov/parasites/toxoplasmosis/epi.html]
32. Hsu PC, Groer M, Beckie T: **New findings: depression, suicide, and toxoplasma gondii infection.** *J Am Assoc Nurse Prac* 2014, [http://dx.doi.org/10.1002/2327-6924.12129]
33. Munoz M, Liesenfeld O, Heimesaat MM: **Immunology of toxoplasma gondii.** *Immunol Rev* 2011, **240**:269–285.
34. Lester D: **Brain parasites and suicide.** *Psychol Rep* 2010, **107**:424.
35. Arling TA, Yolken RH, Lapidus M, Langenberg P, Dickerson FB, Zimmerman SA, Balis T, Cabassa JA, Scrandis DA, Tonelli LH, Postolache TT: **Toxoplasma gondii antibody titers and history of suicide attempts in patients with recurrent mood disorders.** *J Nerv Ment Dis* 2009, **197**:905–908.
36. Sudo N, Chida Y, Aiba Y, Sonoda J, Oyama N, Yu XN, Kubo C, Koga Y: **Postnatal microbial colonization programs the hypothalamic-pituitary-adrenal system for stress response in mice.** *J Physiol* 2004, **558**:263–275.
37. Desbonnet L, Garrett L, Clarke G, Bienenstock J, Dinan TG: **The probiotic Bifidobacteria infantis: an assessment of potential antidepressant properties in the rat.** *J Psychiatr Res* 2008, **43**:164–174.
38. Bravo JA, Forsythe P, Chew MV, Escaravage E, Savignac HM, Dinan TG, Bienenstock J, Cryan JF: **Ingestion of lactobacillus strain regulates emotional behavior and central GABA receptor expression in a mouse via the vagus nerve.** *Proc Natl Acad Sci U S A* 2011, **108**:16050–16055.

39. Maes M, Kubera M, Leunis JC, Berk M: **Increased IgA and IgM responses against gut commensals in chronic depression: further evidence for increased bacterial translocation or leaky gut.** *J Affect Disord* 2012, **141**:55–62.
40. Maes M, Kubera M, Leunis JC: **The gut-brain barrier in major depression: intestinal mucosal dysfunction with an increased translocation of LPS from gram negative enterobacteria (leaky gut) plays a role in the inflammatory pathophysiology of depression.** *Neuro endocrinol Letters* 2008, **29**:117–124.
41. Wang X, Zhang L, Lei Y, Liu X, Zhou X, Liu Y, Wang M, Yang L, Zhang L, Fan S, Xie P: **Meta-analysis of infectious agents and depression.** *Sci Reports* 2014, **4**:4530.
42. Haga S, Yoshimura M, Motoi Y, Arima K, Aizawa T, Ikuta K, Tashiro M, Ikeda K: **Detection of Borna disease virus genome in normal human brain tissue.** *Brain Res* 1997, **770**:307–309.
43. Czygan M, Hallensleben W, Hofer M, Pollak S, Sauder C, Bilzer T, Blumcke I, Riederer P, Bogerts B, Falkai P, Schwarz MJ, Masliah E, Staeheli P, Hufert FT, Lieb K: **Borna disease virus in human brains with a rare form of hippocampal degeneration but not in brains of patients with common neuropsychiatric disorders.** *J Infect Dis* 1999, **180**:1695–1699.
44. Dietrich DE, Bode L: **Human Borna disease virus-infection and its therapy in affective disorders.** *APMIS Suppl* 2008, **124**:61–65.
45. Stevens J, Bies RR, Shekhar A, Anand A: **Bayesian model of Hamilton depression rating score (HDRS) with memantine augmentation in bipolar depression.** *Br J Clin Pharmacol* 2013, **75**:791–798.
46. Berman RM, Cappiello A, Anand A, Oren DA, Heninger GR, Charney DS, Krystal JH: **Antidepressant effects of ketamine in depressed patients.** *Biol Psychiatry* 2000, **47**:351–354.
47. Li N, Lee B, Liu RJ, Banasr M, Dwyer JM, Iwata M, Li XY, Aghajanian G, Duman RS: **mTOR-dependent synapse formation underlies the rapid antidepressant effects of NMDA antagonists.** *Science* 2010, **329**:959–964.
48. Na KS, Tae SH, Song JW, Kim YK: **Failure to detect Borna disease virus antibody and RNA from peripheral blood mononuclear cells of psychiatric patients.** *Psychiatry Investig* 2009, **6**:306–312.
49. Hornig M, Briese T, Licinio J, Khabbaz RF, Altshuler LL, Potkin SG, Schwemmle M, Siemetzki U, Mintz J, Honkavuori K, Kraemer HC, Egan MF, Whybrow PC, Bunney WE, Lipkin WI: **Absence of evidence for bornavirus infection in schizophrenia, bipolar disorder and major depressive disorder.** *Mol Psychiatry* 2012, **17**:486–493.
50. Iwata Y, Takahashi K, Peng X, Fukuda K, Ohno K, Ogawa T, Gonda K, Mori N, Niwa S, Shigeta S: **Detection and sequence analysis of borna disease virus p24 RNA from peripheral blood mononuclear cells of patients with mood disorders or schizophrenia and of blood donors.** *J Virol* 1998, **72**:10044–10049.
51. Kim YK, Kim SH, Choi SH, Ko YH, Kim L, Lee MS, Suh KY, Kwak DI, Song KJ, Lee YJ, Yanagihara R, Song JW: **Failure to demonstrate Borna disease virus genome in peripheral blood mononuclear cells from psychiatric patients in Korea.** *J Neurovirol* 1999, **5**:196–199.
52. Lewis CM, Ng MY, Butler AW, Cohen-Woods S, Uher R, Pirlo K, Weale ME, Schosser A, Paredes UM, Rivera M, Craddock N, Owen MJ, Jones L, Jones I, Korszun A, Aitchison KJ, Shi J, Quinn JP, Mackenzie A, Vollenweider P, Waeber G, Heath S, Lathrop M, Muglia P, Barnes MR, Whittaker JC, Tozzi F, Holsboer F, Preisig M, Farmer AE, *et al*: **Genome-wide association study of major recurrent depression in the U.K. population.** *Am J Psychiatry* 2010, **167**:949–957.
53. Verbeek EC, Bakker IM, Bevova MR, Bochdanovits Z, Rizzu P, Sondervan D, Willemsen G, de Geus EJ, Smit JH, Penninx BW, Boomsma DI, Hoogendijk WJ, Heutink P: **A fine-mapping study of 7 top scoring genes from a GWAS for major depressive disorder.** *PLoS One* 2012, **7**:e37384.
54. Lander ES, Linton LM, Birren B, Nusbaum C, Zody MC, Baldwin J, Devon K, Dewar K, Doyle M, FitzHugh W, Funke R, Gage D, Harris K, Heaford A, Howland J, Kann L, Lehoczky J, LeVine R, McEwan P, McKernan K, Meldrim J, Mesirov JP, Miranda C, Morris W, Naylor J, Raymond C, Rosetti M, Santos R, Sheridan A, Sougnez C, *et al*: **Initial sequencing and analysis of the human genome.** *Nature* 2001, **409**:860–921.
55. Kurdyukov SG, Lebedev YB, Artamonova II, Gorodentseva TN, Batrak AV, Mamedov IZ, Azhikina TL, Legchilina SP, Efimenko IG, Gardiner K, Sverdlov ED: **Full-sized HERV-K (HML-2) human endogenous retroviral LTR sequences on human chromosome 21: map locations and evolutionary history.** *Gene* 2001, **273**:51–61.
56. Belyi VA, Levine AJ, Skalka AM: **Unexpected inheritance: multiple integrations of ancient bornavirus and ebolavirus/marburgvirus sequences in vertebrate genomes.** *PLoS Pathog* 2010, **6**:e1001030.
57. Gilbert C, Schaack S, Pace JK 2nd, Brindley PJ, Feschotte C: **A role for host-parasite interactions in the horizontal transfer of transposons across phyla.** *Nature* 2010, **464**:1347–1350.
58. Cryan JF, Dinan TG: **Mind-altering microorganisms: the impact of the gut microbiota on brain and behaviour.** *Nat Rev Neurosci* 2012, **13**:701–712.
59. Yatsunenko T, Rey FE, Manary MJ, Trehan I, Dominguez-Bello MG, Contreras M, Magris M, Hidalgo G, Baldassano RN, Anokhin AP, Heath AC, Warner B, Reeder J, Kuczynski J, Caporaso JG, Lozupone CA, Lauber C, Clemente JC, Knights D, Knight R, Gordon JI: **Human gut microbiome viewed across age and geography.** *Nature* 2012, **486**:222–227.
60. Wylie KM, Mihindukulasuriya KA, Sodergren E, Weinstock GM, Storch GA: **Sequence analysis of the human virome in febrile and afebrile children.** *PLoS One* 2012, **7**:e27735.
61. Dantzer R, O'Connor JC, Freund GG, Johnson RW, Kelley KW: **From inflammation to sickness and depression: when the immune system subjugates the brain.** *Nat Rev Neurosci* 2008, **9**:46–56.
62. Johnson DR, O'Connor JC, Hartman ME, Tapping RI, Freund GG: **Acute hypoxia activates the neuroimmune system, which diabetes exacerbates.** *J Neurosci* 2007, **27**:1161–1166.
63. Ohayon MM: **The effects of breathing-related sleep disorders on mood disturbances in the general population.** *J Clin Psychiatry* 2003, **64**:1195–1200. quiz, 1274–1196.
64. Regvat J, Zmitek A, Vegnuti M, Kosnik M, Suskovic S: **Anxiety and depression during hospital treatment of exacerbation of chronic obstructive pulmonary disease.** *J Int Med Res* 2011, **39**:1028–1038.
65. VanElzakker MB: **Chronic fatigue syndrome from vagus nerve infection: a psychoneuroimmunological hypothesis.** *Med Hypotheses* 2013, **81**:414–423.
66. Hoge EA, Brandstetter K, Moshier S, Pollack MH, Wong KK, Simon NM: **Broad spectrum of cytokine abnormalities in panic disorder and posttraumatic stress disorder.** *Depress Anxiety* 2009, **26**:447–455.
67. Pace TWW, Heim CM: **A short review on the psychoneuroimmunology of posttraumatic stress disorder: from risk factors to medical comorbidities.** *Brain Behav Immun* 2011, **25**:6–13.
68. Kuczynski J, Lauber CL, Walters WA, Parfrey LW, Clemente JC, Gevers D, Knight R: **Experimental and analytical tools for studying the human microbiome.** *Nat Rev Genet* 2012, **13**:47–58.
69. Human Microbiome Project C: **A framework for human microbiome research.** *Nature* 2012, **486**:215–221.
70. Barber RM, Porter BF, Li Q, May M, Claiborne MK, Allison AB, Howerth EW, Butler A, Wei S, Levine JM, Levine GJ, Brown DR, Schatzberg SJ: **Broadly reactive polymerase chain reaction for pathogen detection in canine granulomatous meningoencephalomyelitis and necrotizing meningoencephalitis.** *J Vet Intern Med* 2012, **26**:962–968.
71. Allen LZ, Ishoey T, Novotny MA, McLean JS, Lasken RS, Williamson SJ: **Single virus genomics: a new tool for virus discovery.** *PLoS One* 2011, **6**:e17722.
72. Zeigler Allen L, Ishoey T, Novotny MA, McLean JS, Lasken RS, Williamson SJ: **Isolation and genome analysis of single virions using 'single virus genomics'.** *J Vis Exp* 2013, **75**:e3899. doi:10.3791/3899.
73. Cook S, Chung BY, Bass D, Moureau G, Tang S, McAlister E, Culverwell CL, Glucksman E, Wang H, Brown TD, Gould EA, Harbach RE, de Lamballerie X, Firth AE: **Novel virus discovery and genome reconstruction from field RNA samples reveals highly divergent viruses in dipteran hosts.** *PLoS One* 2013, **8**:e80720.
74. Tang P, Chiu C: **Metagenomics for the discovery of novel human viruses.** *Future Microbiol* 2010, **5**:177–189.
75. Kreuze JF, Perez A, Untiveros M, Quispe D, Fuentes S, Barker I, Simon R: **Complete viral genome sequence and discovery of novel viruses by deep sequencing of small RNAs: a generic method for diagnosis, discovery and sequencing of viruses.** *Virology* 2009, **388**:1–7.
76. Barzon L, Lavezzo E, Costanzi G, Franchin E, Toppo S, Palu G: **Next-generation sequencing technologies in diagnostic virology.** *J Clin Virol* 2013, **58**:346–350.

18

Neurocognitive therapeutics: from concept to application in the treatment of negative attention bias

David M Schnyer[1*], Christopher G Beevers[1], Megan T deBettencourt[2], Stephanie M Sherman[3], Jonathan D Cohen[4], Kenneth A Norman[4] and Nicholas B Turk-Browne[4]

Abstract

There is growing interest in the use of neuroimaging for the direct treatment of mental illness. Here, we present a new framework for such treatment, neurocognitive therapeutics. What distinguishes neurocognitive therapeutics from prior approaches is the use of precise brain-decoding techniques within a real-time feedback system, in order to adapt treatment online and tailor feedback to individuals' needs. We report an initial feasibility study that uses this framework to alter negative attention bias in a small number of patients experiencing significant mood symptoms. The results are consistent with the promise of neurocognitive therapeutics to improve mood symptoms and alter brain networks mediating attentional control. Future work should focus on optimizing the approach, validating its effectiveness, and expanding the scope of targeted disorders.

Keywords: Attention bias, Real-time neurofeedback, Multivoxel pattern analysis (MVPA), Mood disorders, fMRI

Background

Neurocognitive therapeutics combines cognitive training with state-of-the-art neural-monitoring techniques in order to facilitate neuroplasticity. By combining behavioral paradigms with brain imaging, specific mental states of interest can be targeted directly and effectively. A particularly promising approach combines real-time functional magnetic resonance imaging (fMRI) with multivoxel pattern analysis (MVPA): a classifier can be trained to measure the presence of a mental state in brain activity patterns [1]; this measure can then be used to dynamically alter the behavioral paradigm, in essence adapting it to the personal ability of the individual. We have begun to apply this kind of approach in depressed adults with negatively biased attention, and our preliminary results are promising. The chief purpose of this article is to outline the methodological approach we have developed, rather than to report conclusive findings. Before doing so, however, we first describe some relevant prior work involving (1) behavioral-attention-training paradigms and (2) real-time fMRI neurofeedback.

* Correspondence: schnyer@utexas.edu
[1]Department of Psychology & Institute for Mental Health Research, University of Texas at Austin, Austin, TX 78712, USA
Full list of author information is available at the end of the article

Behavioral attention training

The ability to control attentional capture and disengagement from affective stimuli is a crucial element of adaptive self-regulation [2]. For example, excessive attention to negative affective information has been identified as a fundamental process observed across diagnosis that may underlie the development of multiple disorders [3,4]. As a result, a number of investigators have developed and tested cognitive paradigms to train attentional control in an effort to diminish attentional bias to negative content. In prior work, we have shown that changes in attentional bias mediated the effect of attention training on depression symptom change [5,6]. Similar results have been found with depressed [7] and depression-vulnerable [8] individuals and in other psychiatric conditions [9-11], although null findings have also been reported [12]. One possible reason for the mixed results of prior attention-training work may be that it has involved delivering feedback based on behavior, and often without tailoring the feedback to the individual patient.

Real-time fMRI neurofeedback

Real-time fMRI is an approach to brain imaging that involves simultaneously measuring and analyzing the blood-oxygen-level-dependent (BOLD) signal [13]. A number of researchers have used real-time fMRI to provide neurofeedback, by reflecting back to participants the results of the real-time analysis during the scanning session. Participants are encouraged to use this feedback and adjust their cognitive strategy to alter their neural response in real time [14]. Virtually all fMRI neurofeedback studies with clinical populations have used a block design approach in which participants are presented with visual feedback indicating the magnitude of the BOLD signal in a brain region of interest [15]. Frequently in such studies, the signal being measured cannot easily be tied directly to any particular mental state - it is often unclear what participants are actually doing. More recent applications have combined multiple brain-imaging techniques in an attempt to identify more specific mental states, such as positive emotion induction [16]. However, despite the multiple real-time brain measures (fMRI and EEG), the signals are not employed to directly alter a cognitive task. In particular, no real-time fMRI paradigm has targeted the negative attention bias in depression.

Attention training with closed-loop real-time fMRI neurofeedback

We recently adapted a real-time fMRI neurofeedback approach developed for studying attention in the normal brain [17] to attempt to alter the neurobiology underlying the negative attention bias (Figure 1). In a pilot feasibility study, participants with elevated depression were trained to selectively attend to an emotionally neutral target category (for example, scenes) for a period of time while ignoring an emotionally salient distractor category (for example, sad faces). All experimental parameters were identical to those reported by deBettencourt, *et al.* [15], including scanner make and model and scanning and experimental protocols. Further, all procedures were approved by the Institutional Review Board at the University of Texas at Austin and participants provided written informed consent.

Each training session in this study involved a series of scanning runs in two phases: a classifier-training phase and a testing/feedback phase. During the training phase, fMRI data were collected from participants as they performed a task requiring selective attention to a continuous stream of composite images containing overlaid (neutral) face-and-scene stimuli. Participants alternated between attending to the face or scene while trying to detect rare lure images. These data were used to train a pattern classifier to decode neural activity that reflected attention to face *vs.* attention to scenes.

During the testing/feedback phase, fMRI data were collected and decoded in real time using the trained classifier. Participants were always instructed to attend to scenes, and sad faces were introduced as distractors. The output of the classifier provided evidence about whether participants were attending to the correct category (that is, scene), and this was translated (within 2 s) into feedback for the participant. Feedback took the form of altering the visual display

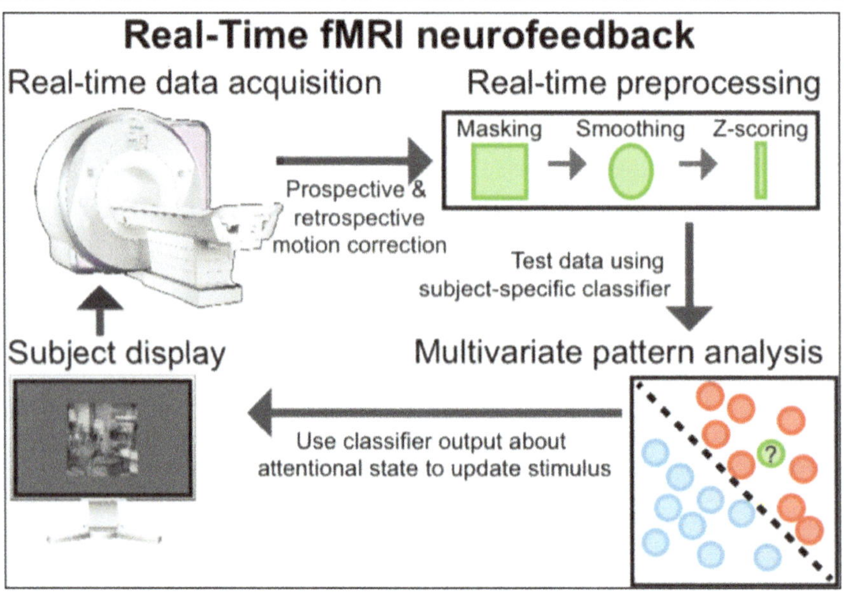

Figure 1 Overview of the real-time fMRI neurofeedback attention-training procedure. A video showing a typical visual display the participant might experience during the neurofeedback phase can be seen here - http://www.nature.com/neuro/journal/v18/n3/abs/nn.3940.html#videos. fMRI, functional magnetic resonance imaging.

to encourage correctly directed attention and discourage incorrectly directed attention. For example, while the participants were supposed to be attending to scenes, if the classifier indicated that sad faces were distracting them, the proportion of the scene stimulus in the composite image was *reduced* (for example, from 50% scene/face to 30% scene/70% face).

This feedback served to 'externalize' participants' attentional state, making their distraction by the sad faces more tangible. This also made the task of attending to scenes more difficult, providing an error signal that distraction was undesirable. The logic was that participants could learn from this tangible feedback about good and bad attentional states and gain an ability to better monitor and control these states. The alternative approach of making the scenes more visible when distraction by the faces occurred might have helped participants in that moment to reorient to the scenes; however, this would potentially incentivize lapses. That is, to simplify the task demands in this regime, the best strategy would be to seek distraction rather than avoid it. Ultimately, the effectiveness of different feedback regimes awaits further empirical study, but the approach used here of making the task more difficult when attention lapsed has proven effective in controls [15] and in depressed individuals, as shown below.

We ran a pilot study to demonstrate that this elaborate fMRI procedure is feasible in patients with depression. Seven adults with elevated symptoms of depression (mean Beck Depression Inventory-II [BDI-II] = 25; 4 female; mean age = 24) completed three sessions of neurofeedback training across a 5-day period, in between two laboratory assessment sessions. We were able to execute this procedure successfully, confirming the feasibility of the approach. Furthermore, the results were consistent with the possibility that this might be a useful approach. Specifically, improvements in attention control with training predicted improvements in mood symptoms across a 4-week follow-up period (Figure 2, left). Moreover, resting-state fMRI connectivity between frontal and parietal nodes of a previously identified attention control network [6] showed increased connectivity from before to after training (Figure 2, right).

These results must be interpreted with caution, as a control group was not included. Any future clinical study

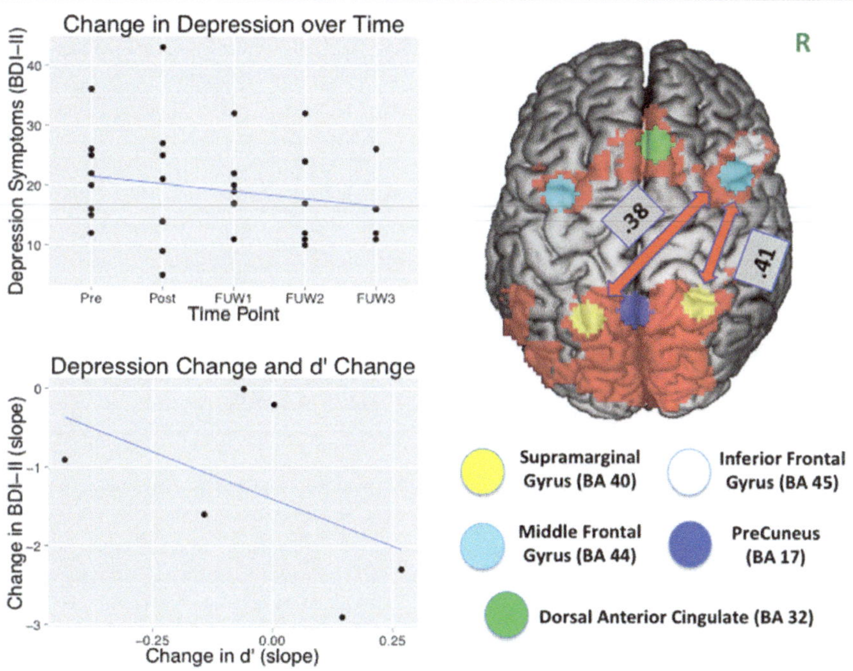

Figure 2 Preliminary results of feasibility study. Upper left panel graph shows BDI scores *pre* and *post* training and at three 1-week follow-ups (*FUW1*, *FUW2*, and *FUW3*). Lower left panel shows that changes in performance accuracy (indexed by d' - a statistic that is calculated from hit and false alarm rates and hence reflects detection sensitivity) during training were associated with changes in BDI across this 4-week period. Mean d' and standard deviation for performance across the 3 days were 1.06(.718), 1.32(.720), and 1.59(.871), respectively. The right panel shows the attention control network that was tested for pre-post changes in resting-state connectivity. This network was identified in previous work as associated with attention control and amenable to change with behavioral training [6]. All participants showed increased connectivity between right middle frontal gyrus (MFG) and bilateral supramarginal gyrus (SMG) of the parietal lobe. The mean and standard deviation in connectivity between right MFG and left SMG pre and post training were 0.11(0.18) and 0.38(0.26), respectively; between right MFG and right SMG 0.17(0.22) and 0.41(0.26), respectively. BA, Brodmann's area; BDI, Beck Depression Inventory.

adopting this approach will need such a group, to ensure that the results cannot be attributed simply to practice with the task or other incidental aspects of the training. One control used in the previous study upon which this task was based [17] involved providing participants with sham feedback that was derived from other participants' feedback sessions - and thus out of sync with their actual attentional state and thus presumably less useful for training. Future empirical work should include an appropriate active control condition.

Conclusions

Neurocognitive therapeutics offers the promise of combining precision neural-monitoring techniques with behavioral training paradigms in order to increase the effectiveness of cognitive training. The critical difference between this approach and typical neurofeedback paradigms is that instead of directly presenting the individual with a measure of their brain activity, neurocognitive therapeutics uses that measure to dynamically alter the cognitive task itself. For attention training, real-time fMRI and multivariate analysis techniques can detect when attention is shifting and use that information to provide an error signal in the visual display being attended to help individuals learn to better control their attentional state. Although a long-term goal is to transition the neural-monitoring component from fMRI to a less costly, field-based technology, the initial use of fMRI is critical because it is currently the best technology for identifying distributed mental states non-invasively and with high fidelity. Our hope is that such translations of cutting-edge methods from cognitive neuroscience will increase the efficacy of cognitive training and clinical treatment.

Abbreviations

BA: Brodmann's area; BDI: Beck Depression Inventory; BOLD: blood-oxygen-level-dependent signal; d': d prime; EEG: electroencephalography; fMRI: functional magnetic resonance imaging; MVPA: multivoxel pattern analysis.

Competing interests

The authors declare that they have no competing interests.

Authors' contributions

DS wrote the article and designed, directed, and participated in the analysis of the treatment feasibility trial; CB assisted with writing the article and designed, directed, and participated in the analysis of the treatment feasibility trial; MD was part of the team that developed the real-time attention-training task, implemented that task at the Austin site, and was involved in the analysis of the treatment feasibility trial; SS collected the data and was involved in the analysis of the treatment feasibility trial; JC was part of the team that developed the real-time attention-training task; KN assisted with writing the article and was part of the team that developed the real-time attention-training task; and NT assisted with writing the article and was part of the team that developed the real-time attention-training task. All authors read and approved the manuscript.

Acknowledgements

The authors thank Seth Disner, Robert Chapman, and Emily Viehman at The University of Texas at Austin for their help with participant recruitment and data collection. We would also like to thank Ray Lee, Princeton University, and Jeff Luci, UT Austin, for their technical assistance. Preparation of this article was supported by the National Institute of Health award numbers R21 MH092430 to CGB and R01EY021755 to NBB, US National Science Foundation (NSF) grant BCS1229597 to NBB, NSF fellowship DGE1148900 to MTD, and the John Templeton Foundation. The opinions expressed in this publication are those of the authors and do not necessarily reflect the views of these funding agencies. The authors report no financial interests or potential conflicts of interest.

Author details

[1]Department of Psychology & Institute for Mental Health Research, University of Texas at Austin, Austin, TX 78712, USA. [2]Princeton Neuroscience Institute, Princeton University, Princeton, NJ 08540-1010, USA. [3]Department of Psychology, University of Texas at Austin, Austin, TX 78712, USA. [4]Department of Psychology and Princeton Neuroscience Institute, Princeton University, Princeton, NJ 08540-1010, USA.

References

1. Norman KA, Polyn SM, Detre GJ, Haxby JV. Beyond mind-reading: multi-voxel pattern analysis of fMRI data. Trends Cogn Sci (Regul Ed). 2006;10(9):424–30. doi:10.1016/j.tics.2006.07.005.
2. Posner MI, Rothbart MK. Developing mechanisms of self-regulation. Dev Psychopathol. 2000;12:427–41.
3. Nolen-Hoeksema S, Watkins ER. A heuristic for developing transdiagnostic models of psychopathology explaining multifinality and divergent trajectories. Perspect Psychol Sci. 2011;6(6):589–609. Available at: http://pps.sagepub.com/content/6/6/589.short.
4. Mclaughlin KA, Nolen-Hoeksema S. Rumination as a transdiagnostic factor in depression and anxiety. Behav Res Ther. 2011;49(3):186–93. doi:10.1016/j.brat.2010.12.006.
5. Wells TT, Beevers CG. Biased attention and dysphoria: manipulating selective attention reduces subsequent depressive symptoms. PCEM. 2010;24(4):719–28.
6. Beevers CG, Clasen PC, Enoch P, Schnyer DM. Attention bias modification for major depressive disorder: effects on attention bias, resting state connectivity, and symptom change. J Abnorm Psychol. (In press).
7. Baert S, De Raedt R, Schacht R, Koster EHW. Attentional bias training in depression: therapeutic effects depend on depression severity. J Behav Ther Exp Psychiatry. 2010;41(3):265–74. doi:10.1016/j.jbtep.2010.02.004.
8. Browning M, Holmes EA, Charles M, Cowen PJ, Harmer CJ. Using attentional bias modification as a cognitive vaccine against depression. Biol Psychiatry. 2012;72(7):572–9. doi:10.1016/j.biopsych.2012.04.014.
9. Amir N, Beard C, Taylor CT, Klumpp H, Elias J, Burns M, et al. Attention training in individuals with generalized social phobia: a randomized controlled trial. J Consult Clin Psychol. 2009;77(5):961–73. doi:10.1037/a0016685.
10. Eldar S. Attention bias modification treatment for pediatric anxiety disorders: a randomized controlled trial. Am J Psychiatry. 2012;169(2):213. doi:10.1176/appi.ajp.2011.11060886.
11. Hallion LS, Ruscio AM. A meta-analysis of the effect of cognitive bias modification on anxiety and depression. Psychol Bull. 2011;137(6):940–58. doi:10.1037/a0024355.
12. Mogoaşe C, David D, Koster EHW. Clinical efficacy of attentional bias modification procedures: an updated meta-analysis. J Clin Psychol. 2014:n/a–n/a. doi:10.1002/jclp.22081.
13. Sulzer J, Haller S, Scharnowski F, Weiskopf N, Birbaumer N, Blefari ML, et al. Real-time fMRI neurofeedback: progress and challenges. Neuroimage. 2013;76:386–99. doi:10.1016/j.neuroimage.2013.03.033.
14. Caria A, Sitaram R, Birbaumer N. Real-time fMRI: a tool for local brain regulation. Neuroscientist. 2012;18(5):487–501. doi:10.1177/1073858411407205.
15. Stoeckel LE, Garrison KA, Ghosh S, Wighton P, Hanlon CA, Gilman JM, et al. Optimizing real time fMRI neurofeedback for therapeutic discovery and development. Neuroimage Clin. 2014;5:245–55. doi:10.1016/j.nicl.2014.07.002.
16. Zotev V, Krueger F, Phillips R, Alvarez RP, Simmons WK, Bellgowan P, et al. Self-regulation of amygdala activation using real-time fMRI neurofeedback. PLoS One. 2011;6(9), e24522. doi:10.1371/journal.pone.0024522.
17. DeBettencourt MT, Cohen JD, Lee RF, Norman KA, Turk-Browne NB. Closed-loop training of attention with real-time brain imaging. Nat Neurosci. 2015;18(3):470–5. doi:10.1038/nn.3940.

19

Brain white matter integrity and association with age at onset in pediatric obsessive-compulsive disorder

Isabelle M Rosso[1,2*], Elizabeth A Olson[1,2], Jennifer C Britton[3], S Evelyn Stewart[4,9], George Papadimitriou[5,6,7], William DS Killgore[1,2], Nikos Makris[5,6,7], Sabine Wilhelm[2,8], Michael A Jenike[2,8,10] and Scott L Rauch[1,2]

Abstract

Background: Obsessive-compulsive disorder (OCD) is a common and debilitating neuropsychiatric illness thought to involve abnormal connectivity of widespread brain networks, including frontal-striatal-thalamic circuits. At least half of OCD cases arise in childhood and their underlying neuropathology may differ at least in part from that of adult-onset OCD. Yet, only a few studies have examined brain white matter (WM) integrity in childhood-onset OCD using diffusion tensor imaging (DTI), and none have examined potential associations with age at onset.

Results: In this study, 17 youth with OCD and 19 healthy control subjects, ages 10 to 19 years, underwent DTI on a 3T Siemens scanner. DSM-IV diagnoses were established with standardized interviews, and OCD symptom severity was evaluated using the Childrens Yale-Brown Obsessive-Compulsive Scale (CY-BOCS). Voxel-wise analyses were conducted on data processed with tract-based spatial statistics (TBSS) to derive measures of fractional anisotropy (FA), axial diffusivity (AD), radial diffusivity (RD), and mean diffusivity (MD). OCD patients had significantly lower FA in seven WM clusters, with over 80% of significant voxels in bilateral frontal cortex and corpus callosum (CC). There were no regions of significantly higher FA in patients compared with controls. Patients also had significantly higher RD in right frontal cortex and right body of the CC. Earlier age at onset of OCD correlated significantly with lower FA in the right thalamus and with higher RD in the right CC. FA and RD were not significantly associated with symptom severity.

Conclusions: These findings point to compromised WM integrity and reduced myelination in some brain regions of children with OCD, particularly the CC and fiber tracts that connect the frontal lobes to widespread cortical and subcortical targets. They also suggest that age at onset may be a moderator of some of the WM changes in pediatric OCD.

Keywords: Obsessive-compulsive disorder, Childhood, Diffusion tensor imaging, Corpus callosum, Thalamus, Age at onset

Background

Obsessive-compulsive disorder (OCD) is a common neuropsychiatric illness characterized by repetitive thoughts and behaviors that are unwanted, distressing, and disabling (DSM-IV; [1]). Onset occurs in childhood for more than half of OCD patients, with about 40% of pediatric cases achieving remission and the remaining persisting into adulthood [2,3]. Epidemiological studies show that pediatric OCD has typical onset between 7 and 13 years [2] and that it differs from its adult-onset counterpart in a number of ways, including male preponderance, high familial loading, and more frequent comorbidity with developmental disorders [2,4]. Based on these correlates, it has been speculated that pediatric OCD may be a developmental subtype that is discontinuous from adult OCD, or a developmentally moderated expression of etiologic processes that are shared with the adult clinical phenotype [5,6].

* Correspondence: irosso@hms.harvard.edu
[1]Center for Depression, Anxiety and Stress Research, McLean Hospital, 115 Mill Street, mailstop 334, Belmont, MA 02478, USA
[2]Department of Psychiatry, Harvard Medical School, Boston, MA, USA
Full list of author information is available at the end of the article

Neuroimaging research has provided converging evidence that OCD symptoms arise from alterations in widespread brain networks. Abnormalities in frontal-striatal-thalamo-cortical loops are central to prevailing conceptual models of the disorder [7,8]. Pathological obsessions and compulsions are proposed to involve insufficient inhibitory control of striatal and thalamic nuclei by prefrontal cortical regions, particularly the anterior cingulate and lateral orbitofrontal cortices [9], and neuroimaging findings of altered regional brain volumes and function largely support these models (e.g., [10,11]). In addition, there is growing evidence implicating brain regions outside of the frontal-subcortical loops, including the posterior parietal and occipital regions [12]. Similarly, neuropsychological findings identify deficits across multiple domains of cognitive functioning, including set shifting, response inhibition, memory, and attention [13-17].

Most of the imaging literature to date is in adult rather than pediatric OCD. This is especially the case for studies that have used diffusion tensor imaging (DTI) to identify changes in brain white matter (WM) [18]. DTI is a magnetic resonance method that estimates the magnitude and direction of water diffusion, which is dependent on the underlying structure of brain tissue. In particular, highly organized myelinated axon fibers will constrain and direct water diffusion, such that DTI parameters allow inferences about WM organization and integrity. Mean diffusivity (MD) is the DTI parameter that reflects *magnitude* of diffusion at each voxel, which varies with tissue density regardless of fiber orientation [19]. Fractional anisotropy (FA) is the DTI parameter reflecting *directionality* of diffusion in each voxel, such that FA is higher along fiber bundles that are more coherent or organized [20]. FA can also be separated into components reflecting diffusion parallel and perpendicular to the WM tracts, referred to as the axial diffusivity (AD) and radial diffusivity (RD), respectively. FA values decrease when AD decreases and/or RD increases. Interestingly, RD and AD may be biomarkers of different cellular developmental or pathological processes. Specifically, changes in RD appear to be associated with cell membrane alterations (myelination), whereas variations in AD may be more related to axonal injuries (volume and organization) [21].

In DTI studies of adult OCD, FA has been the most commonly studied diffusion parameter. FA alterations have been observed most consistently in the corpus callosum (CC), cingulum bundle, internal capsule, and anterior thalamic radiation, as well as the parietal cortex (e.g., [22-25]). However, the directionality of FA alterations has varied, with reports of lower [23,24,26,27], higher [25,28], or comparable FA values when comparing adult OCD patients with healthy control (HC) subjects [22,29,30]. These seemingly disparate findings likely reflect true regional brain variability in hypo- and hyper-connectivity across fiber tracts implicated in OCD, as well as methodological differences across studies. For instance, although all studies have reported on FA, fewer have incorporated other diffusivity measures that can help contextualize FA findings. In addition, findings may relate to certain patient variables, such as psychiatric comorbidity, illness duration, and medication use. Notably, investigation of childhood OCD can help reduce some of these confounding influences including those related to illness chronicity [6] and can also isolate neurobehavioral features that relate to an early age at onset. Most adult OCD studies have combined patients with childhood and adult onset, which may introduce neurobiological variability. For instance, whereas meta-analyses of functional imaging findings indicate a central role of the caudate nucleus in adult OCD, neuroimaging studies of pediatric OCD point to more prominent involvement of other basal ganglia structures and the thalamus [5]. Thus, age at onset may be associated with neurobiological variability in OCD and could help parse disease heterogeneity.

As in the adult literature, studies of pediatric OCD have provided evidence of diffusion abnormalities in multiple WM tracts, although the nature and directionality of diffusion changes have varied, as have their associations with clinical features of illness. Two pediatric OCD DTI studies have reported FA as the main measure of diffusion [16,31]. Zarei et al. [31] found increased FA across a number of WM tracts in adolescent OCD patients, changes more widespread than those found in many adult OCD studies. Moreover, OCD symptom severity was positively correlated with FA in several of these tracts. Similarly, Gruner and colleagues [16] found that children with OCD had FA increases, though these were localized to four WM tracts, namely the left dorsal cingulum bundle, splenium of the CC, right corticospinal tract, and left inferior fronto-occipital fasciculus. Interestingly, increased FA in the cingulum bundle predicted better executive functioning within the OCD group, suggesting that it may reflect a compensatory process. Another two pediatric OCD studies found no group differences in FA, but examination of AD and RD revealed significant diffusivity differences [32,33]. Specifically, Silk et al. [33] found lower AD in the genu and splenium of the CC of children with OCD compared with controls, and lower AD correlated with greater severity of symptoms. In contrast, Jayarajan et al. [32] found significantly higher AD and RD, and neither was significantly correlated with symptom severity, medication dosage, or treatment duration. No pediatric OCD study has yet reported on whether diffusion changes are significantly associated with age at onset.

In this study, we used DTI to compare brain WM microstructure in youth with OCD compared with healthy matched controls, examining four diffusion parameters (MD, FA, AD, and RD). We hypothesized that pediatric

OCD would be associated with altered FA, without an *priori* prediction concerning the directionality of alteration (i.e., increased or decreased) due to scant published data in pediatric samples and inconsistent adult OCD DTI findings. Based on theoretical and empirical indications that age at onset may be relevant to the variability of DTI findings in OCD, we also tested the hypothesis that diffusion differences would be associated with age at onset of OCD.

Methods

Subjects

Thirty-six youth were enrolled in this neuroimaging experiment as paid volunteers. OCD subjects were treatment-seeking children presenting to an OCD clinic, and control subjects were recruited in the surrounding Boston metropolitan community via advertisements. The subjects were selected to be between 10 and 19 years old, similar to the age range in prior imaging studies of pediatric OCD. Participants were excluded if they reported current medical or neurological illness, or a history of head injury with loss of consciousness. Prior to enrollment, written informed consent was obtained from a parent/legal guardian and written informed assent was obtained from the child/adolescent participant. All study procedures were performed in accordance with the Human Research Committees at McLean Hospital and Partners Healthcare System.

The Kiddie Schedule for Affective Disorders and Schizophrenia (KSADS) was administered to all participants and their parents by doctoral-level psychologists [34]. Individuals included in the OCD group met DSM-IV criteria for this disorder based on the KSADS [1]. In addition, OCD symptom severity scores were determined using the Childrens Yale-Brown Obsessive-Compulsive Scale (CY-BOCS) [35]. To recruit a representative and generalizable OCD sample, the inclusion criteria for the OCD group allowed for comorbid psychiatric disorders, with the exception of psychotic disorders, bipolar disorder, mental retardation, substance use disorders, and pervasive developmental disorders. Neuroleptic and anti-hypertensive medications were exclusionary. All individuals included in the HC group were free from any current Axis I psychiatric disorder and psychotropic medications. All subjects completed the Child Depression Inventory (CDI) [36], and the Yale Global Tic Severity Scale (YGTSS) was used to rule out subjects with Tourettes syndrome and other tic-related disorders [37].

The participants consisted of 17 children with OCD and 19 HC youth. This sample was obtained after excluding data from participants for excessive head movement (1 OCD) and poor head coverage (1 HC). The patient group endorsed the following types of OCD symptoms across previously identified clusters [38]: contamination/washing ($N = 4$); symmetry/arranging/counting/repeating ($N = 10$); and aggression, sexual, religious, and/or somatic obsessions/checking ($N = 14$). No hoarding symptoms were reported. Nine (9) of the patients had no comorbid Axis I diagnosis. The following comorbidities were present in the remaining eight OCD patients, based on KSADS interviews: generalized anxiety disorder ($N = 1$), specific phobia ($N = 2$), agoraphobia ($N = 1$), major depressive disorder ($N = 2$), depression not otherwise specified ($N = 2$), oppositional defiant disorder ($N = 1$), and attention-deficit hyperactivity disorder ($N = 2$). Three (3) of the OCD patients were not taking any psychotropic medication. Primary medications taken by the remaining 14 OCD subjects were antidepressants: selective serotonin reuptake inhibitors ($N = 13$) and tricyclic agents ($N = 1$). In addition, some patients were taking secondary medications, namely stimulants ($N = 4$), mood stabilizers ($N = 3$), and benzodiazepines ($N = 1$).

Diffusion tensor imaging

Image acquisition

DTI scans were acquired using a Siemens Tim Trio 3T scanner at the McLean Hospital Imaging Center. Diffusion weighted imaging data were obtained in 60 directions with the following parameters: echo time = 98 ms, bandwidth = 1,396 Hz/pixel, matrix = 128 mm 128 mm, FOV = 256 mm 256 mm, NEX = 1, voxel size = 2.0 mm ^{3} 2.0 mm^3 2.0 mm ^{3}, 10 T2 low b ($b = 0$ s/mm^2), and 60 DWI (diffusion sensitivity $b = 700$ s/mm^2), and 60 axial slices with 2-mm thickness.

Image processing and analysis

The analysis of DTI data was done using the FMRIB Diffusion Toolbox from the FSL processing software package (http://www.fmrib.ox.ac.uk/fsl) [39,40]. The first step was motion and eddy current distortion correction, applied using FSLs *eddy_correct* tool, which ran with its default options. The raw data were skull-stripped using FSLs Brain Extraction Tool (BET) [41]. A diffusion tensor model was fit at each voxel using a least squares fit to the diffusion signal with FSLs *dtifit* tool; this generated maps for each of the diffusivity measures (FA, MD, AD, and RD). At this point, a mathematical correction for systematic vibration artifact was applied [42]. Voxel-wise processing of diffusivity measures was carried out using tract-based spatial statistics (TBSS) [43], which is part of FSL [44]. Images from all subjects were aligned to each other using nonlinear registration in order to determine the most representative individual (i.e., the closest to the mean of the group) to be defined as the target image. This target image was then aligned, using affine registration, to MNI152 standard space. Each individual subject was then registered into the Montreal Neurological Institute (MNI) space by combining the nonlinear transform (generated via FSLs FNIRT) from the subject to the target image with the affine transform from the target image into the MNI space. A mean FA image was created by averaging all aligned FA maps and was thresholded with an FA ≥ 0.2 to generate a mean FA skeleton, which represents the centers of all fiber tracts common to all subjects. Each subjects aligned FA image was projected onto the mean FA skeleton and served as the input to the TBSS. Group statistical analysis was then conducted only on voxels within the white matter skeleton mask, therefore restricting the voxel-wise analysis only to voxels with high confidence of lying within equivalent major white matter pathways in each individual. After completing the above procedures for FA, the nonlinear warps and skeleton projection were applied to MD, RD, and AD using tbss_non_FA. Differences in FA, MD, and axial and radial diffusivity between the OCD and control groups were assessed using voxel-wise independent two-sample *t*-tests by randomization, the nonparametric analysis tool in FSL. The Threshold-Free Cluster Enhancement (TFCE [45]) option was employed at family-wise error-corrected $p < 0.05$ to obtain cluster inferences.

Statistical analyses

Group differences in demographic characteristics were examined using χ^2 tests for categorical variables and independent *t*-tests for continuous variables. DTI parameters (FA, RD, MD, and AD) were analyzed using permutation testing and TFCE in FSL by applying an independent *t*-test to the data for between-group comparisons. The significance level was $p < 0.05$, family-wise error-corrected. Within significant clusters, the mean values were computed. Correlations of DTI variables with demographic and clinical variables were performed in SPSS version 20.

Results

Demographic and clinical data are summarized in Table 1. CY-BOCS total scores ranged from 8 to 32, spanning the mild to extreme severity range of obsessive and compulsive symptoms. In addition, OCD patients endorsed significantly higher levels of depression than HC subjects on the CDI (ps < 0.01).

Table 1 Demographic and clinical characteristics of the sample (mean SD or *N* (%))

Variable	OCD ($n = 17$)	Controls ($n = 19$)	*p*
Female	6 (35%)	6 (32%)	0.8
Age (years)	14.06 2.56	13.58 2.12	0.54
Education (years)	8.65 2.40	8.37 1.95	0.70
CDI (total)	8.94 7.16	3.47 3.79	<0.01
CY-BOCS (total)	17.06 8.17	-	
Obsessions	8.12 4.47	-	
Compulsions	8.94 4.19	-	
Age at onset (years)	8.82 3.36	-	
Duration of illness (years)	5.24 2.97	-	

Between-group differences in diffusion

OCD youth had significantly lower FA than HC subjects in widespread areas across seven separate clusters, numbered 1 7 in Table 2 and Figures 1 and 2. Nearly 98% of the significant voxels localized to clusters 1 and 2. Cluster 1 was a bilateral cluster (9,022 voxels) encompassing areas of the frontal lobes and CC (genu, body, and splenium). Cluster 2 (1,454 voxels) encompassed areas of the anterior cingulate cortex and extended into several subcortical regions including the putamen, amygdala, and thalamus. Cluster 3 (132 voxels) localized to the right angular and lateral occipital gyri. Cluster 4 (50 voxels) was in the right inferior frontal cortex, more specifically the subcallosal cortex. Cluster 5 was also a right inferior frontal cluster but more anteriorly, corresponding to the orbitofrontal cortex. Cluster 6 corresponded to 14 voxels in the right thalamus, and cluster 7 comprised 6 voxels in the right caudate and anterior internal capsule. There were no significant clusters where FA was higher in OCD patients than in HC subjects. Compared with HC subjects, OCD patients also had significantly increased RD in areas of the right frontal cortex and body of the CC, across three clusters that overlapped with the first FA cluster (Table 3; Figure 3). There were no significant clusters where RD was lower in OCD patients than in HC subjects. There were no statistically significant group differences in MD or AD.

Post hoc analyses showed that the mean FA and RD of clusters that differed between the diagnostic groups did not differ significantly between OCD patients with and without current comorbid disorders.

Clinical correlates of diffusion changes

Age at onset

To examine relationships with age at onset, the mean FA and mean RD were extracted from the seven FA clusters and the three RD clusters characterized above. Lower age at onset was associated with significantly decreased FA in FA cluster 6 (right thalamus: Figure 2), $r(15) = 0.691$, $p = 0.002$, and with significantly increased RD in RD cluster 2 (right body of the CC), $r(15) =$ 0.552, $p = 0.022$. The correlation between age at onset and FA in the thalamus remained significant after partialing out age, $r(14) = 0.636$, $p = 0.008$, though the correlation between age at onset and RD in the right body of the CC was reduced to a trend level after partialing out age, $r(14) =$ 0.435, $p = 0.093$. After partialing out duration of illness, the correlations between both DTI variables and age at onset remained significant: for the FA cluster, $r(14) = 0.556$ and $p = 0.022$; for the RD cluster, $r(14) =$ 0.520 and $p = 0.039$.

Table 2 White matter clusters with reduced fractional anisotropy (FA) in pediatric OCD patients versus healthy controls

Cluster label and anatomical localization	Voxels	MNI coordinates			FA		
		x	*y*	*z*	OCD	HC	*p*
1. Bilateral frontal (ATR, UF, IFOF, forceps minor, anterior corona radiata) and corpus callosum (genu, body, splenium)	9,022	20	37	6	0.533 0.191	0.573 0.188	0.026
2. Right cingulate and basal ganglia: anterior cingulate cortex (UF), anterior limb of IC (ATR), putamen (UF), amygdala (ILF), cerebral peduncle (CST), thalamus, and posterior limb of IC (ATR)	1,454	23	0	−9	0.419 0.157	0.460 0.158	0.035
3. Right posterior cerebral cortex: lateral occipital and angular gyri (SLF)	132	36	−56	33	0.423 0.100	0.500 0.098	0.048
4. Right inferior frontal lobe (subcallosal cortex)	50	8	21	−19	0.296 0.067	0.370 0.107	0.049
5. Right inferior frontal: orbitofrontal cortex	36	8	37	−22	0.267 0.067	0.323 0.073	0.050
6. Right thalamus	14	18	−5	11	0.639 0.041	0.668 0.038	0.050
7. Right caudate, anterior IC (ATR)	6	22	−4	24	0.430 0.056	0.493 0.081	0.050

ATR anterior thalamic radiation, *CST* corticospinal tract, *IC* internal capsule, *IFOF* inferior fronto-occipital fasciculus, *ILF* inferior longitudinal fasciculus, *SLF* superior longitudinal fasciculus, *UF* uncinate fasciculus.

Symptom severity

The mean FA and mean RD from the identified clusters were also examined in relation to symptom severity. There were no significant correlations with CY-BOCS total scores, CY-BOCS compulsive symptom scores, or CY-BOCS obsessive symptom scores. CY-BOCS total scores were not significantly correlated with age, age at onset, or duration of illness.

Discussion

These findings add to emerging evidence of abnormal integrity of brain WM tracts in pediatric OCD. This is the first DTI study to report that children with OCD compared with healthy youth show regional brain *reductions* in FA. Over 84% of the significant voxels localized to a single cluster that encompassed a large expanse of bilateral frontal cortex and extended into the CC. Smaller clusters of FA reduction were seen in the right posterior parietal and occipital cortices and the subcallosal and orbitofrontal cortices, as well as the thalamus and putamen. Youth with OCD also had significantly increased RD in areas that overlapped with the largest cluster of FA reduction, including the right anterior cingulate cortex and right body of the CC, suggesting deficient myelination in these areas. Finally, an earlier onset of OCD was associated with more pronounced FA reductions in the right thalamus and greater RD increases in the right body of the CC. Overall, our results are in line with increasing evidence that brain WM alterations are present in pediatric OCD and support a possible moderating role of age at onset on some aspects of OCD pathophysiology.

We found prominent alterations of frontal WM in subjects with OCD, affecting fiber tracts that connect the frontal lobe to both cortical and subcortical regions. Thus, OCD youth exhibited lower FA in a large cluster of bilateral frontal cortex, including anterior cingulate cortex (BA 32) and orbital-frontal cortex (BA 11), areas that are considered central to OCD pathophysiology [4,7]. This cluster overlapped with multiple WM tracts, including projection and association fibers that extend to the thalamus, anterior temporal-limbic regions, and parietal and occipital cortices. Consistent with frontal-subcortical models of OCD, FA reductions were also seen in the putamen, caudate, and thalamus of OCD youth. In adult DTI studies, both increased and decreased frontal FA have been found in OCD (e.g., [22,24]) and this may relate in part to illness heterogeneity. One source of variance in DTI studies of adult OCD appears to be the relative predominance of genetic versus environmental etiologic factors [29]. In their adult sample of monozygotic twins concordant and discordant for OCD, den Braber et al. [29] found that some WM tracts (including frontal tracts) show FA alterations that are in the opposite direction in subjects at high genetic risk compared with subjects at high environmental risk for OCD. Although neither the

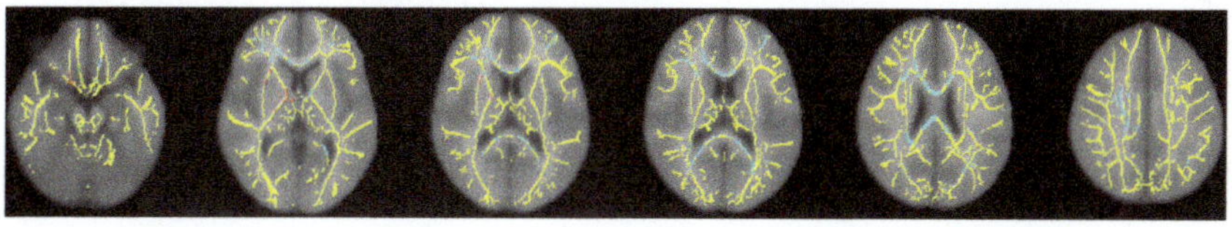

Figure 1 Clusters of significantly lower fractional anisotropy in youth with obsessive-compulsive disorder compared with healthy controls (skeleton: yellow; cluster 1: light blue; cluster 2: red; cluster 3: dark blue; cluster 4: bright green; cluster 5: copper; cluster 6: magenta; cluster 7: light green).

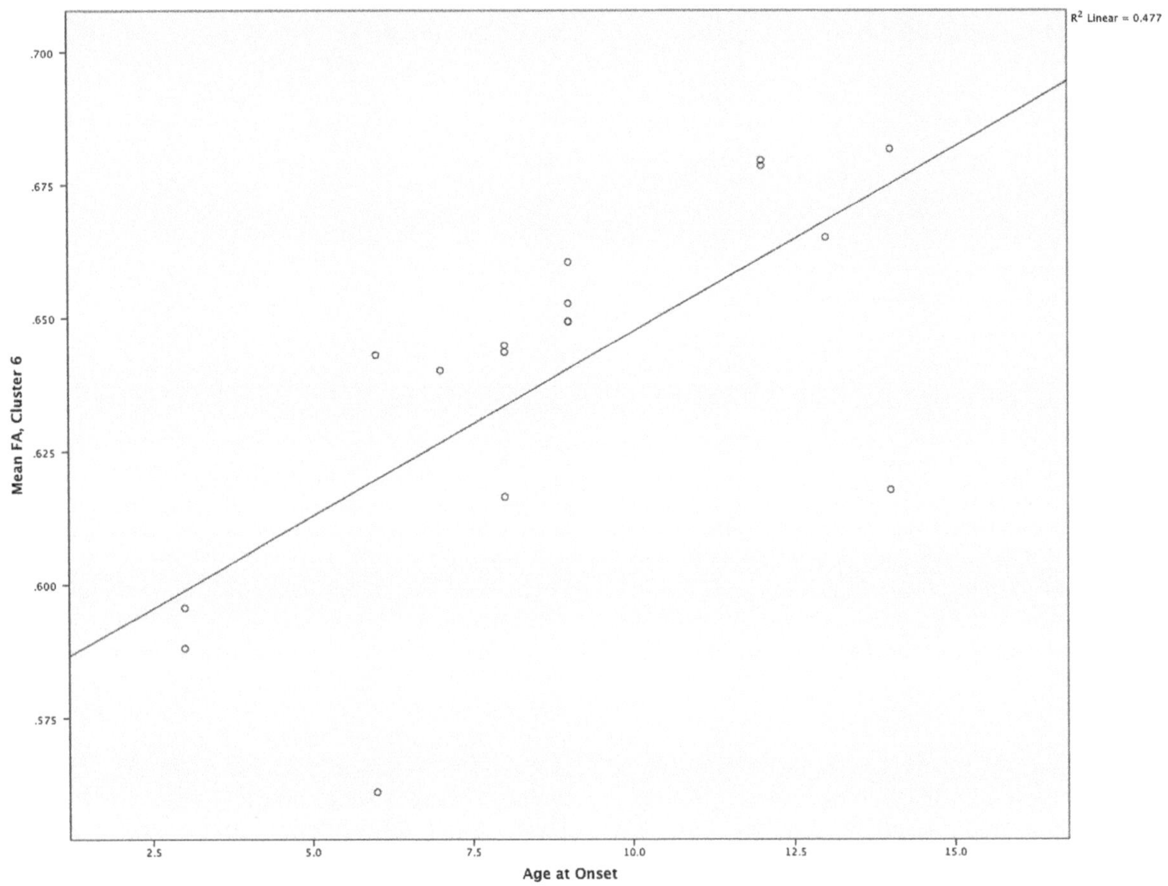

Figure 2 Association of age at onset with fractional anisotropy (FA) in youth with OCD in cluster 6.

current nor prior DTI studies of pediatric OCD formally assessed family history, it is possible that our sample was relatively high on genetic loading given its particularly early age at onset (averaging several years earlier than in prior studies [31,32]) and that this would explain findings of reduced FA in our sample but not prior pediatric OCD studies. Future DTI studies could be designed to parse the influences of genetic and environmental influences on WM in pediatric OCD.

Consistent with a growing body of neurobehavioral evidence that posterior association cortices are implicated in OCD, we found reduced WM integrity in the angular and lateral occipital gyri. A number of functional imaging studies have found abnormalities of glucose metabolism, cerebral blood flow, and brain activation in the posterior cortices of adult OCD patients [12]. Neuropsychological studies have shown that adults with OCD are impaired on visuospatial and decision-making functions that rely on the integrity of the parietal lobe [46-48]. In addition, a magnetic resonance spectroscopy study found increased choline in the parietal lobe WM of OCD, indicative of increased phospholipid turnover of myelinated axons in this

Table 3 White matter clusters with increased radial diffusivity (RD) in pediatric OCD patients versus healthy controls

Cluster label and anatomical localization	Voxels	MNI coordinates			RD				
		x	*y*	*z*	OCD		HC		*p*
1. Right frontal (anterior corona radiata, forceps minor, ATR; overlaps FA cluster 1)	406	19	32	12	0.000655	0.000085	0.000594	0.000089	0.042
2. Right body of the corpus callosum (overlaps FA cluster 1)	81	12	4	28	0.000421	0.000085	0.000358	0.000083	0.049
3. Right body of the corpus callosum (close to midline; overlaps FA cluster 1)	49	3	4	23	0.000474	0.000084	0.000399	0.000077	0.049

ATR anterior thalamic radiation.

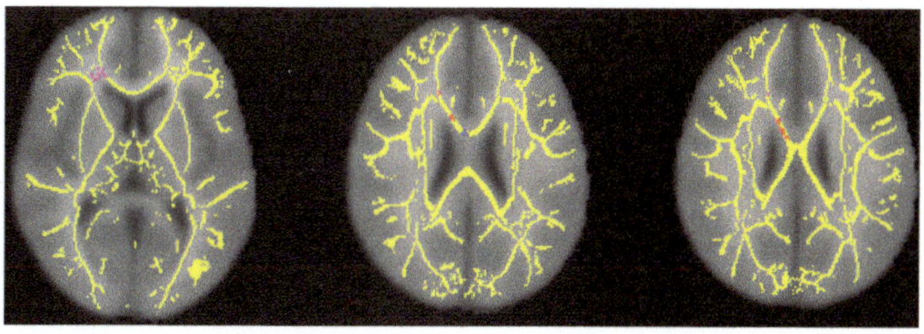

Figure 3 Clusters of significantly higher radial diffusivity in youth with obsessive-compulsive disorder compared with healthy controls (skeleton: yellow; cluster 1: magenta; cluster 2: red; cluster 3: blue).

region [49]. Although prior childhood OCD DTI studies found evidence of CC alterations suggestive of posterior association cortex involvement, the current study is the first to identify a cluster of altered FA in parietal cortex of pediatric patients. In DTI studies of adult OCD, reduced FA in parietal WM also has been found to distinguish patients from healthy control subjects (e.g., [12,24]). Thus, our results extend those of adult DTI studies by indicating that reduced parietal WM integrity is present in pediatric patients. This finding converges with a report of reduced parietal WM volume in adolescents with OCD compared with healthy youth [50]. Neurodevelopmental studies have shown that increases in FA and other maturational changes occur in parietal-occipital WM structure from the earliest years of childhood [51], such that disruption of this process could relate to early-onset pathophysiology [52]. In adult studies, visuospatial deficits and intrusive visual imagery are prominent features of OCD and have been documented premorbidly in adults prior to their onset of OCD symptoms [53]. Altogether, this suggests that abnormal parietal-occipital lobe structure and its behavioral manifestations are present in childhood OCD and early in the course of adult OCD.

Findings of diffusion alterations in the CC add to growing evidence of interhemispheric abnormalities in OCD, evident in both the pediatric and adult literatures [18,54]. In this study, OCD compared with healthy youth had reduced FA in portions of the genu, body, and splenium, which implicates fibers that connect bilateral frontal, parietal, and temporal-occipital association cortices [55,56]. There was a prominent cluster of FA reduction in the middle to posterior body of the CC, which connects bilateral somatosensory cortices and posterior parietal regions [57]. We also found decreased FA in the anterior portion of the genu, where small axons connect bilateral prefrontal cortex and ventral prefrontal cortex to the striatum. In an earlier study of pediatric OCD, Zarei et al. [31] had found increased FA in somewhat different CC areas corresponding to the posterior genu and anterior body of the CC, where larger axons connect primary motor cortices. Thus, it is possible that directional coherence of fiber tracts is differentially altered across different sections of the genu and body of the CC in childhood OCD, indicating variable pathology across topographically distinct association cortices.

Our finding of decreased splenium FA conflicts with two prior reports on youth with OCD [16,31]. Both investigations found higher splenium FA, which correlated with significantly greater OCD symptom severity [16,31]. Both of these prior studies had a lower proportion of medicated OCD patients (61%, 52%) than the current study (82%). Moreover, significantly elevated splenium FA was seen only among the subgroup of unmedicated patients in one of those studies [16]. Thus, it may be that our finding of lower splenium FA reflects the effects of medication treatment. Our study design does not allow us to test this question, but there is some prior evidence that treatment-nave OCD patients, including pediatric patients, have higher FA, greater WM density, and larger size of the CC [57]. Moreover, in a longitudinal study of adults with OCD, Yoo et al. [25] found that drug-nave patients had multiple areas of increased FA (including in the posterior CC) and that these normalized after a course of clinically effective citalopram treatment. Another possible source of conflicting findings across DTI studies is heterogeneity of OCD clinical features (e.g., our sample included a minority of washers relative to checkers). The adult OCD literature has begun to explore neural correlates of symptom dimensions in OCD [58]. Similar studies could be designed in pediatric OCD by selecting more homogeneous patient samples.

Alterations in diffusion anisotropy (FA) can result from changes in either RD (perpendicular) and/or AD (parallel), and these subcomponents are differentially modulated by myelin and axonal degeneration mechanisms, respectively [59]. In this study, we found concomitant decreases in FA and increases in RD in the right frontal cortex and right body of the CC, a pattern thought to reflect deficient myelination [59-62]. Abnormal myelination also has been implicated in OCD by other lines of research, including magnetic resonance spectroscopy findings of increased levels of cell membrane breakdown products in OCD youth [63,64], and genetic evidence of an association between OCD and a gene (OLIG2) involved in the development of oligodendrocytes [65]. Similar to our study, Jayarajan and colleagues [32] also had found significantly increased RD in a DTI in children with OCD compared with controls, although FA did not differ significantly between groups. Because increased RD was accompanied by increased AD in their patient sample, Jayarajan et al. [32] interpreted this as indicative of hyperconnected yet insufficiently myelinated WM tracts in affected regions. In contrast, Gruner et al. [16] found decreased RD in the context of significantly increased FA in four WM regions of pediatric OCD compared with control subjects, pointing to excessive myelination of certain axon fibers. Finally, Silk et al. [33] found significantly decreased AD in the genu and splenium of the CC of OCD youth, which could indicate less coherently organized callosal axons; FA was not significantly different between the groups in the CC or any other WM tract of that study. Thus, in the relatively small literature to date, there are different patterns of FA/RD/AD findings across pediatric OCD DTI studies. This could indicate involvement of multiple possible combinations of WM microstructure alterations in pediatric OCD wherein both myelin and axonal changes may be present in the context of either reduced or increased coherence of fiber tracts. The pattern of abnormalities may vary across brain regions, due to age-related maturational processes [16,31] and/or as a function of clinical phenomenology. These questions will need to be disentangled by conducting additional studies in this relatively young area of study.

Our findings suggest that age at onset may be an influential moderating factor on some of the WM changes in pediatric OCD. On average, our patients had an earlier onset of illness (average 8 years) than those in the two earlier pediatric OCD studies that reported on age at onset (11 years [31] and 13 years [32] on average). Moreover, within our patient sample, earlier onset was associated with significantly lower FA in the right thalamus and significantly higher RD in the right CC. The former association remained significant even after controlling for age, suggesting that earlier onset of OCD disease-related processes is associated with reduced integrity of WM in the thalamus. Involvement of the thalamus in early-onset OCD is consistent with the conclusions of a literature review that prominent thalamic abnormalities may be a component of a slightly different neuropathological substrate of childhood-onset versus adult-onset OCD [54].

Studying pediatric patients near the onset of their illness helps identify neurobiological changes that may be more primary than those arising later on in the course of illness, although developmental and disease effects may still be influential. Brain alterations noted during childhood and adolescence may change in their nature due to ongoing maturation of both gray matter and WM, which may contribute to variable findings across studies. In addition, compulsively engaging in a particular type of behavior or cognitive process can change brain structure [4,66,67]. Thus, even in pediatric OCD, anatomical brain differences may reflect a consequence rather than a precursor of the disorder. In the only study of neuropsychological correlates of DTI measures in pediatric OCD, the pattern of results found by Gruner et al. [16] suggested that certain FA increases might reflect compensatory increases in WM coherence to mitigate neuropsychological deficits. This highlights the usefulness of studying patients with OCD as close to symptom onset as possible, when such epiphenomenal changes may be less prominent.

Our findings should be interpreted in the context of the studys limitations. This was a cross-sectional investigation, and our results are therefore correlational in nature. We cannot rule out that these findings were affected by comorbidity within our OCD sample, particularly depression and other anxiety disorders present in a third of the patients. However, in *post hoc* analyses, severity of depression and anxiety symptoms was not associated with FA or RD in any of the significant clusters. Moreover, only a small percentage of the sample had any particular comorbid condition, making it implausible that the group findings were driven by a particular comorbidity. Similarly, we cannot exclude the possibility of medication effects, since most of our patients were medicated; although none of the previous pediatric OCD studies found any indication that DTI parameters were affected by medication use [16,31,32], it is possible that this reflected limited power to detect such effects. Finally, this and other pediatric OCD studies to date have not had sufficient power to examine the relationship of DTI WM measures with OCD symptom profile, which have been found to differentially relate to regional brain abnormalities in adult OCD [68].

Conclusions

Our findings of significantly lower FA and higher RD in childhood OCD are consistent with compromised WM integrity and reduced myelination, particularly involving the CC and fiber tracts that connect the frontal lobes to widespread cortical and subcortical targets. Our findings also suggest that age at onset may be a moderator of some of the WM changes in children with OCD. DTI research in childhood OCD is still in its infancy, and future studies should incorporate examination of how genetic and environmental risk factors, as well as aspects of illness phenomenology, may help parse divergent findings across studies.

Abbreviations

AD: Axial diffusivity; CC: Corpus callosum; CDI: Child Depression Inventory; CY-BOCS: Children s Yale-Brown Obsessive-Compulsive Scale; DTI: Diffusion tensor imaging; FA: Fractional anisotropy; HC: Healthy control; KSADS: Kiddie

Schedule for Affective Disorders and Schizophrenia; MD: Mean diffusivity; RD: Radial diffusivity; OCD: Obsessive-compulsive disorder; TBSS: Tract-based spatial statistics; TFCE: Threshold-Free Cluster Enhancement; WM: White matter; YGTSS: Yale Global Tic Severity Scale.

Competing interests
The authors declare that they have no competing interests.

Authors contributions
IMR was involved in data collection and analysis and wrote the first draft of the manuscript. EAO analyzed the imaging data and contributed to writing of the methods and results. JCB, SES, and SLR designed the study and were involved in subject recruitment and data interpretation. GP and NM contributed to the processing, analysis, and interpretation of the imaging data. WDSK was involved in data collection. SW and MAJ assisted with subject recruitment. All authors contributed to and have approved the final manuscript.

Acknowledgements
This research was supported by an anonymous donor. We would like to acknowledge the contributions of Jennifer Ragan, Anne Chosak, Adriane Alpern, Elizabeth Flamm, Sarah Glaser, and Elizabeth Sadock for their assistance in conducting assessments and the McLean Hospital Imaging Center MRI technologists for their assistance with scanning.

Author details
[1]Center for Depression, Anxiety and Stress Research, McLean Hospital, 115 Mill Street, mailstop 334, Belmont, MA 02478, USA. [2]Department of Psychiatry, Harvard Medical School, Boston, MA, USA. [3]Department of Psychology, University of Miami, 5665 Ponce de Leon Blvd, Flipse Building, Coral Gables, Miami, FL 33146, USA. [4]British Columbia Mental Health and Addictions Research Institute, University of British Columbia, Vancouver, BC, Canada. [5]Center for Morphometric Analysis, Massachusetts General Hospital, Bldg 149, 13th Street, Charlestown, MA 02129, USA. [6]Department of Neurology, Harvard Medical School, Boston, MA, USA. [7]Department of Radiology, Harvard Medical School, Boston, MA, USA. [8]Department of Psychiatry, Massachusetts General Hospital, Simches Research Building, 185 Cambridge Street, Suite 2282, Boston, MA 02114, USA. [9]UBC Psychiatry A3-118, 938 West 28th Ave, Vancouver, BC V5Z 4H4, Canada. [10]Department of Psychiatry, University of Arizona, Tucson, AZ, USA.

References

1. American Psychiatric Association: *Diagnostic and Statistical Manual of Mental Disorders, Fourth Edition (DSM-IV)*. Washington, D.C.: American Psychiatric Association; 1994.
2. Geller DA: **Obsessive-compulsive and spectrum disorders in children and adolescents.** *Psychiatr Clin North Am* 2006, **29:**353 370.
3. Stewart SE, Geller DA, Jenike M, Pauls D, Shaw D, Mullin B, Faraone SV: **Long-term outcome of pediatric obsessive-compulsive disorder: a meta-analysis and qualitative review of the literature.** *Acta Psychiatr Scand* 2004, **110:**4 13.
4. Maia TV, Cooney RE, Peterson BS: **The neural bases of obsessive-compulsive disorder in children and adults.** *Dev Psychopathol* 2008, **20:**1251 1283.
5. Huyser C, Veltman DJ, de Haan E, Boer F: **Paediatric obsessive-compulsive disorder, a neurodevelopmental disorder? Evidence from neuroimaging.** *Neurosci Biobehav Rev* 2009, **33:**818 830.
6. Rosenberg DR, Keshavan MS: **A.E. Bennett Research Award. Toward a neurodevelopmental model of obsessive compulsive disorder.** *Biol Psychiatry* 1998, **43:**623 640.
7. Graybiel AM, Rauch SL: **Toward a neurobiology of obsessive-compulsive disorder.** *Neuron* 2000, **28:**343 347.
8. Saxena S, Brody AL, Schwartz JM, Baxter LR: **Neuroimaging and frontal-subcortical circuitry in obsessive-compulsive disorder.** *Br J Psychiatry Suppl* 1998, **35:**26 37.
9. Fineberg NA, Potenza MN, Chamberlain SR, Berlin HA, Menzies L, Bechara A, Sahakian BJ, Robbins TW, Bullmore ET, Hollander E: **Probing compulsive and impulsive behaviors, from animal models to endophenotypes: a narrative review.** *Neuropsychopharmacology* 2010, **35:**591 604.
10. Radua J, van den Heuvel OA, Surguladze S, Mataix-Cols D: **Meta-analytical comparison of voxel-based morphometry studies in obsessive-compulsive disorder vs other anxiety disorders.** *Arch Gen Psychiatry* 2010, **67:**701 711.
11. Rotge JY, Guehl D, Dilharreguy B, Tignol J, Bioulac B, Allard M, Burbaud P, Aouizerate B: **Meta-analysis of brain volume changes in obsessive-compulsive disorder.** *Biol Psychiatry* 2009, **65:**75 83.
12. Menzies L, Chamberlain SR, Laird AR, Thelen SM, Sahakian BJ, Bullmore ET: **Integrating evidence from neuroimaging and neuropsychological studies of obsessive-compulsive disorder: the orbitofronto-striatal model revisited.** *Neurosci Biobehav Rev* 2008, **32:**525 549.
13. Abramovitch A, Dar R, Schweiger A, Hermesh H: **Neuropsychological impairments and their association with obsessive-compulsive symptom severity in obsessive-compulsive disorder.** *Arch Clin Neuropsychol* 2011, **26:**364 376.
14. Bannon S, Gonsalvez CJ, Croft RJ, Boyce PM: **Response inhibition deficits in obsessive-compulsive disorder.** *Psychiatry Res* 2002, **110:**165 174.
15. Chamberlain SR, Blackwell AD, Fineberg NA, Robbins TW, Sahakian BJ: **The neuropsychology of obsessive compulsive disorder: the importance of failures in cognitive and behavioural inhibition as candidate endophenotypic markers.** *Neurosci Biobehav Rev* 2005, **29:**399 419.
16. Gruner P, Vo A, Ikuta T, Mahon K, Peters BD, Malhotra AK, Ulug AM, Szeszko PR: **White matter abnormalities in pediatric obsessive-compulsive disorder.** *Neuropsychopharmacology* 2012, **37:**2730 2739.
17. Penades R, Catalan R, Rubia K, Andres S, Salamero M, Gasto C: **Impaired response inhibition in obsessive compulsive disorder.** *Eur Psychiatry* 2007, **22:**404 410.
18. Fontenelle LF, Harrison BJ, Yucel M, Pujol J, Fujiwara H, Pantelis C: **Is there evidence of brain white-matter abnormalities in obsessive-compulsive disorder?: A narrative review.** *Top Magn Reson Imaging* 2009, **20:**291 298.
19. Olson EA, Collins PF, Hooper CJ, Muetzel R, Lim KO, Luciana M: **White matter integrity predicts delay discounting behavior in 9- to 23-year-olds: a diffusion tensor imaging study.** *J Cogn Neurosci* 2009, **21:**1406 1421.
20. Beaulieu C: **The basis of anisotropic water diffusion in the nervous system - a technical review.** *NMR Biomed* 2002, **15:**435 455.
21. Harsan LA, Poulet P, Guignard B, Steibel J, Parizel N, de Sousa PL, Boehm N, Grucker D, Ghandour MS: **Brain dysmyelination and recovery assessment by noninvasive in vivo diffusion tensor magnetic resonance imaging.** *J Neurosci Res* 2006, **83:**392 402.
22. Cannistraro PA, Makris N, Howard JD, Wedig MM, Hodge SM, Wilhelm S, Kennedy DN, Rauch SL: **A diffusion tensor imaging study of white matter in obsessive-compulsive disorder.** *Depress Anxiety* 2007, **24:**440 446.
23. Garibotto V, Scifo P, Gorini A, Alonso CR, Brambati S, Bellodi L, Perani D: **Disorganization of anatomical connectivity in obsessive compulsive disorder: a multi-parameter diffusion tensor imaging study in a subpopulation of patients.** *Neurobiol Dis* 2010, **37:**468 476.
24. Szeszko PR, Ardekani BA, Ashtari M, Malhotra AK, Robinson DG, Bilder RM, Lim KO: **White matter abnormalities in obsessive-compulsive disorder: a diffusion tensor imaging study.** *Arch Gen Psychiatry* 2005, **62:**782 790.
25. Yoo SY, Jang JH, Shin YW, Kim DJ, Park HJ, Moon WJ, Chung EC, Lee JM, Kim IY, Kim SI, Kwon JS: **White matter abnormalities in drug-naive patients with obsessive-compulsive disorder: a diffusion tensor study before and after citalopram treatment.** *Acta Psychiatr Scand* 2007, **116:**211 219.
26. Nakamae T, Narumoto J, Sakai Y, Nishida S, Yamada K, Nishimura T, Fukui K: **Diffusion tensor imaging and tract-based spatial statistics in obsessive-compulsive disorder.** *J Psychiatr Res* 2011, **45:**687 690.
27. Saito Y, Nobuhara K, Okugawa G, Takase K, Sugimoto T, Horiuchi M, Ueno C, Maehara M, Omura N, Kurokawa H, Ikeda K, Tanigawa N, Sawada S, Kinoshita T: **Corpus callosum in patients with obsessive-compulsive disorder: diffusion-tensor imaging study.** *Radiology* 2008, **246:**536 542.
28. Li F, Huang X, Yang Y, Li B, Wu Q, Zhang T, Lui S, Kemp GJ, Gong Q: **Microstructural brain abnormalities in patients with obsessive-compulsive disorder: diffusion-tensor MR imaging study at 3.0 T.** *Radiology* 2011, **260:**216 223.
29. den Braber A, van t D, Boomsma DI, Cath DC, Veltman DJ, Thompson PM, de Geus EJ: **White matter differences in monozygotic twins discordant or concordant for obsessive-compulsive symptoms: a combined diffusion tensor imaging/voxel-based morphometry study.** *Biol Psychiatry* 2011, **70:**969 977.
30. Menzies L, Williams GB, Chamberlain SR, Ooi C, Fineberg N, Suckling J, Sahakian BJ, Robbins TW, Bullmore ET: **White matter abnormalities in**

patients with obsessive-compulsive disorder and their first-degree relatives. *Am J Psychiatry* 2008, **165**:1308 1315.
31. Zarei M, Mataix-Cols D, Heyman I, Hough M, Doherty J, Burge L, Winmill L, Nijhawan S, Matthews PM, James A: **Changes in gray matter volume and white matter microstructure in adolescents with obsessive-compulsive disorder.** *Biol Psychiatry* 2011, **70**:1083 1090.
32. Jayarajan RN, Venkatasubramanian G, Viswanath B, Janardhan Reddy YC, Srinath S, Vasudev MK, Chandrashekar CR: **White matter abnormalities in children and adolescents with obsessive-compulsive disorder: a diffusion tensor imaging study.** *Depress Anxiety* 2012, **29**:780 788.
33. Silk T, Chen J, Seal M, Vance A: **White matter abnormalities in pediatric obsessive-compulsive disorder.** *Psychiatry Res* 2013, **213**:154 160.
34. Kaufman J, Birmaher B, Brent D, Rao U, Flynn C, Moreci P, Williamson D, Ryan N: **Schedule for affective disorders and schizophrenia for school-Age children-present and lifetime version (K-SADS-PL): initial reliability and validity data.** *J Am Acad Child Adolesc Psychiatry* 1997, **36**:980 988.
35. Goodman WK, Price LH, Rasmussen SA, Mazure C, Fleischmann RL, Hill CL, Heninger GR, Charney DS: **The Yale-Brown Obsessive Compulsive Scale. I. Development, use, and reliability.** *Arch Gen Psychiatry* 1989, **46**:1006 1011.
36. Kovacs M: *Childrens Depression Inventory Manual.* North Tonawanda: Multi-Health Systems; 1992.
37. Leckman JF, Riddle MA, Hardin MT, Ort SI, Swartz KL, Stevenson J, Cohen DJ: **The Yale Global Tic Severity Scale: initial testing of a clinician-rated scale of tic severity.** *J Am Acad Child Adolesc Psychiatry* 1989, **28**:566 573.
38. Stewart SE, Rosario MC, Baer L, Carter AS, Brown TA, Scharf JM, Illmann C, Leckman JF, Sukhodolsky D, Katsovich L, Rasmussen S, Goodman W, Delorme R, Leboyer M, Chabane N, Jenike MA, Geller DA, Pauls DL: **Four-factor structure of obsessive-compulsive disorder symptoms in children, adolescents, and adults.** *J Am Acad Child Adolesc Psychiatry* 2008, **47**:763 772.
39. Andersson JLR, Jenkinson M, Smith S: **Non-linear optimisation.** [www.fmrib.ox.ac.uk/analysis/techrep]
40. Andersson JLR, Jenkinson M, Smith S: **Non-linear registration, aka spatial normalisation.** [www.fmrib.ox.ac.uk/analysis/techrep]
41. Smith SM: **Fast robust automated brain extraction.** *Hum Brain Mapp* 2002, **17**:143 155.
42. Gallichan D, Scholz J, Bartsch A, Behrens TE, Robson MD, Miller KL: **Addressing a systematic vibration artifact in diffusion-weighted MRI.** *Hum Brain Mapp* 2010, **31**:193 202.
43. Smith SM, Jenkinson M, Johansen-Berg H, Rueckert D, Nichols TE, Mackay CE, Watkins KE, Ciccarelli O, Cader MZ, Matthews PM, Behrens TE: **Tract-based spatial statistics: voxelwise analysis of multi-subject diffusion data.** *Neuroimage* 2006, **31**:1487 1505.
44. Smith SM, Jenkinson M, Woolrich MW, Beckmann CF, Behrens TE, Johansen-Berg H, Bannister PR, De Luca M, Drobnjak I, Flitney DE, Niazy RK, Saunders J, Vickers J, Zhang Y, De Stefano N, Brady JM, Matthews PM: **Advances in functional and structural MR image analysis and implementation as FSL.** *Neuroimage* 2004, **23**(Suppl 1):S208 S219.
45. Nichols TE, Holmes AP: **Nonparametric permutation tests for functional neuroimaging: a primer with examples.** *Hum Brain Mapp* 2002, **15**:1 25.
46. Chamberlain SR, Fineberg NA, Blackwell AD, Clark L, Robbins TW, Sahakian BJ: **A neuropsychological comparison of obsessive-compulsive disorder and trichotillomania.** *Neuropsychologia* 2007, **45**:654 662.
47. Menzies L, Achard S, Chamberlain SR, Fineberg N, Chen CH, del Campo N, Sahakian BJ, Robbins TW, Bullmore E: **Neurocognitive endophenotypes of obsessive-compulsive disorder.** *Brain* 2007, **130**:3223 3236.
48. Okasha A, Rafaat M, Mahallawy N, El Nahas G, El Dawla AS, Sayed M, El Kholi S: **Cognitive dysfunction in obsessive-compulsive disorder.** *Acta Psychiatr Scand* 2000, **101**:281 285.
49. Kitamura H, Shioiri T, Kimura T, Ohkubo M, Nakada T, Someya T: **Parietal white matter abnormalities in obsessive-compulsive disorder: a magnetic resonance spectroscopy study at 3-Tesla.** *Acta Psychiatr Scand* 2006, **114**:101 108.
50. Lazaro L, Bargallo N, Castro-Fornieles J, Falcon C, Andres S, Calvo R, Junque C: **Brain changes in children and adolescents with obsessive-compulsive disorder before and after treatment: a voxel-based morphometric MRI study.** *Psychiatry Res* 2009, **172**:140 146.
51. Giedd JN, Blumenthal J, Jeffries NO, Castellanos FX, Liu H, Zijdenbos A, Paus T, Evans AC, Rapoport JL: **Brain development during childhood and adolescence: a longitudinal MRI study.** *Nat Neurosci* 1999, **2**:861 863.
52. Barnea-Goraly N, Menon V, Eckert M, Tamm L, Bammer R, Karchemskiy A, Dant CC, Reiss AL: **White matter development during childhood and adolescence: a cross-sectional diffusion tensor imaging study.** *Cereb Cortex* 2005, **15**:1848 1854.
53. Grisham JR, Anderson TM, Poulton R, Moffitt TE, Andrews G: **Childhood neuropsychological deficits associated with adult obsessive-compulsive disorder.** *Br J Psychiatry* 2009, **195**:138 141.
54. MacMaster FP, O Neill J, Rosenberg DR: **Brain imaging in pediatric obsessive-compulsive disorder.** *J Am Acad Child Adolesc Psychiatry* 2008, **47**:1262 1272.
55. Giedd JN, Rumsey JM, Castellanos FX, Rajapakse JC, Kaysen D, Vaituzis AC, Vauss YC, Hamburger SD, Rapoport JL: **A quantitative MRI study of the corpus callosum in children and adolescents.** *Brain Res Dev Brain Res* 1996, **91**:274 280.
56. Mac Master FP, Keshavan MS, Dick EL, Rosenberg DR: **Corpus callosal signal intensity in treatment-naive pediatric obsessive compulsive disorders.** *Prog Neuropsychopharmacol Biol Psychiatry* 1999, **23**:601 612.
57. Rosenberg DR, Keshavan MS, Dick EL, Bagwell WW, MacMaster FP, Birmaher B: **Corpus callosal morphology in treatment-naive pediatric obsessive compulsive disorder.** *Prog Neuropsychopharmacol Biol Psychiatry* 1997, **21**:1269 1283.
58. Mataix-Cols D, Cullen S, Lange K, Zelaya F, Andrew C, Amaro E, Brammer MJ, Williams SC, Speckens A, Phillips ML: **Neural correlates of anxiety associated with obsessive-compulsive symptom dimensions in normal volunteers.** *Biol Psychiatry* 2003, **53**:482 493.
59. Song SK, Sun SW, Ramsbottom MJ, Chang C, Russell J, Cross AH: **Dysmyelination revealed through MRI as increased radial (but unchanged axial) diffusion of water.** *Neuroimage* 2002, **17**:1429 1436.
60. Basser PJ: **Inferring microstructural features and the physiological state of tissues from diffusion-weighted images.** *NMR Biomed* 1995, **8**:333 344.
61. Song SK, Sun SW, Ju WK, Lin SJ, Cross AH, Neufeld AH: **Diffusion tensor imaging detects and differentiates axon and myelin degeneration in mouse optic nerve after retinal ischemia.** *Neuroimage* 2003, **20**:1714 1722.
62. Song SK, Yoshino J, Le TQ, Lin SJ, Sun SW, Cross AH, Armstrong RC: **Demyelination increases radial diffusivity in corpus callosum of mouse brain.** *Neuroimage* 2005, **26**:132 140.
63. Rosenberg DR, MacMillan SN, Moore GJ: **Brain anatomy and chemistry may predict treatment response in paediatric obsessive compulsive disorder.** *Int J Neuropsychopharmacol* 2001, **4**:179 190.
64. Smith EA, Russell A, Lorch E, Banerjee SP, Rose M, Ivey J, Bhandari R, Moore GJ, Rosenberg DR: **Increased medial thalamic choline found in pediatric patients with obsessive-compulsive disorder versus major depression or healthy control subjects: a magnetic resonance spectroscopy study.** *Biol Psychiatry* 2003, **54**:1399 1405.
65. Stewart SE, Platko J, Fagerness J, Birns J, Jenike E, Smoller JW, Perlis R, Leboyer M, Delorme R, Chabane N, Rauch SL, Jenike MA, Pauls DL: **A genetic family-based association study of OLIG2 in obsessive-compulsive disorder.** *Arch Gen Psychiatry* 2007, **64**:209 214.
66. Lazar SW, Kerr CE, Wasserman RH, Gray JR, Greve DN, Treadway MT, McGarvey M, Quinn BT, Dusek JA, Benson H, Rauch SL, Moore CI, Fischl B: **Meditation experience is associated with increased cortical thickness.** *Neuroreport* 2005, **16**:1893 1897.
67. Schlaug G: **The brain of musicians. A model for functional and structural adaptation.** *Ann N Y Acad Sci* 2001, **930**:281 299.
68. van den Heuvel OA, Remijnse PL, Mataix-Cols D, Vrenken H, Groenewegen HJ, Uylings HB, van Balkom AJ, Veltman DJ: **The major symptom dimensions of obsessive-compulsive disorder are mediated by partially distinct neural systems.** *Brain* 2009, **132**:853 868.

Aberrant amygdala functional connectivity at rest in pediatric anxiety disorders

Lisa L Hamm[1], Rachel H Jacobs[1], Meghan W Johnson[1], Daniel A Fitzgerald[1], Kate D Fitzgerald[2], Scott A Langenecker[1], Christopher S Monk[2,3] and K Luan Phan[1,2,4,5*]

Abstract

Background: Childhood onset of anxiety disorders is associated with greater functional impairment and burden across the lifespan. Recent work suggests that generalized anxiety disorder (GAD) is characterized by dysfunctional connectivity in amygdala-based circuits at rest in adolescents, consistent with adults. However, neural mechanisms underlying a broad spectrum of often-comorbid anxiety disorders in children remains unclear and understudied. The current study examines amygdala functional connectivity at rest in children and adolescents across comorbid anxiety disorders (ADs) including youth with primary diagnoses of GAD and social phobia (SP).

Results: Compared with healthy controls (HCs), AD youth exhibited hyperconnectivity between the right amygdala and the insula and hypoconnectivity between the left amygdala and the ventromedial prefrontal cortex (vmPFC) and posterior cingulate cortex (PCC). Within the AD group, connectivity was not correlated with anxiety severity and only the amygdala-PCC connectivity was positively correlated with age.

Conclusions: Our findings indicate that youth with comorbid ADs demonstrate aberrant connectivity in the anterior limbic network (ALN) as well as the PCC at rest. This extends upon previous work suggesting alterations in amygdala circuits underlying fear learning, emotion regulation, and the processing of interoceptive states. Presence of these findings within this young, comorbid sample points to underlying common mechanisms across ADs and illuminates future targets for prevention and intervention in childhood.

Keywords: Children, Adolescent, Anxiety, Amygdala, Connectivity, Resting state, fMRI

Background

Anxiety disorders (ADs) are among the most prevalent and disabling psychiatric disorders to occur in youth [1-4] and set children on a negative trajectory towards continued and additional comorbid psychological disorders during adulthood [5-7]. When left untreated, pediatric anxiety disorders can result in severe ongoing social impairment, decreased educational achievement, and interrupted employment [7-9]. The three most common anxiety disorders among youth include generalized anxiety disorder (GAD), social phobia (SP), and separation anxiety disorder (SAD) and are collectively referred to as the "pediatric anxiety triad" [10,11]. High rates of comorbidity across these diagnoses suggest greater similarities than differences [12], including sensitivity to perceived or actual negative life events [13] and debilitating worry leading to avoidance patterns (DSM-5, 2013). Additionally, these three disorders respond to similar treatments [12,14,15], further implicating diagnostic overlap and, perhaps, common neural mechanisms. Recent examinations of pediatric anxiety have moved towards a more dimensional approach by including children with comorbid ADs to evaluate neural correlates [16], as well as the effectiveness of treatments, such as cognitive behavioral therapy (CBT), in reducing the severity of anxiety symptoms [17].

Despite the prevalence and negative sequelae of the pediatric anxiety triad, research examining the underlying neural mechanisms is in its infancy. The amygdala is the most frequently studied region of interest in pediatric anxiety, given the robust human neuroimaging literature documenting amygdala activity and connectivity as it relates to emotional processing and regulation [18,19]. Indeed, amygdala hyperactivation to perceived threat is a

* Correspondence: klphan@uic.edu
[1]Department of Psychiatry, University of Illinois at Chicago, 1747 W. Roosevelt Road, IJR/WROB Rm. 244, Chicago, IL 60608, USA
[2]Department of Psychiatry, University of Michigan, Ann Arbor, Michigan, USA
Full list of author information is available at the end of the article

defining neuropathophysiological feature of anxiety disorders [20-22] and frontal regions are known to have dense bidirectional structural connections with the amygdala [23,24]. The amygdala is one region contributing to what has been labeled the anterior limbic network (ALN; [18]). This network encompasses connections between the amygdala, medial prefrontal cortex (mPFC), insula, anterior cingulate cortex (ACC), as well as the ventrolateral and dorsolateral prefrontal cortexes (vlPFC, dlPFC) [18]. These regions modulate complex social and emotional behaviors and share architectural and functional features [25]. Reciprocal connections within this network are hypothesized to contribute to monitoring of internal and external sensory information in order to maintain emotional equilibrium [26].

The strongest evidence implicating aberrant ALN function in anxiety disorders derives from several task-based fMRI studies that measure connectivity of networks during emotional tasks. Altered functional connectivity patterns have been observed during emotional processing and fear responding in regions composing the ALN among adults with anxiety [27,28] as well as among youth [19,22,29,30]. Adults with ADs have demonstrated decreased connectivity between the amygdala and the rostral ACC and dlPFC while viewing fearful faces [27]. An examination of functional connectivity during a face-emotion rating task found greater connectivity between the right amygdala and the insula in youth with GAD compared to healthy controls (HCs). Anxiety symptom severity (as measured by the Pediatric Anxiety Rating Scale (PARS)) was correlated with extent of with amygdala-insula connectivity [29]. Functional connectivity studies of both adults and youth support the notion that ALN disruption contributes to symptoms of anxiety. Disruptions in this network may underlie core phenotypic features of the disorder across the lifespan [31].

Functional connectivity can also be measured during the resting state (labeled rs-fMRI) and allows for the examination of the intrinsic functional connectivity (iFC) *in the absence of a specific emotional task.* Rs-fMRI has proven useful in interrogating neural circuits implicated in anxiety-related processes, with several studies demonstrating the existence of disrupted connectivity *at baseline* in amygdala-based networks among adults with anxiety disorders [27,32]. Importantly, iFC methods have yielded reliable individual differences in neural connectivity that are correlated with self-report of behavior and symptoms [33-36]. This technique has been utilized in recent studies of healthy adults to demonstrate several iFC patterns that covaried with positive and negative affect [35], and trait levels of anxiety modulated amygdala-mPFC connectivity [37]. These results implicate the relevance of functional connectivity in the affective domain *even in the absence of an emotional challenge* among adults with anxiety disorders. In addition, recent rs-fMRI studies have demonstrated altered resting state connectivity in regions considered part of the ALN, including the ACC, mPFC, and insula [27,38,39].

A region outside of the ALN that has been implicated in social and general anxiety is the posterior cingulate cortex (PCC) and the adjacent precuneus. The PCC in particular may play a role in emotional evaluation [40] and social behavior [41]. The PCC may also contribute to modulation of the amygdala [42]. Rs-fMRI data collected from adults with anxiety disorders found that reduced connectivity between the amygdala and the PCC/precuneus was associated with higher state anxiety [43]. Among adolescents with GAD, one study that has examined connectivity of the amygdala during a task of emotional and neutral images found altered connectivity between the right amygdala and the posterior cingulate [19]. In sum, task-based fMRI studies have identified abnormalities in the PCC among youth with anxiety disorders [19,29], but limited work has examined this region at rest among youth.

Examinations of connectivity among youth with anxiety disorders is understudied to date, partly due to the difficulty in recruiting this population and acclimatizing them to the fMRI environment. However, the altered connectivity patterns observed among adults may not be applicable to pediatric populations due to the important structural and functional developmental changes known to occur in the brain during childhood and adolescence [44-46]. Examining the developmental trajectory of neural network abnormalities among youth with anxiety may elucidate predictive or modifiable biomarkers of anxiety in addition to illustrating the long-term effects of anxiety on neurodevelopment [47]. To the best of our knowledge, only one study to date has used rs-fMRI to examine functional connectivity in youth with anxiety [48]. This study documented perturbations in connectivity between the amygdala and the following regions: ACC, striatum, insula, superior temporal gyrus, as well as prefrontal regions including the ventromedial prefrontal cortex (vmPFC), dmPFC, vlPFC, and dlPFC among fifteen youth between 12 and 17 with a diagnosis of GAD. These differences support a more widespread disruption of network function than previously identified.

In the present study, we sought to contribute to the literature by examining rs-fMRI using bilateral amygdala seeds in a sample of 33 youth with primary ADs of GAD and/or SP with several comorbidity profiles and compared them to data for 23 healthy controls (ages 7 to 19). We chose to examine both the left and right amygdala seeds separately given the only pediatric anxiety rs-fMRI study to date detected laterality in amygdala connectivity [48]. We sought to study a representative heterogeneous diagnostic group that would allow for greater generalizability of findings consistent with epidemiologic and intervention trials that demonstrate comorbidity across these disorders and commonality in treatment response [14,49]. In line with emotion regulation models of ADs [50], we hypothesized that relative to healthy peers, youth with ADs would demonstrate hyperconnectivity between the amygdala and insula. We also hypothesized that youth with AD would demonstrate hypoconnectivity between the amygdala and regions included in the ALN such as the ACC and mPFC. We also sought to explore amygdala-PCC connectivity but did not hypothesize a direction based on the paucity of findings to date.

Methods

Subjects

Participants included 33 children (mean age 13.9 ± 3.1 years; 22 female) with a DSM-IV (1) primary diagnosis of GAD, SP, and SAD (collectively referred to as ADs) who were compared to 23 matched HCs (14.6 ± 3.9 years; 13 female; Table 1). All participants were medication-free at the time of testing and were recruited from the University of Michigan Pediatric Anxiety Disorders Clinic as well as advertisements posted in the local community. All subjects had negative urine drug test (and pregnancy test for females) which were administered immediately prior to the fMRI scan. Exclusion criteria included an IQ below 70, a lifetime diagnosis of bipolar disorder, schizophrenia, and/or a pervasive developmental disorder. Healthy comparison youth were required to be free of lifetime diagnoses of DSM-IV Axis I and II disorders. All participants provided written informed consent/assent. The study was approved by the University of Michigan Institutional Review Board.

Both groups of participants (HCs and ADs) were interviewed by clinically trained mental health professionals using the Kiddie-Schedule for Affective Disorders-Present and Lifetime Version (K-SADS-PL) [51], and diagnoses were confirmed by a board-certified psychiatrist. A second rater conducted reliability on 20% of cases to establish inter-rater reliability. Within the primary GAD group, 10 participants (30%) received a comorbid SP/SAD diagnosis. Within the primary SP group, 6 participants (40%) received a comorbid GAD/SAD diagnosis. Current anxiety symptom severity and impairment was assessed by a clinician using the PARS [52] which has demonstrated high inter-rater reliability (The Research Units On Pediatric Psychopharmacology Anxiety Study Group, 2002).

Table 1 Sample demographic data and clinical features

	Anxiety disorder	Healthy controls	*p value*
Total (*n*)	33	23	
Sex, female, *n* (%)	22 (67)	13 (57)	
Age, mean ± SD	13.9 ± 3.1	14.6 ± 3.9	n.s.
Race	29 C, 2 AA, 2 multi	16 C, 1 AA, 1 As, 4 multi, 1 unknown	n.s.
Primary anxiety diagnoses (*n*) (percent of total)			
Generalized anxiety disorder	23 (70%)		
Social phobia	10 (30%)		
PARS ± SD	22 ± 3.9	2 ± 2.5	$p < 0.001$

C Caucasian, *AA* African-American, *As* Asian, *Multi* multiracial, *PARS* Pediatric Anxiety Rating Scale, *n.s.* non-significant ($p > 0.05$).

fMRI acquisition

Functional imaging was performed with blood-oxygen-level-dependent (BOLD) sensitive whole-brain fMRI on a 3.0 Tesla GE Signa System (General Electric; Milwaukee, WI) using a four-channel GE Quadrature sending and receiving head coil. Images were acquired with 30 axial, 5-mm-thick slices using a standard T2*-sensitive gradient echo reverse spiral acquisition sequence (2 s repetition time; 25 ms echo time; 64 × 64 matrix; 24 cm field of view; flip angle 77°; 3.75 × 3.75 × 5 mm final voxel size). A high-resolution, T1-weighted volumetric anatomical scan was also acquired in the axial plane (9 ms repetition time, 1.8 ms echo time; 256 × 256 matrix; 256 mm field of view; flip angle 15°; 124 slices; 1.2 mm slice thickness) at the same position as the functional images for anatomical localization and spatial normalization. Resting-state functional imaging included one 8-min scan during which participants were instructed to look at a fixation cross and let their mind wander without falling asleep.

fMRI analysis

Images were preprocessed and analyzed with the CONN: functional connectivity toolbox (http://www.nitrc.org/projects/conn), with preprocessing steps implemented in SPM8 (http://www.fil.ion.ucl.ac.uk/spm/) running on the MATLAB (Math Works, Natick, MA) platform. Images were segmented into gray matter, white matter, and cerebrospinal fluid (CSF) for use during removal of temporal confounds. Data were then motion corrected, coregistered with a high resolution T1 image, normalized to the Montreal Neurological Institute (MNI) space, and smoothed with an 8-mm Gaussian kernel of full width at half-maximum. Importantly, patients and healthy controls did not significantly differ in either total ($p = 0.255$), maximum ($p = 0.443$) or average ($p = 0.170$) head motion. Connectivity preprocessing followed the CompCor method [53] for removal of non-neuronal sources of noise, as opposed to relying on global signal regression, which subsequently allows for interpretation of anticorrelations. Amygdala connectivity maps were generated for each subject using a seed-driven approach in which the left and right amygdala were defined by the Automated

Anatomical Labeling (AAL) atlas based on the Talairach Daemon database [54]. The entire BOLD time course was extracted from the amygdala seeds, and Pearson's correlation coefficients were calculated between these entire time courses and the time courses of all other voxels across the brain and a mean time course across the entire region of interest. Fisher transformation was used to convert the resulting correlation coefficients into *Z*-scores which were then used in second-level general linear model analyses. Group differences in amygdala connectivity were examined using two-tailed independent samples *t* tests. To determine significance within *a priori* regions in which we had a strong hypothesis within both the ALN (mPFC, ACC, and insula) and PCC given the extant literature, we restricted our analyses to these relevant regions using an anatomically derived (AAL atlas) partial brain mask of the mPFC, ACC, PCC, and insula (search volume = 131,272 mm^3) inclusive of these four anatomical areas. For each between-group analysis in the right and left amygdala connectivity, cluster-based significance thresholding was used to adjust for multiple comparisons within the search volume. Cluster-based significance thresholding was determined via simulation using the ClusterSim utility (10,000 iterations; http://afni.nimh.nih.gov/pub/dist/doc/program_help/3dClustSim.html). Given smoothness estimates of the data (11.2 mm × 11.1 mm × 10.0 mm) across our region of interest mask with a volume of 131.3 cm^3, a family-wise error correction at $\alpha < 0.05$ is realized with a voxel threshold of $p < 0.001$ with minimum cluster size of 44 voxels (352 mm^3).

Statistics

For *a priori* areas showing group differences, we extracted parameter estimates/beta weights (connectivity values, arbitrary units) from a 10-mm spherical region of interest surrounding peak from each subject to illustrate the direction of effects. To investigate the relationship between connectivity differences and clinical symptom severity, PARS scores were correlated with connectivity values extracted from regions in which significant group differences were observed. A similar correlational analysis was conducted with age. To ensure findings did not differ by primary diagnoses, we used independent samples *t* tests to examine whether significant findings differed based on a primary diagnosis of GAD versus a primary diagnosis of SP.

Results and discussion

Group differences in right amygdala connectivity

The AD group exhibited hyperconnectivity from the right amygdala to the left insula (BA 47, *Z*-score = 3.34, $p < 0.05$, corrected), compared to the HC group (Table 2; Figure 1A). In contrast, the AD group did not exhibit hypoconnectivity between the right amygdala to any *a priori* regions of interest, compared with the HC group. Table 2 also displays group differences in areas outside of *a priori* regions for completeness, to obviate bias and to promote new hypotheses for future studies.

Table 2 Group differences in right amygdala functional connectivity at rest

	Region	MNI coordinates			Volume	*T* value
		x	*y*	*z*	(mm^3)	
AD > HC						
	Pallidum	−12	6	0	536	3.67
	Superior temporal cortex	−54	16	−14	536	3.62
	Rectus	−4	12	−22	624	3.55
	Insula	−28	20	−24	688	3.34
	Brainstem/pons	−6	−10	−24	176	3.32
HC > AD						
	Cerebellum	28	−62	−40	1,512	4.10
	Fusiform cortex	−38	−48	−18	280	3.13

All listed clusters are significant at $p < 0.005$ (uncorrected) with a cluster extent threshold of greater than 20 contiguous voxels.
Areas showing *a priori* hypothesized group differences italicized.
MNI Montreal Neurological Institute, *AD* anxiety disorder, *HC* healthy control.

Group differences in left amygdala connectivity

The AD group exhibited hypoconnectivity between the left amygdala and the mPFC (BA 10/11, *Z*-score = 3.18, $p < 0.05$, corrected) and the PCC (BA 26, *Z*-score = 3.69, $p < 0.05$, corrected), as compared with the HC group (Table 3; Figure 1B). In contrast, the AD group did not exhibit hyperconnectivity between the left amygdala to any *a priori* regions of interest, compared with the HC group (Table 3). Table 3 also displays group differences in areas outside of *a priori* regions for completeness, to obviate bias, and to promote new hypotheses for future studies.

Amygdala connectivity and correlations with symptom severity and age

No significant correlations were observed between seed-cluster connectivity values from the insula, vmPFC, and PCC with anxiety severity among youth with ADs (all *ps* > 0.5). However, when looking across the entire sample, PARS scores were significantly negatively correlated with amygdala-PCC ($r = -0.37$, $p < 0.01$) and amygdala-vmPFC ($r = -0.37$, $p < 0.01$) connectivity values and positively correlated with amygdala-insula ($r = 0.36$, $p < 0.01$) connectivity.

In terms of age, the correlation between left amygdala-PCC connectivity and age was significant ($r = 0.48$; $p < 0.01$) among youth with AD; the correlation was not significant within the healthy control group. Increasing age was

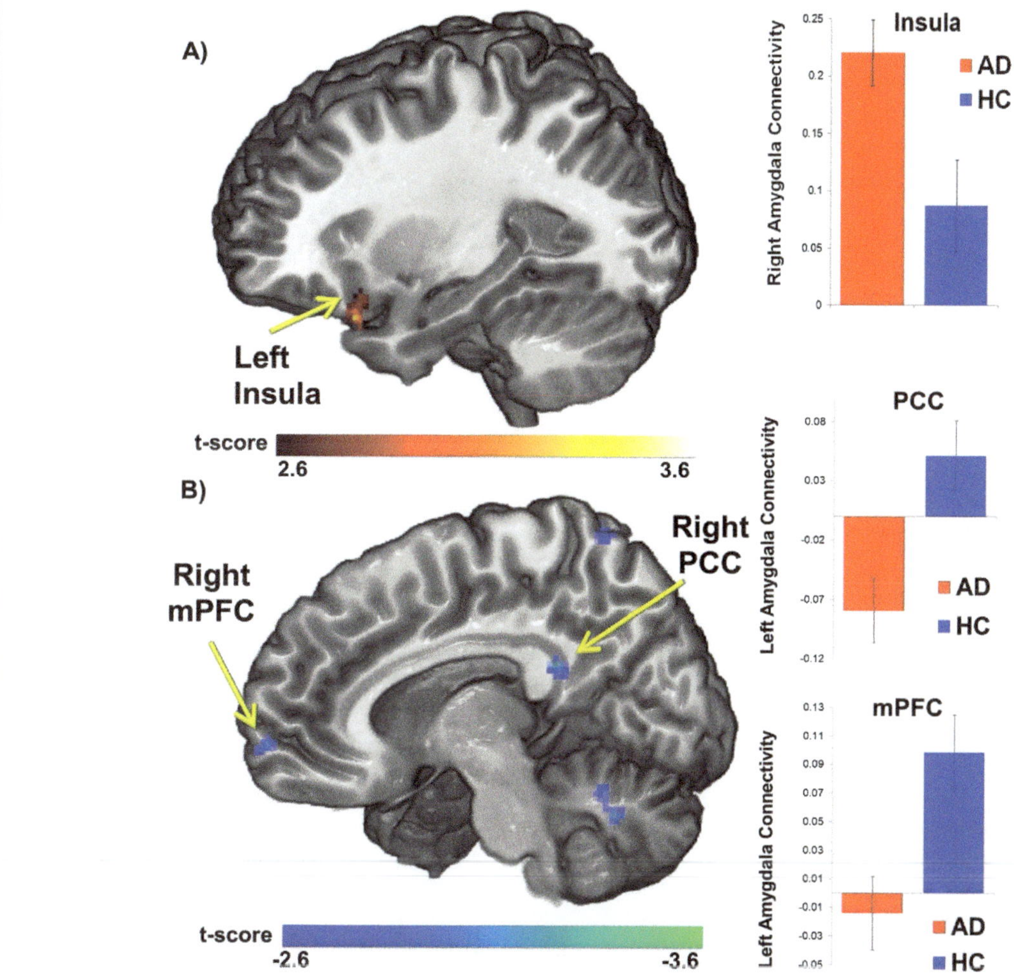

Figure 1 Between-group whole-brain voxel-wise statistical *t* map of *a priori* hypothesized group differences overlaid on a canonical brain rendering showing: (A) greater right amygdala connectivity to the insula (anxiety disorder (AD) group > healthy control (HC) group; and (B) decreased amygdala connectivity to the medial prefrontal cortex (mPFC) and posterior cingulate cortex (PCC) (AD < HC). Statistical *t* map thresholded at whole-brain voxel-wise ($p < 0.005$, cluster volume > 352 mm^3, representing corrected $\alpha < 0.05$); color bar represents statistical *t* scores. Bar graph shows mean extracted parameter estimate β weights in arbitrary units (±SEM) within each group from 10 mm spherical region of interest surrounding peak.

associated with increased connectivity between the amygdala and the PCC, whereas among younger children decreased connectivity between these regions was observed. Of note, even when controlling for age, the previously identified connectivity differences between groups remained.

Comorbidity profiles

Our analysis included 10 participants (30% of the AD group) with a primary diagnosis of SP compared to 70% with a primary diagnosis of GAD; as such, we examined for group differences in connectivity between GAD and SP. The youth with a primary diagnosis of GAD did not differ from those with a primary diagnosis of SP for connectivity between the amygdala and the insula ($t(31) = -0.05$, $p = 0.96$), left PCC ($t(31) = -0.74$, $p = 0.47$), or the left vmPFC ($t(31) = 1.47$, $p = 0.15$).

Discussion

Consistent with our hypotheses, the youth with AD demonstrated aberrant amygdala connectivity with regions of the ALN including the vmPFC and insula when compared to HCs. Surprisingly, we did not find connectivity differences with the ACC but did observe amygdala-PCC hypoconnectivity among AD compared to HC youth. Our results replicate previous observations and extend upon the only study to date that has examined resting-state iFC in adolescents with AD [48], suggesting

Table 3 Group differences in left amygdala functional connectivity at rest

	Region	MNI coordinates			Volume	*T* value
		x	*y*	*z*	(mm³)	
AD > HC						
	Cerebellum	6	−64	−46	1,128	4.02
	Brainstem–midbrain	−4	−32	−2	272	3.40
	Precentral cortex	−62	−12	40	192	3.38
	Cuneus	−8	−96	14	440	3.32
	Thalamus	−18	−24	8	168	3.14
	Ventro-lateral prefrontal cortex	56	38	10	192	3.06
HC > AD						
	Posterior cingulate cortex	10	−40	24	456	3.69
	Superior parietal cortex	16	−58	72	832	3.38
	Medial prefrontal cortex	6	62	−4	376	3.18
	Inferior parietal cortex	−36	−80	44	1,424	3.15

All listed clusters significant at $p < 0.005$ (uncorrected) with a cluster extent threshold of greater than 20 contiguous voxels.
Areas showing *a priori* hypothesized group differences italicized.
MNI Montreal Neurological Institute, *AD* anxiety disorder, *HC* healthy control.

these findings may be reliable and could even generalize across diagnostic categories - from GAD to SP and their comorbidities.

Specifically, we found hyperconnectivity between the right amygdala seed and the left insula among anxious youth compared to HC peers, consistent with the previous literature [34,55-57]. Insula and amygdala involvement in the detection of salience, emotion, and attention is well established [34] and task-based fMRI findings have indicated the hyperactivity of these regions may be a key neural mechanism underlying anxiety-related processes [34,58,59]. The amygdala has been found to be structurally connected to the insula [60], and our results contribute to emerging evidence of a functional connection between the structures [27,34,48]. Altered functional connectivity between the amygdala and insula has been previously observed in groups with anxiety disorders during task [27,29] and more recently during rest [27,38,39,48]. Given the insula's role in interoceptive processing, increased connectivity with the amygdala at rest may reflect increased interactions between a region implicated in fear perception-expression (amygdala) and another implicated in anxious arousal-anticipation (insula).

The extant literature implicates dysfunction in amygdala connections to the prefrontal cortex [19]. Our finding of decreased iFC between the amygdala and frontal regions such as the vmPFC among youth with ADs is consistent with prior findings in adult and pediatric resting-state studies. Specifically, previous research in healthy adults has demonstrated positive coupling between the amygdala and vmPFC at rest [37,61] and has also found this relationship to be compromised in those with higher levels of self-reported anxiety [37]. The latter study found those with high levels of anxiety displayed negative coupling between the amygdala and vmPFC. These findings have since been replicated within a sample of adolescents with GAD [48]. This study documented perturbed amygdala-PFC circuitry, finding negative connectivity between amygdala and vmPFC and positive connectivity between amygdala and dmPFC, in the group of adolescents with GAD. The healthy control adolescents showed opposite patterns of coupling between the amygdala and these regions. Our findings of negative connectivity between the amygdala and vmPFC within the AD group contribute to the growing body of evidence implicating disruption of the dynamic interplay within amygdala-PFC circuitry among individuals with anxiety disorders. Further, our results suggest this aberrant connectivity pattern can be observed at rest. Taken together, these findings suggest inefficient crosstalk between the amygdala and mPFC may lead to increased anxiety levels. Additional research will be needed in order to determine if this compromised connectivity is a defining feature of the underlying neurocircuitry of anxiety disorders.

In the current study, we observed altered connectivity between the amygdala and PCC, which is consistent with the growing body of literature linking disruption of this functional connection to mood and anxiety disorders [42,43,62]. Recent studies have implicated functional connections between the amygdala and posterior regions, such as the PCC and precuneus [19,29], in the implementation of emotional processing [62]. In addition, the PCC is a hub in the default mode network (DMN), a network that subserves processes such as mentalization and self-referential thinking [19,29], which may contribute to hypervigilance to interoceptive cues of anxiety. Indeed, prior studies have observed altered amygdala-PCC connectivity in pediatric GAD cohorts during emotional processing tasks [19,29] and at rest [48]. Taken together, these convergent findings suggest a tonic (task-independent) versus phasic (task-dependent) disruption in amygdala-PCC connectivity and future research will be needed to elucidate whether this is a defining neural underpinning of pediatric anxiety disorders. Recent work in depression has shown that treatment normalizes posterior cingulate-amygdala connectivity [52] and our findings suggest treatment targets for ADs and depression may overlap.

Amygdala-based connectivity correlated with PARS anxiety score across the entire sample, but this correlation was not significant within the AD group or HC group when considered independently, likely due to restriction of range. However, within the AD group, connectivity between the amygdala and PCC was positively correlated with age. Given this is the first documentation of this finding among youth and a cross-sectional study, we hesitate to over-interpret this finding. However, among HC youth, decreased connectivity between the amygdala and PCC has been observed across development [63]. The PCC is a key node in the DMN and default mode regions are known to functionally connect in a more integrated fashion across development [64], which may contribute to the current finding.

The current study is not without limitation. Although the sample size represents the largest to date, replication with a larger cohort of youth is necessary. However, the comorbidity profile of the current cohort may make our findings more generalizable, while noting that most patients (70%) had a GAD diagnosis. Participants in the current study met criteria for multiple ADs, similar to children presenting in clinical settings for treatment and to more recent clinical trials testing the efficacy of interventions in reducing overall anxiety. Moreover, although we observed one finding was significantly correlated with age, our sample size is underpowered for these analyses within the AD group. We captured a relatively wide age range in line with our desire to cast a wider net than previous studies. Data collection is ongoing, and a larger sample will allow for greater exploration of potential developmental effects. This larger sample may also allow for greater variability in anxiety levels within the AD group, making it more likely that variability in network functioning can be linked to severity of symptoms. We did not collect state anxiety symptoms at the time of the fMRI scan to relate to resting-state amygdala iFC. An additional limitation of the current data is that adolescent network functioning may differ from that of children and we look forward to future studies that can explore the nuances of healthy and disordered brain development. Clearly, the examination of the developmental trajectories of resting state networks among youth with and without ADs will be a groundbreaking work. Lastly, this is a cross-sectional observation and emotional face processing tasks (findings reported elsewhere) administered before the resting-state scan may have influenced connectivity in unexpected ways. Future work should address multiple resting state collection periods, acute influences of a preceding "emotional" task, as well as test order effects across tasks and rest, in order to determine the reliability of these networks.

Conclusions

The current findings indicate that youth with ADs demonstrate altered intrinsic functional connectivity patterns, which has several implications. First, these results suggest dysfunction in the ALN, even in the absence of a specific anxiogenic task. Second, our results of aberrant connectivity are consistent with the adult literature. If network dysfunction is detectable early in the course of illness across youth with multiple ADs, then this may be a useful target for existing and novel treatments. This also opens the possibility that aberrant amygdala-frontal iFC is present early in the pathophysiology of pediatric anxiety and thus can serve as a potential biomarker of risk or illness development. Lastly, the examination of a brain marker across distinct primary AD diagnoses takes a step towards new dimensional construct of developmental psychopathology consistent with the Research Domain Criteria (RDoC) [65,66].

Abbreviations

GAD: generalized anxiety disorder; AD: anxiety disorder; SP: social phobia; HC: healthy control; vmPFC: ventromedial prefrontal cortex; PCC: posterior cingulate cortex; ALN: anterior limbic network; SAD: separation anxiety disorder; CBT: cognitive behavioral therapy; mPFC: medial prefrontal cortex; ACC: anterior cingulate cortex; vlPFC: ventrolateral prefrontal cortex; dlPFC: dorsolateral prefrontal cortex; PARS: Pediatric Anxiety Rating Scale; rs-fMRI: resting-state functional magnetic resonance imaging; iFC: intrinsic functional connectivity; BOLD: blood-oxygen-level-dependent; AAL: automated anatomical labeling; DMN: default mode network.

Competing interests

The authors declare that they have no competing interests.

Authors' contributions

LH participated in the acquisition, analysis, and interpretation of the data, along with drafting and revising the manuscript. RJ participated in the analysis and interpretation of the data, along with drafting and revising the manuscript. DF participated in the analysis and interpretation of the data, along with revising the manuscript. MJ participated in the acquisition and interpretation of the data, along with drafting the manuscript. KF participated in the conception and design of the study, along with revising the manuscript. SL participated in the analysis and interpretation of the data and in the revision of the manuscript. CM participated in the conception and design of the study, along with revising the manuscript. KLP participated in the conception and design of the study, along with interpretation of the data and drafting of the manuscript. All authors read and approved the final manuscript.

Acknowledgements

This study was supported by the National Institutes of Health (R01MH086517 to KLP and CSM). RHJ was supported by the National Institutes of Health (UL1TR00050). The content is solely the responsibility of the authors and does not necessarily represent the official views of the National Institutes of Health.

Author details
[1]Department of Psychiatry, University of Illinois at Chicago, 1747 W. Roosevelt Road, IJR/WROB Rm. 244, Chicago, IL 60608, USA. [2]Department of Psychiatry, University of Michigan, Ann Arbor, Michigan, USA. [3]Department of Psychology, University of Michigan, Ann Arbor, Michigan, USA. [4]Department of Psychology, University of Illinois at Chicago, Chicago, Illinois, USA. [5]Department of Anatomy and Cell Biology, University of Illinois at Chicago, Chicago, Illinois, USA.

References

1. Pine DS, Cohen P, Gurley D, Brook J, Ma Y: **The risk for early-adulthood anxiety and depressive disorders in adolescents with anxiety and depressive disorders.** *Arch Gen Psychiatry* 1998, **55:**56–64.
2. Costello EJ, Angold A, Burns BJ, Stangl DK, Tweed DL, Erkanli A, Worthman CM: **The Great Smoky Mountains Study of Youth. Goals, design, methods, and the prevalence of DSM-III-R disorders.** *Arch Gen Psychiatry* 1996, **53:**1129–1136.
3. Beesdo K, Bittner A, Pine DS, Stein MB, Höfler M, Lieb R, Wittchen H-U: **Incidence of social anxiety disorder and the consistent risk for secondary depression in the first three decades of life.** *Arch Gen Psychiatry* 2007, **64:**903–912.
4. Merikangas KR, He J-P, Burstein M, Swanson SA, Avenevoli S, Cui L, Benjet C, Georgiades K, Swendsen J: **Lifetime prevalence of mental disorders in U.S. adolescents: results from the National Comorbidity Survey Replication–Adolescent Supplement (NCS-A).** *J Am Acad Child Adolesc Psychiatry* 2010, **49:**980–989.
5. Labellarte MJ, Ginsburg GS, Walkup JT, Riddle MA: **The treatment of anxiety disorders in children and adolescents.** *Biol Psychiatry* 1999, **46:**1567–1578.
6. Stein MB: **Disability and quality of life in social phobia: epidemiologic findings.** *Am J Psychiatry* 2000, **157:**1606–1613.
7. Safren SA, Heimberg RG, Brown EJ, Holle C: **Quality of life in social phobia.** *Depress Anxiety* 1996, **4:**126–133.
8. Hambrick JP, Turk CL, Heimberg RG, Schneier FR, Liebowitz MR: **The experience of disability and quality of life in social anxiety disorder.** *Depress Anxiety* 2003, **18:**46–50.
9. Safren SA, Heimberg RG, Juster HR: **Clients' expectancies and their relationship to pretreatment symptomatology and outcome of cognitive-behavioral group treatment for social phobia.** *J Consult Clin Psychol* 1997, **65:**694–698.
10. Beesdo K, Pine DS, Lieb R, Wittchen H-U: **Incidence and risk patterns of anxiety and depressive disorders and categorization of generalized anxiety disorder.** *Arch Gen Psychiatry* 2010, **67:**47–57.
11. Kessler RC, Avenevoli S, Costello EJ, Georgiades K, Green JG, Gruber MJ, He J, Koretz D, McLaughlin KA, Petukhova M, Sampson NA, Zaslavsky AM, Merikangas KR: **Prevalence, persistence, and sociodemographic correlates of DSM-IV disorders in the National Comorbidity Survey Replication Adolescent Supplement.** *Arch Gen Psychiatry* 2012, **69:**372–380.
12. Verduin TL, Kendall PC: **Differential occurrence of comorbidity within childhood anxiety disorders.** *J Clin Child Adolesc Psychol* 2003, **32:**290–295.
13. Silverman WK, Ollendick TH: **Evidence-based assessment of anxiety and its disorders in children and adolescents.** *J Clin Child Adolesc Psychol* 2005, **34:**380–411.
14. Compton SN, Walkup JT, Albano AM, Piacentini JC, Birmaher B, Sherrill JT, Ginsburg GS, Rynn MA, McCracken JT, Waslick BD, Iyengar S, Kendall PC, March JS: **Child/Adolescent Anxiety Multimodal Study (CAMS): rationale, design, and methods.** *Child Adolesc Psychiatry Ment Health* 2010, **4:**1.
15. Kendall PC, Compton SN, Walkup JT, Birmaher B, Albano AM, Sherrill J, Ginsburg G, Rynn M, McCracken J, Gosch E, Keeton C, Bergman L, Sakolsky D, Suveg C, Iyengar S, March J, Piacentini J: **Clinical characteristics of anxiety disordered youth.** *J Anxiety Disord* 2010, **24:**360–365.
16. Van den Bulk BG, Meens PHF, van Lang NDJ, de Voogd EL, van der Wee NJA, Rombouts SARB, Crone EA, Vermeiren RRJM: **Amygdala activation during emotional face processing in adolescents with affective disorders: the role of underlying depression and anxiety symptoms.** *Front Hum Neurosci* 2014, **8:**393.
17. Walkup JT, Albano AM, Piacentini J, Birmaher B, Compton SN, Sherrill JT, Ginsburg GS, Rynn MA, McCracken J, Waslick B, Iyengar S, March JS, Kendall PC: **Cognitive behavioral therapy, sertraline, or a combination in childhood anxiety.** *N Engl J Med* 2008, **359:**2753–2766.
18. Strawn JR, Dominick KC, Doyle CD, Picard LS, Phan KL: **Neurobiology of pediatric anxiety disorders.** *Curr Behav Neurosci Rep* 2014, **1:**154–160.
19. Strawn JR, Bitter SM, Weber WA, Chu W-J, Whitsel RM, Adler C, Cerullo MA, Eliassen J, Strakowski SM, DelBello MP: **Neurocircuitry of generalized anxiety disorder in adolescents: a pilot functional neuroimaging and functional connectivity study.** *Depress Anxiety* 2012, **29:**939–947.
20. Monk CS, Nelson EE, McClure EB, Mogg K, Bradley BP, Leibenluft E, Blair RJR, Chen G, Charney DS, Ernst M, Pine DS: **Ventrolateral prefrontal cortex activation and attentional bias in response to angry faces in adolescents with generalized anxiety disorder.** *Am J Psychiatry* 2006, **163:**1091–1097.
21. Beesdo K, Lau JYF, Guyer AE, McClure-Tone EB, Monk CS, Nelson EE, Fromm SJ, Goldwin MA, Wittchen H-U, Leibenluft E, Ernst M, Pine DS: **Common and distinct amygdala-function perturbations in depressed vs anxious adolescents.** *Arch Gen Psychiatry* 2009, **66:**275–285.
22. Guyer AE, Lau JYF, McClure-Tone EB, Parrish J, Shiffrin ND, Reynolds RC, Chen G, Blair RJR, Leibenluft E, Fox NA, Ernst M, Pine DS, Nelson EE: **Amygdala and ventrolateral prefrontal cortex function during anticipated peer evaluation in pediatric social anxiety.** *Arch Gen Psychiatry* 2008, **65:**1303–1312.
23. Ghashghaei HT, Hilgetag CC, Barbas H: **Sequence of information processing for emotions based on the anatomic dialogue between prefrontal cortex and amygdala.** *Neuroimage* 2007, **34:**905–923.
24. Petrides M, Pandya D: **Association pathways of the prefrontal cortex and functional observations.** In *Princ Front Lobe Funct.* Oxford: Oxford University Press; 2002:31–50.
25. Cerullo MA, Adler CM, Delbello MP, Strakowski SM: **The functional neuroanatomy of bipolar disorder.** *Int Rev Psychiatry* 2009, **21:**314–322.
26. Strakowski SM, Eliassen JC, Lamy M, Cerullo MA, Allendorfer JB, Madore M, Lee J-H, Welge JA, DelBello MP, Fleck DE, Adler CM: **Functional magnetic resonance imaging brain activation in bipolar mania: evidence for disruption of the ventrolateral prefrontal-amygdala emotional pathway.** *Biol Psychiatry* 2011, **69:**381–388.
27. Prater KE, Hosanagar A, Klumpp H, Angstadt M, Phan KL: **Aberrant amygdala–frontal cortex connectivity during perception of fearful faces and at rest in generalized social anxiety disorder.** *Depress Anxiety* 2013, **30:**234–241.
28. Etkin A, Prater KE, Hoeft F, Menon V, Schatzberg AF: **Failure of anterior cingulate activation and connectivity with the amygdala during implicit regulation of emotional processing in generalized anxiety disorder.** *Am J Psychiatry* 2010, **167:**545–554.
29. McClure EB, Monk CS, Nelson EE, Parrish JM, Adler A, Blair RJR, Fromm S, Charney DS, Leibenluft E, Ernst M, Pine DS: **Abnormal attention modulation of fear circuit function in pediatric generalized anxiety disorder.** *Arch Gen Psychiatry* 2007, **64:**97–106.
30. Monk CS, Telzer EH, Mogg K, Bradley BP, Mai X, Louro HMC, Chen G, McClure-Tone EB, Ernst M, Pine DS: **Amygdala and ventrolateral prefrontal cortex activation to masked angry faces in children and adolescents with generalized anxiety disorder.** *Arch Gen Psychiatry* 2008, **65:**568–576.
31. Casey BJ, Ruberry EJ, Libby V, Glatt CE, Hare T, Soliman F, Duhoux S, Frielingsdorf H, Tottenham N: **Transitional and translational studies of risk for anxiety.** *Depress Anxiety* 2011, **28:**18–28.
32. Etkin A, Prater KE, Schatzberg AF, Menon V, Greicius MD: **Disrupted amygdalar subregion functional connectivity and evidence of a compensatory network in generalized anxiety disorder.** *Arch Gen Psychiatry* 2009, **66:**1361–1372.
33. Bijsterbosch J, Smith S, Forster S, John OP, Bishop SJ: **Resting state correlates of subdimensions of anxious affect.** *J Cogn Neurosci* 2014, **26:**914–926.
34. Baur V, Hänggi J, Langer N, Jäncke L: **Resting-state functional and structural connectivity within an insula-amygdala route specifically index state and trait anxiety.** *Biol Psychiatry* 2013, **73:**85–92.
35. Rohr CS, Okon-Singer H, Craddock RC, Villringer A, Margulies DS: **Affect and the brain's functional organization: a resting-state connectivity approach.** *PLoS One* 2013, **8:**e68015.
36. Li Y, Qin W, Jiang T, Zhang Y, Yu C: **Sex-dependent correlations between the personality dimension of harm avoidance and the resting-state functional connectivity of amygdala subregions.** *PLoS One* 2012, **7:**e35925.
37. Kim MJ, Gee DG, Loucks RA, Davis FC, Whalen PJ: **Anxiety dissociates dorsal and ventral medial prefrontal cortex functional connectivity with the amygdala at rest.** *Cereb Cortex* 2011, **21:**1667–1673.

38. Rabinak CA, Angstadt M, Welsh RC, Kenndy AE, Lyubkin M, Martis B, Phan KL: **Altered amygdala resting-state functional connectivity in post-traumatic stress disorder.** *Front Psychiatry* 2011, **2**:62.
39. Sripada RK, King AP, Garfinkel SN, Wang X, Sripada CS, Welsh RC, Liberzon I: **Altered resting-state amygdala functional connectivity in men with posttraumatic stress disorder.** *J Psychiatry Neurosci* 2012, **37**:241–249.
40. Wright P, Albarracin D, Brown RD, Li H, He G, Liu Y: **Dissociated responses in the amygdala and orbitofrontal cortex to bottom-up and top-down components of emotional evaluation.** *Neuroimage* 2008, **39**:894–902.
41. Adolphs R: **Cognitive neuroscience of human social behaviour.** *Nat Rev Neurosci* 2003, **4**:165–178.
42. Pessoa L, Padmala S, Morland T: **Fate of unattended fearful faces in the amygdala is determined by both attentional resources and cognitive modulation.** *Neuroimage* 2005, **28**:249–255.
43. Hahn A, Stein P, Windischberger C, Weissenbacher A, Spindelegger C, Moser E, Kasper S, Lanzenberger R: **Reduced resting-state functional connectivity between amygdala and orbitofrontal cortex in social anxiety disorder.** *Neuroimage* 2011, **56**:881–889.
44. Gee DG, Humphreys KL, Flannery J, Goff B, Telzer EH, Shapiro M, Hare TA, Bookheimer SY, Tottenham N: **A developmental shift from positive to negative connectivity in human amygdala-prefrontal circuitry.** *J Neurosci* 2013, **33**:4584–4593.
45. Andreescu C, Sheu LK, Tudorascu D, Walker S, Aizenstein H: **The ages of anxiety–differences across the lifespan in the default mode network functional connectivity in generalized anxiety disorder.** *Int J Geriatr Psychiatry* 2014, **29**:704–712.
46. Perlman SB, Pelphrey KA: **Developing connections for affective regulation: age-related changes in emotional brain connectivity.** *J Exp Child Psychol* 2011, **108**:607–620.
47. Qin S, Young CB, Duan X, Chen T, Supekar K, Menon V: **Amygdala subregional structure and intrinsic functional connectivity predicts individual differences in anxiety during early childhood.** *Biol Psychiatry* 2014, **75**:892–900.
48. Roy AK, Fudge JL, Kelly C, Perry JSA, Daniele T, Carlisi C, Benson B, Xavier Castellanos F, Milham MP, Pine DS, Ernst M: **Intrinsic functional connectivity of amygdala-based networks in adolescent generalized anxiety disorder.** *J Am Acad Child Adolesc Psychiatry* 2013, **52**:290–299. e2.
49. Salum GA, Desousa DA, do Rosário MC, Pine DS, Manfro GG: **Pediatric anxiety disorders: from neuroscience to evidence-based clinical practice.** *Rev Bras Psiquiatr* 2013, **35**(Suppl 1):S03–S21.
50. Mennin DS, Heimberg RG, Turk CL, Fresco DM: **Preliminary evidence for an emotion dysregulation model of generalized anxiety disorder.** *Behav Res Ther* 2005, **43**:1281–1310.
51. Kaufman J, Birmaher B, Brent D, Rao U, Flynn C, Moreci P, Williamson D, Ryan N: **Schedule for Affective Disorders and Schizophrenia for School-Age Children-Present and Lifetime Version (K-SADS-PL): initial reliability and validity data.** *J Am Acad Child Adolesc Psychiatry* 1997, **36**:980–988.
52. Research Units on Pediatric Psychopharmacology Anxiety Study Group, (RUPP): **The Pediatric Anxiety Rating Scale (PARS): development and psychometric properties.** *J Am Acad Child Adolesc Psychiatry* 2002, **41**:1061–1069.
53. Behzadi Y, Restom K, Liau J, Liu TT: **A component based noise correction method (CompCor) for BOLD and perfusion based fMRI.** *Neuroimage* 2007, **37**:90–101.
54. Tzourio-Mazoyer N, Landeau B, Papathanassiou D, Crivello F, Etard O, Delcroix N, Mazoyer B, Joliot M: **Automated anatomical labeling of activations in SPM using a macroscopic anatomical parcellation of the MNI MRI single-subject brain.** *Neuroimage* 2002, **15**:273–289.
55. LeDoux JE: **Emotion: clues from the brain.** *Annu Rev Psychol* 1995, **46**:209–235.
56. Menon V, Uddin LQ: **Saliency, switching, attention and control: a network model of insula function.** *Brain Struct Funct* 2010, **214**:655–667.
57. Craig ADB: **How do you feel–now? The anterior insula and human awareness.** *Nat Rev Neurosci* 2009, **10**:59–70.
58. Etkin A, Wager TD: **Functional neuroimaging of anxiety: a meta-analysis of emotional processing in PTSD, social anxiety disorder, and specific phobia.** *Am J Psychiatry* 2007, **164**:1476–1488.
59. Etkin A: **Functional neuroanatomy of anxiety: a neural circuit perspective.** *Curr Top Behav Neurosci* 2010, **2**:251–277.
60. Reynolds SM, Zahm DS: **Specificity in the projections of prefrontal and insular cortex to ventral striatopallidum and the extended amygdala.** *J Neurosci* 2005, **25**:11757–11767.
61. Roy AK, Shehzad Z, Margulies DS, Kelly AMC, Uddin LQ, Gotimer K, Biswal BB, Castellanos FX, Milham MP: **Functional connectivity of the human amygdala using resting state fMRI.** *Neuro Image* 2009, **45**:614–626.
62. Fang Z, Zhu S, Gillihan SJ, Korczykowski M, Detre JA, Rao H: **Serotonin transporter genotype modulates functional connectivity between amygdala and PCC/PCu during mood recovery.** *Front Hum Neurosci* 2013, **7**:704.
63. Gabard-Durnam LJ, Flannery J, Goff B, Gee DG, Humphreys KL, Telzer E, Hare T, Tottenham N: **The development of human amygdala functional connectivity at rest from 4 to 23 years: a cross-sectional study.** *Neuroimage* 2014, **95**:193–207.
64. Fair DA, Cohen AL, Dosenbach NUF, Church JA, Miezin FM, Barch DM, Raichle ME, Petersen SE, Schlaggar BL: **The maturing architecture of the brain's default network.** *Proc Natl Acad Sci U S A* 2008, **105**:4028–4032.
65. Cuthbert BN, Kozak MJ: **Constructing constructs for psychopathology: the NIMH research domain criteria.** *J Abnorm Psychol* 2013, **122**:928–937.
66. Insel T, Cuthbert B, Garvey M, Heinssen R, Pine DS, Quinn K, Sanislow C, Wang P: **Research domain criteria (RDoC): toward a new classification framework for research on mental disorders.** *Am J Psychiatry* 2010, **167**:748–751.

Permissions

All chapters in this book were first published in BMAD, by BioMed Central; hereby published with permission under the Creative Commons Attribution License or equivalent. Every chapter published in this book has been scrutinized by our experts. Their significance has been extensively debated. The topics covered herein carry significant findings which will fuel the growth of the discipline. They may even be implemented as practical applications or may be referred to as a beginning point for another development.

The contributors of this book come from diverse backgrounds, making this book a truly international effort. This book will bring forth new frontiers with its revolutionizing research information and detailed analysis of the nascent developments around the world.

We would like to thank all the contributing authors for lending their expertise to make the book truly unique. They have played a crucial role in the development of this book. Without their invaluable contributions this book wouldn't have been possible. They have made vital efforts to compile up to date information on the varied aspects of this subject to make this book a valuable addition to the collection of many professionals and students.

This book was conceptualized with the vision of imparting up-to-date information and advanced data in this field. To ensure the same, a matchless editorial board was set up. Every individual on the board went through rigorous rounds of assessment to prove their worth. After which they invested a large part of their time researching and compiling the most relevant data for our readers.

The editorial board has been involved in producing this book since its inception. They have spent rigorous hours researching and exploring the diverse topics which have resulted in the successful publishing of this book. They have passed on their knowledge of decades through this book. To expedite this challenging task, the publisher supported the team at every step. A small team of assistant editors was also appointed to further simplify the editing procedure and attain best results for the readers.

Apart from the editorial board, the designing team has also invested a significant amount of their time in understanding the subject and creating the most relevant covers. They scrutinized every image to scout for the most suitable representation of the subject and create an appropriate cover for the book.

The publishing team has been an ardent support to the editorial, designing and production team. Their endless efforts to recruit the best for this project, has resulted in the accomplishment of this book. They are a veteran in the field of academics and their pool of knowledge is as vast as their experience in printing. Their expertise and guidance has proved useful at every step. Their uncompromising quality standards have made this book an exceptional effort. Their encouragement from time to time has been an inspiration for everyone.

The publisher and the editorial board hope that this book will prove to be a valuable piece of knowledge for researchers, students, practitioners and scholars across the globe.

List of Contributors

Melissa L Murphy and Thomas Frodl
Department of Psychiatry and Institute of Neuroscience, School of Medicine, Trinity College Dublin, University of Dublin, College Green, Dublin 2, Ireland

Quentin JM Huys
Gatsby Computational Neuroscience Unit, UCL, London, UK
Wellcome Trust Centre for Neuroimaging, UCL, London, UK
Translational Neuromodeling Unit, University of Zurich and ETH Zurich, Switzerland
Department ofPsychiatry, Psychotherapy and Psychosomatics, University Hospital of Psychiatry, Zurich, Switzerland

Diego A Pizzagalli
Department of Psychiatry, Harvard Medical School, MA, USA

Ryan Bogdan
Department of Psychology and Neuroscience, Duke University, NC, USA

Peter Dayan
Gatsby Computational Neuroscience Unit, UCL, London, UK

Christian E Waugh
Department of Psychology, Wake Forest University, P.O. Box 7778, Winston Salem, NC 27109, USA

J Paul Hamilton, Michael C Chen, and Ian H Gotlib
Department of Psychology, Stanford University, Stanford, CA, USA

Jutta Joormann
Department of Psychology, University of Miami, Coral Gables, FL, USA

Jared D Minkel and Kristin McNealy
Laboratory of NeuroGenetics, Department of Psychology & Neuroscience, Duke University, 417 Chapel Dr., Durham, NC 27708, USA

Peter J Gianaros and Stephen B Manuck
Department of Psychology, University of Pittsburgh, Pittsburgh, Pennsylvania, USA

Emily M Drabant and James J Gross
Department of Psychology, Stanford University, Stanford, CA, USA

Ahmad R Hariri
Institute for Genome Sciences & Policy, Duke University, Durham, NC 27708, USA

Heide Klumpp, David Post and Daniel A Fitzgerald
Mood and Anxiety Disorders Research Program, Department of Psychiatry (HK, DP, DAF, KLP), University of Illinois at Chicago, 1747 W. Roosevelt Rd, Chicago, IL 60608, USA

Mike Angstadt
Department of Psychiatry (MA, KLP), University of Michigan, Ann Arbor, MI, USA

K Luan Phan
Mood and Anxiety Disorders Research Program, Department of Psychiatry (HK, DP, DAF, KLP), University of Illinois at Chicago, 1747 W. Roosevelt Rd, Chicago, IL 60608, USA
Department of Psychiatry (MA, KLP), University of Michigan, Ann Arbor, MI, USA
Neuropsychiatric Research Program (KLP), Mental Health Service, Jesse Brown VA Medical Center, Chicago, IL, USA

Clas Linnman, Roger K Pitman and Mohammed R Milad
Department of Psychiatry, Harvard Medical School & Massachusetts General Hospital, 149 13th street, Charlestown, MA, USA

Thomas A Zeffiro
Neural Systems Group, Massachusetts General Hospital, 149 13th street, Charlestown, MA, USA

Michal Ziv , Philippe R Goldin, Hooria Jazaieri, Kevin S Hahn and James J Gross
Department of Psychology, Stanford University, Jordan Hall, Bldg. 420, 94305-2130 Stanford, CA, USA

Elena L Goetz and Timothy J Strauman
Department of Psychology & Neuroscience, Duke University, Durham, NC, USA

Ahmad R Hariri
Department of Psychology & Neuroscience, Duke University, Durham, NC, USA
Institute for Genome Sciences and Policy, Duke University, Durham, NC, USA

Diego A Pizzagalli
Department of Psychiatry, Harvard University Medical School, Boston, MA, USA

Michael T Treadway and Diego A Pizzagalli
Center for Depression Anxiety and Stress Research, McLean Hospital/Harvard Medical School, 115 Mill Street, Belmont, MA 02478, USA

Lori Lowthert, Janine Leffert, Kathleen Maloney, Anjana Muralidharan, Rajita Sinha,Boris Lorberg and Robert Beech
Department of Psychiatry, New Haven, CT 06511, USA

Aiping Lin
Keck Foundation Biotechnology Biostatistics Resource, New Haven, CT 06511, USA

Sheila Umlauf and Shrikant Mane
Center for Genome Analysis, New Haven, CT 06511, USA

Hongyu Zhao
Department of Epidemiology and Public Health, Yale University School of Medicine, New Haven, CT 06511, USA

Zubin Bhagwagar
Department of Psychiatry, New Haven, CT 06511, USA
Neuroscience Global Clinical Research, Bristol-Myers Squibb, Wallingford, CT 06492-1996, USA

Jonathan B Savitz and Wayne C Drevets
Section on Neuroimaging in Mood and Anxiety Disorders, NIH/NIMH, Bethesda, MD, USA
Laureate Institute for Brain Research, Tulsa University, and University of Oklahoma, Tulsa, OK, USA

Omer Bonne
Department of Psychiatry, Hadassah-Hebrew University Medical Center, Jerusalem, Israel

Allison C Nugent
Section on Neuroimaging in Mood and Anxiety Disorders, NIH/NIMH, Bethesda, MD, USA
Experimental Therapeutics and Pathophysiology Branch, NIH/NIMH, Bethesda, MD, USA

Meena Vythilingam
Section on Neuroimaging in Mood and Anxiety Disorders, NIH/NIMH, Bethesda, MD, USA
Psychological Health Strategic Operations, Force Health Protection & Readiness, Office of the Assistant Secretary of Defense, Falls Church, VA, USA

Wendy Bogers
Section on Neuroimaging in Mood and Anxiety Disorders, NIH/NIMH, Bethesda, MD, USA

Dennis S Charney
Mount Sinai School of Medicine, New York, NY, USA

Erin L Maresh, Joseph P Allen and James A Coan
Department of Psychology, University of Virginia, 314 Gilmer Hall, P.O. Box 400400, Charlottesville, VA 22904, USA

Karen G Martínez, José A Franco-Chaves and Brenda Ojeda-Arce
Department of Psychiatry, University of Puerto Rico School of Medicine, P.O. Box 365067, San Juan, PR 00936, USA

Melissa Castro-Couch
Clinical Psychology Program, Ponce School of Medicine, Ponce, PR, USA

Gustavo Segura
Clinical Psychology Program, Carlos Albizu University, San Juan, PR, USA

Mohammed R Milad
Department of Psychiatry, Massachusetts General Hospital and Harvard Medical School, Charlestown, MA, USA

Gregory J Quirk
Department of Psychiatry, University of Puerto Rico School of Medicine, P.O. Box 365067, San Juan, PR 00936, USA
Department of Anatomy & Neurobiology, University of Puerto Rico School of Medicine, San Juan, PR, USA

Kelimer Lebron-Milad and Mohammed R Milad
Department of Psychiatry, Harvard Medical School & Massachusetts General Hospital, Boston, MA, USA

Reid Offringa, Kathryn Handwerger Brohawn, Lindsay K Staples, Stacey J Dubois, Michael B VanElzakker, F Caroline Davis and Lisa M Shin
Department of Psychology, Tufts University, Medford, MA, USA
Department of Psychiatry, Massachusetts General Hospital, Charlestown, MA, USA

Katherine C Hughes
Department of Psychiatry, Massachusetts General Hospital, Charlestown, MA, USA

Danielle L Pfaff
Department of Psychology, Tufts University, Medford, MA, USA

Carly Kiselycznyk and Andrew Holmes
Laboratory of Behavioral and Genomic Neuroscience, National Institute on Alcohol Abuse and Alcoholism, NIH, Bethesda, MD, USA

Dax A Hoffman
Molecular Neurophysiology and Biophysics Unit, Laboratory of Cellular and Synaptic Neurophysiology, Eunice Kennedy Shriver National Institute of Child Health and Human Development, NIH, Bethesda, MD, USA

Turhan Canli
Department of Psychology, Stony Brook University, Stony Brook, NY 11794, USA
Department of Radiology, Stony Brook University, Stony Brook, NY 11794, USA
Program in Genetics, Stony Brook University, Stony Brook, NY 11794, USA
Program in Neuroscience, Stony Brook University, Stony Brook, NY 11794, USA

David M Schnyer and Christopher G Beevers
Department of Psychology & Institute for Mental Health Research, University of Texas at Austin, Austin, TX 78712, USA

Megan T deBettencourt
Princeton Neuroscience Institute, Princeton University, Princeton, NJ 08540-1010, USA

Stephanie M Sherman
Department of Psychology, University of Texas at Austin, Austin, TX 78712, USA

Jonathan D Cohen, Kenneth A Norman and Nicholas B Turk-Browne
Department of Psychology and Princeton Neuroscience Institute, Princeton University, Princeton, NJ 08540-1010, USA

Isabelle M Rosso, Elizabeth A Olson, William DS Killgore and Scott L Rauch
Center for Depression, Anxiety and Stress Research, McLean Hospital, 115 Mill Street, mailstop 334, Belmont, MA 02478, USA
Department of Psychiatry, Harvard Medical School, Boston, MA, USA

Jennifer C Britton
Department ofPsychology, University of Miami, 5665 Ponce de Leon Blvd, Flipse Building, Coral Gables, Miami, FL 33146, USA

S Evelyn Stewart
British Columbia Mental Health and Addictions Research Institute, University of British Columbia, Vancouver, BC, Canada
UBC Psychiatry A3-118, 938 West 28th Ave, Vancouver, BC V5Z 4H4, Canada

George Papadimitriou and Nikos Makris
Center for Morphometric Analysis, Massachusetts General Hospital, Bldg 149, 13th Street, Charlestown, MA 02129, USA
Department of Neurology, Harvard Medical School, Boston, MA, USA
Department of Radiology, Harvard Medical School, Boston, MA, USA

Sabine Wilhelm
Department of Psychiatry, Harvard Medical School, Boston, MA, USA
Department of Psychiatry, Massachusetts General Hospital, Simches Research Building, 185 Cambridge Street, Suite 2282, Boston, MA 02114, USA

Michael A Jenike
Department of Psychiatry, Harvard Medical School, Boston, MA, USA
Department of Psychiatry, Massachusetts General Hospital, Simches Research Building, 185 Cambridge Street, Suite 2282, Boston, MA 02114, USA
Department of Psychiatry, University of Arizona, Tucson, AZ, USA

Index

A

Aberrant Amygdala Functional Connectivity, 199, 201, 203, 205

Anhedonia, 5, 13-17, 19-23, 25-27, 97, 105, 107-108, 111-113

Anticipation, 22, 27, 30, 37, 43, 54, 60, 66, 69, 107-108, 130-137, 139-141, 202

Apoptosis, 10, 114-115, 117-119, 124

Attention Bias, 183-186

B

Biological Mechanisms, 44, 50

Bipolar Disorder (bpd), 13

Blood Oxygen-level Dependent (bold) Signal, 74

Brain Imaging, 61, 149, 158, 183, 186, 196

Brain White Matter Integrity, 187, 189, 191, 193, 195

C

Caudate Activity, 62

Cerebral Blood Flow, 73, 125, 161, 167

Comorbidity, 11, 26, 29-32, 42, 60, 62, 123, 141, 187-188, 194, 197-199, 204

Conditioned Stimulus (cs), 62, 67, 142, 172, 175

Corpus Callosum, 2, 7-9, 11-12, 164, 187-188, 191-192, 194-196

D

Default Mode Network, 130-131, 133, 135, 137, 139-141, 202-203, 205

Diffusion Tensor Imaging, 1, 3, 5, 7-9, 11-12, 187-188, 195-196

Dopaminergic Challenge, 13

Dysfunction of Cognitive Reappraisal, 74

E

Emotion Regulation, 26, 44-45, 47-49, 51, 54, 74-75, 77, 79, 81, 83, 85, 87-90, 103, 110, 113, 141, 176, 181, 197, 199

Emotional Faces, 42, 53-55, 58-60, 89

Emotional Interference, 61, 149, 162-163, 166-167

Estrus Cycle, 150

Etiology of Mdd, 101, 178

F

Fear Conditioning, 62, 71-72, 142-143, 145, 147-149, 151-152, 156-159, 171

Fmri Study, 42, 61-63, 65, 67, 69, 71-73, 89, 99, 110-111, 158-159, 167

Fractional Anisotropy, 1-5, 7-9, 11, 187-188, 191-192, 194

G

Gene Expression, 114-115, 121-122, 124, 156, 177

Generalized Social Anxiety Disorder (gsad), 53

Genetic Deletion, 168-169, 171, 173, 175, 177

Genetic Moderation, 93, 95, 97, 99

Glutamate, 10, 101, 103-104, 106, 109, 112, 174, 176-177

Gonadal Hormones, 150-151, 153, 155, 157, 159, 161

Gray Matter Volume, 125, 196

H

Habenula Volume, 125-129

Healthy Caucasians, 91

High-resolution Mri, 125, 127, 129

I

Infectious Disease, 178-179, 181

Insula Response, 53, 55, 57, 59, 61

K

Kv4.2 Voltagegated, 168-169, 171, 173, 175, 177

L

Lithium-response, 114 M

Major Depressive Disorder (mdd), 1, 13, 16, 101, 125

Medial Prefrontal Cortical Regions, 150

Menstrual Cycle, 150, 152-153, 159-160

Meta-analysis, 1-11, 13, 15, 17, 19, 21, 23-27, 51, 60, 90, 99, 106, 110, 112, 123, 141, 166, 178-179, 181-182, 186, 195, 205

Microarray, 114, 116-117, 123-124

Microstructural Changes, 1-2, 9

Mitochondria, 118-119
Murine Anxiety, 168

N
Neural Circuit Function, 45, 47, 49, 51, 106
Neural Temporal Dynamics, 31, 33, 35, 37, 39, 41, 43
Neurobiological Research, 29
Neurocognitive Therapeutics, 183, 185-186
Neuroimaging, 1-3, 11-13, 24, 42-43, 52, 54, 56, 60, 62, 65, 71, 73-75, 89-90, 98, 101-103, 105-108, 110, 113, 125, 129, 141, 151, 153, 157-158, 161-162, 166-167, 183, 188-189, 195, 197, 204-205
Neurotransmitter Systems, 101, 104, 106, 109

O
Obsessive-compulsive Disorder (ocd), 187
Occipital Cortex, 29, 34-36, 134-135, 137-138

P
Pathophysiology of Mdd, 102, 105
Pediatric Anxiety Disorders, 197, 199, 201, 203, 205
Personality Traits, 142, 149
Physiological Responses, 10, 30, 54, 142-143, 145, 147, 149, 157
Pittsburgh Sleep Quality Index, 49, 52
Post-traumatic Stress Disorder (ptsd), 62, 67, 69, 125, 128, 157
Potassium Channel, 168-169, 171, 173, 175-177
Prediction Error, 13-14, 17, 22, 25, 66, 71
Progesterone, 150, 152-153, 156, 160-161
Proof-of-concept Study, 91, 96
Psychological Tests, 143, 145, 147, 149
Punishment, 15, 18-20, 28, 130-131, 133, 135, 138, 140-141

R
Racc Activation, 162-163, 165-166
Real-time Neurofeedback, 183
Reappraisal, 44-48, 50-51, 74-76, 79-81, 83-90, 110, 181
Regulatory Focus, 91-95, 97-99
Reinforcement Learning, 13-17, 19, 21, 23-27, 103
Reward Learning, 13-14, 25-27, 93
Reward Processing, 103-104, 111, 130-131, 133, 135, 137, 139-141, 179
Reward Responsiveness, 26, 91, 93, 95-100
Robust Structural Changes, 125

S
Sex Hormones, 150, 152-153, 157, 161
Skin Conductance, 63, 71, 142, 144-145, 147
Sleep Problems, 45
Socio-emotional Tasks, 74, 77
Statistical Power, 125, 129
Stress-related Behaviors, 168

T
Temporal Dynamics, 29, 31, 33, 35, 37, 39, 41, 43, 74-75, 80-81, 83-84, 86-88
Threat Processing, 53-54

U
Unconditioned Responses, 62-63, 65, 67, 69, 71-73, 146, 159

V
Ventral Striatum Reactivity, 130
Vigilance-avoidance Activation Pattern, 29
Voxel-based Diffusion Tensor Imaging, 1, 3